Exploring and Exploiting Genetic Risk for Psychiatric Disorders

Strüngmann Forum Reports

Julia R. Lupp, series editor

The Ernst Strüngmann Forum is made possible through the generous support of the Ernst Strüngmann Foundation, inaugurated by Dr. Andreas and Dr. Thomas Strüngmann.

This Forum was supported by the Deutsche Forschungsgemeinschaft

Exploring and Exploiting Genetic Risk for Psychiatric Disorders

Edited by

Joshua A. Gordon and Elisabeth B. Binder

Program Advisory Committee:

Elisabeth B. Binder, Joshua A. Gordon, Cathryn M. Lewis, Julia R. Lupp, Elise B. Robinson, Stephan J. Sanders, and Nenad Sestan

The MIT Press

Cambridge, Massachusetts
London, England

Series Editor: J. R. Lupp
Editorial Assistance: C. Stephen, A. Ducey-Gessner,
Lektorat: BerlinScienceWorks

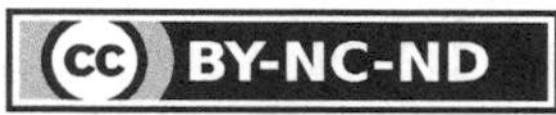

The book was set in TimesNewRoman and Arial.
Printed and bound in the United States of America.

Library of Congress Cataloging-in-Publication Data

Names: Gordon, Joshua A., editor. | Binder, Elisabeth (Elisabeth B.), editor.
Title: Exploring and exploiting genetic risk for psychiatric disorders / edited by Joshua A. Gordon and Elisabeth B. Binder.
Description: Cambridge, Massachusetts : The MIT Press, [2023] | Series: Strüngmann forum reports | Includes bibliographical references and index.
Identifiers: LCCN 2023021101 (print) | LCCN 2023021102 (ebook) | ISBN 9780262547383 (paperback) | ISBN 9780262377430 (epub) | ISBN 9780262377423 (pdf)
Subjects: LCSH: Mental illness--Genetic aspects.
Classification: LCC RC455.4.G4 E97 2023 (print) | LCC RC455.4.G4 (ebook)
| DDC 616.89/042--dc23/eng/20230527
LC record available at https://lccn.loc.gov/2023021101
LC ebook record available at https://lccn.loc.gov/2023021102

Ernst Strüngmann Forum (31st : 2022 : Frankfurt am Main, Germany)

10 9 8 7 6 5 4 3 2 1

Contents

List of Contributors

Andlauer, Till F. M. Global Computational Biology and Digital Sciences, Boehringer Ingelheim Pharma GmbH & Co. KG, 88400 Biberach an der Riss and Dept. of Neurology, Klinikum rechts der Isar, School of Medicine, Technical University of Munich, 81675 Munich, Germany

Appelbaum, Paul S. Center for Research on Ethical, Legal, and Social Implications of Psychiatric, Neurologic, and Behavioral Genetics, New York State Psychiatric Institute and Columbia University, New York, NY 10032, U.S.A.

Atwoli, Lukoye Medical College East Africa, and Brain and Mind Institute, The Aga Khan University, Nairobi, Kenya

Austin, Jehannine C. Depts. of Psychiatry and Medical Genetics, University of British Columbia, Vancouver, BC V5Z 4H4, Canada

Bearden, Carrie E. Semel Institute of Neuroscience and Human Behavior, Depts. of Psychiatry and Biobehavioral Sciences and Psychology, and Brain Research Institute, University of California, Los Angeles, Los Angeles, CA 90095, U.S.A.

Binder, Elisabeth B. Dept. of Genes and Environment, Max Planck Institute of Psychiatry, 80804 Munich, Germany

Brennand, Kristen J. Depts. of Psychiatry and Genetics, Yale University School of Medicine, New Haven, CT 06511, U.S.A.

Cai, Na Helmholtz Pioneer Campus, Helmholtz Zentrum München, 85764 Neuherberg, Germany

Chattarji, Sumantra CHINTA, Centers for Research and Education in Science and Technology (CREST), Kolkata 700091, India

Davis, Lea K. Dept. of Medicine, Vanderbilt University Medical Center, Nashville, TN 37232, U.S.A.

Degenhardt, Franziska Dept. of Child and Adolescent Psychiatry, Psychosomatics and Psychotherapy, University Hospital Essen, University of Duisburg-Essen, 45147 Duisburg, Germany

Dolmetsch, Ricardo uniQure N.V., 1105 BP, Amsterdam, The Netherlands

Franke, Barbara Dept. of Cognitive Neuroscience, Dept. of Human Genetics, and Dept. of Psychiatry, Donders Institute for Brain, Cognition and Behaviour, Radboud University Medical Center, 6525 GA Nijmegen, The Netherlands

Gandal, Michael J. Depts. of Psychiatry and Genetics and the Lifespan Brain Institute, Children's Hospital of Philadelphia and Penn Medicine, University of Pennsylvania, Philadelphia, PA 19104, U.S.A.

Gordon, Joshua A. National Institute of Mental Health, Bethesda, MD 20892, U.S.A.

Hu, Ellen Department of Biostatistics, University of North Carolina at Chapel Hill, NC 27599, U.S.A.

Iakoucheva, Lilia M. Dept. of Psychiatry, School of Medicine, University of California San Diego, La Jolla, CA 92093, U.S.A.

Jacquemont, Sébastien Dept. of Pediatrics, University of Montréal, CHU Sainte-Justine, Montréal, QC H3T 1C5, Canada

Kim, Heesu Broad Institute of MIT and Harvard, Cambridge, MA 02142, U.S.A.

Kushner, Steven A. Dept. of Psychiatry, Erasmus MC, 3015 GD Rotterdam, The Netherlands

Lehner, Thomas Neuropsychiatric Disease Genomics, New York Genome Center, New York, NY 10013, U.S.A.

Lewis, Cathryn M. Dept. of Social, Genetic and Developmental Psychiatry Centre, King's College London, London SE5 8AF, U.K.

Ljungdahl, Alicia Institute of Developmental and Regenerative Medicine, Dept. of Paediatrics, University of Oxford, Oxford, OX3 7TY, U.K. and Dept. of Psychiatry and Behavioral Sciences, UCSF Weill Institute for Neurosciences, University of California San Francisco, San Francisco, CA 94158, U.S.A.

Nivard, Michel G. Dept. of Biological Psychology, VU Amsterdam, 1081 BT Amsterdam, The Netherlands

Penninx, Brenda W. J. H. Dept. of Psychiatry, Amsterdam UMC, Vrije Universiteit, 1081 HL Amsterdam, The Netherlands

Robinson, Elise B. Harvard T. H. Chan School of Public Health, Broad Institute of MIT and Harvard, Cambridge, MA 02142, U.S.A.

Roeder, Kathryn Dept. of Statistics and Data Science, Carnegie Mellon University, Pittsburgh, PA 15213, U.S.A.

Ronald, Angelica School of Psychology, University of Surrey, Guildford, GU2 7XH and Dept. of Psychological Sciences, Birkbeck, University of London, London WC1E 7HX, U.K.

Sahin, Mustafa Rosamund Stone Zander Translational Neuroscience Center, Dept. of Neurology, Boston Children's Hospital, Harvard Medical School, Boston, MA 02115, U.S.A.

Sanders, Stephan J. Institute of Developmental and Regenerative Medicine, Dept. of Paediatrics, University of Oxford, Oxford, OX3 7TY, U.K. and Dept. of Psychiatry and Behavioral Sciences, UCSF Weill Institute for Neurosciences, University of California San Francisco, San Francisco, CA 94158, U.S.A.

Sestan, Nenad Kavli Institute for Neuroscience, Yale University, New Haven, CT 06520-8001, U.S.A.

Shimogori, Tomomi Center for Brain Science, Wako, Saitama, 351-0198, Japan

Smoller, Jordan W. Center for Precision Psychiatry, Dept. of Psychiatry, Psychiatric and Neurodevelopmental Genetics Unit, Center for Genomic Medicine, Massachusetts General Hospital, Boston, MA 02114, U.S.A.

Stevens, Beth Stanley Center, The Broad Institute, Cambridge, MA 02142, Dept. of Neurology, Boston Childrens Hospital, Harvard Medical School, Boston, MA 02115, and Howard Hughes Medical Institute, Chevy Chase, MD 20815-6789, U.S.A.

Streit, Fabian Department of Genetic Epidemiology in Psychiatry, Central Institute of Mental Health, Medical Faculty Mannheim, Heidelberg University, 68159 Mannheim, Germany

Südhof, Thomas Molecular and Cellular Physiology (MCP), Stanford University, Stanford, CA 94305, U.S.A

Weiner, Daniel Dept. of Biomedical Informatics, Harvard Medical School, Boston, MA 0211, U.S.A.

Won, Hyejung UNC Neuroscience Center and Department of Genetics, University of North Carolina at Chapel Hill, Chapel Hill, NC 27599, U.S.A.

Wray, Naomi R. Institute for Molecular Bioscience and Queensland Brain Institute, University of Queensland, Brisbane QLD 4072, Australia

Ziller, Michael J. Translational Psychiatry, Max Planck Institute of Psychiatry, 80804 Munich, Germany

Preface

Science is a highly specialized enterprise—one that enables areas of enquiry to be minutely pursued, establishes working paradigms and normative standards, and supports rigor in experimental research. All too often, however, "problems" encountered in research fall outside the scope of any one area of study, and to enable progress, new perspectives are needed to expand conceptualization, increase understanding, and identify pathways for research to pursue.

The Ernst Strüngmann Forum was established in 2006 to address these types of topics. Founded on the tenets of scientific independence and the inquisitive nature of the human mind, we provide a platform for experts to scrutinize topics that require input from multiple areas of expertise. Our gatherings (or Forums) are best thought of as intellectual retreats: existing perspectives are questioned, gaps in knowledge exposed, and strategies are sought collectively to fill these gaps. The results of the entire process are made available to the broad scientific community through the Strüngmann Forum Report series.

In 2019, preparations for this project began when Josh Gordon and Elisabeth Binder approached us with this topic. Cathryn Lewis, Elise Robinson, Stephan Sanders, and Nenad Sestan joined the Program Advisory Committee, which met to transform the proposal into a framework that would support an extended, multidisciplinary discussion. The committee worked together to delineate discussion topics, identify potential participants, and formulate the overarching goals: to identify areas in the translation of genomics to neurobiology where a systematic, consensus-based, and collaborative approach to experimental science could help reveal the key neurobiological mechanisms associated with genetic risk for mental illness and foster translation of this knowledge into clinically useful approaches.

To focus discussion, thematic areas were selected and questions posed for participants to consider (for details, see Binder and Gordon, this volume). To maximize in-person interactions, invited "background papers" were circulated in advance, and from June 26–July 1, 2022, experts from psychiatric and statistical genetics, neurobiology, and clinical psychiatry gathered in Frankfurt.

This volume is organized around the four main thematic areas that guided the Forum: gene discovery, understanding rare variation, understanding common variation, and clinical considerations. Each section contains the background papers in their finalized form (i.e., after peer review and revision) as well as the summary reports of the discussions (Chapters 2, 5, 8, and 12). As one might imagine, a Forum is not a linear process. The initial framework put into place triggered lively debate and helped expose the "gaps" in knowledge. To summarize these, Gordon and Binder highlight open issues that remain to be addressed (see Chapter 16).

An endeavor of this kind—especially one convened during COVID lockdowns—creates unique group dynamics and puts demands on everyone. I wish to thank each person who participated in this Forum for their time, effort, and positive outlook. A special word of thanks goes to the Program Advisory Committee as well as to the authors and reviewers of the background papers. Importantly, the work of the discussion groups' moderators—Josh Gordon, Naomi Wray, Stephan Sanders, and Cathryn Lewis—and rapporteurs—Angelica Ronald, Hyejung Won, Carrie Bearden, and Lea Davis—deserves special recognition. To support lively debate and transform this into a coherent, multiauthor report is no simple matter. Finally, I extend my appreciation to Josh Gordon and Elisabeth Binder, whose expertise and leadership accompanied the entire project.

The Ernst Strüngmann Forum is able to conduct its work in the service of science and society due to the backing of the Ernst Strüngmann Foundation, established by Dr. Andreas and Dr. Thomas Strüngmann in honor of their father. I also wish to acknowledge the support received from our Scientific Advisory Board as well as the Deutsche Forschungsgemeinschaft, which provided supplemental financial support for this project.

It is never easy to extend the boundaries to knowledge, and long-held views are often difficult to put aside. Yet once such limitations are recognized, the act of formulating strategies to go beyond this point becomes a most invigorating activity. On behalf of everyone involved in this 31st Ernst Strüngmann Forum, I hope this volume will help assist the delineation of strategic approaches that will lead to further discovery and accelerate scientific and clinical progress.

Julia R. Lupp, Director, Ernst Strüngmann Forum
Frankfurt Institute for Advanced Studies
Ruth-Moufang-Str. 1, 60438 Frankfurt am Main, Germany
https://esforum.de/

1

Exploring and Exploiting Genetic Risk for Psychiatric Disorders

Elisabeth B. Binder and Joshua A. Gordon

Even before a basic understanding of genetic principles became widely available, careful clinical observation identified the hereditary underpinnings of mental illness (Kendler 2021). Building on these early observations, large-scale twin, adoption, and family studies ultimately solidified the notion that genetic factors contribute strongly to psychiatric illness. With the advent of robust molecular tools and large-scale collaborative consortia, the structure of genetic risk as well as many of the individual genetic factors conferring this risk have been elucidated. Indeed, the pace of progress in psychiatric genetics has been dizzying. No sooner is an article published that identifies yet another tranche of loci or genes linked to a disorder than it is out of date, and new advances have been posted to preprint servers.

Despite this remarkable progress, critics continue to maintain that the genetic revolution has led neither to increased understanding of the nature of mental illness nor to the development of novel therapies for these disabling conditions. Indeed, it is important to recognize the limits of progress in psychiatric genetics and to consider carefully how success in understanding and identifying genetic risk can be translated into understanding and treatment of mental illness. Such was the purpose of the Ernst Strüngmann Forum on Exploring and Exploiting Genetic Risk for Psychiatric Disorders, and such is the purpose of this book which arises from those proceedings. The Forum brought together experts in psychiatric and statistical genetics, neurobiology, and clinical psychiatry to discuss the state of psychiatric genetics and chart a path forward for further discovery and translation in the field. Discussions at the Forum centered around three issues:

- Whether and how to pursue discovery of additional genetic risk factors for mental illnesses.
- How best to use existing knowledge of genetic risk factors to enhance our understanding of the biology underlying mental illnesses.

- How best to use existing knowledge of genetic risk to improve the care of patients with mental illnesses.

Here, we provide an overview of these issues and crystallize the aims and structure of the Forum and this book. In doing so, we hope to inform the reader of the current issues in the field and to foreshadow the principle overarching outcome of the Forum: that a coordinated, strategic approach to further discovery and translation in psychiatric genetics is imperative to accelerate scientific and clinical progress.

Discovering Genetic Loci and Describing Genetic Architecture

Thanks to the combination of technical advances and a shift toward large collaborative efforts, this past decade has seen unprecedented progress in unraveling the genetics of psychiatric disorders. We now have many hundred robust risk loci for psychiatric disorders, including both common as well as rare variants, and a deeper understanding of the genetic architecture of these disorders (for a review, see chapters by Robinson et al., Wray, and Hu and Won, this volume). For array-based genotyping, costs have dropped below 50 USD/sample, covering most common genetic variants with arrays available that can account for the linkage disequilibrium structure of different ethnic backgrounds, which increase diversity. Whole-genome sequencing approaches can now generate data for one individual for less than 500 USD, and new methods allow turnover times of about five hours, so that these results can even be used in critical care medicine (Gorzynski et al. 2022). Meanwhile, the Psychiatric Genomics Consortium (Sullivan et al. 2018) has spearheaded collaborative science in psychiatric genetics, facilitating the gathering of the very large sample sizes required for statistical power to detect variants. The work of the Consortium focuses on attention deficit hyperactivity disorder (ADHD), Alzheimer disease, autism spectrum disorder (ASD), bipolar disorder, eating disorders, major depressive disorder (MDD), obsessive-compulsive disorder/Tourette syndrome (OCD/TS), posttraumatic stress disorder (PTSD), schizophrenia, substance use disorders, and all other anxiety disorders. It includes well over 800 investigators from over 150 institutions and over 40 different countries and data from several 100,000 patients and controls. In addition, there are initiatives and resources for large-scale genetic analyses that focus on discovery of both rare and common variants. These include additional large consortia such as the Autism Sequencing Consortium and the Schizophrenia Exome Meta-Analysis Consortium (SCHEMA), consumer-directed genotyping (e.g., 23andme, GeneDx, Regeneron), large national biobank initiatives (e.g., UK Biobank or iPSYCH), all of which have contributed to the discovery of risk genes.

Thus far, the payoff has been tremendous, especially for disorders such as schizophrenia and intellectual/neurodevelopmental disorders (ID/NDD), which are farthest along in terms of our understanding. These two disorders illustrate different types of observed genetic architecture, with *de novo* variants being the largest contributor of risk for ID/NDD and a mix of common and rare variants contributing to the risk of schizophrenia. The number of risk variants that have been identified for both disorders is high. Common variation at 270 distinct loci have been definitively demonstrated to contribute to the polygenic risk for schizophrenia, each conferring a small amount of risk (with odds ratios well below 1.5×). Meanwhile, with more modest sample sizes, whole-exome and whole-genome sequencing has identified ultra-rare variants in at least ten genes, which have been definitively identified as conferring substantial risk for the disorder, each with an odds ratio of 10× or greater. For ID/NDD, rare (frequently *de novo*) variation in over 80 genes confers substantial genetic risk. Overall, these studies confirm an inverse relationship of disease risk and variant frequency (Robinson et al., this volume; Singh et al. 2022). Both risk scenarios necessitate large sample sizes for discovery, and the range of middle frequency variants located between these common and rare ranges is thus far mostly unchartered territory (Robinson et al., this volume).

Given the hundreds of loci that have already been discovered, the question emerges as to when we will have discovered the majority of genetic risk variants in this field. Currently, we still are far from this point. Across psychiatric and neuropsychiatric disorders, we continue to identify new loci and do not see evidence of plateauing (Robinson et al., this volume), even though current sample sizes for genome-wide association studies now often reach one million subjects, and more exome sequencing studies are being performed in well over 100,000 individuals. Indeed, for most disorders beyond schizophrenia and autism, the field is still very much in discovery mode, with the numbers of identified genetic risk factors merely in the dozens. Moreover, an important limitation of the current body of genetic evidence is the lack of diversity in the samples; by far, most individuals who participate in these genetic studies are of European descent. This lack of diversity has implications for both discovery and translation of genetic risk (see Ronald et al., this volume). Thus, an important aspect of efforts focused on finding additional genetic risk factors needs to be focused on expanding the diversity of our genetic samples.

Understanding Biology

Even if there is still room for discovery, the fact that many genetic associations have been cataloged raises the question whether this has improved our understanding of the biology of psychiatric disorders. At the level of understanding the structure of genetic risk, the field can justifiably claim significant progress for at least some mental illnesses. Schizophrenia, as noted above, demonstrates high levels of polygenicity, well beyond those observed for other common disorders (Zeng et al. 2021). This polygenicity could relate to its intrinsic brain-based biology (with the highest numbers of genes expressed in the brain) or to the potential heterogeneity of the biological disease underpinning the common current diagnostic label (see Hu and Won, this volume). Schizophrenia, however, is also a disorder with very high "genetic correlation with itself"; that is, high genetic correlation between one schizophrenia case-control data set to another (over 0.9), indicating that influences of common variants on schizophrenia are extremely similar, regardless of the circumstances of ascertainment of the individuals with the diagnosis. Other psychiatric disorders, such as ASD or MDD, have lower cross-cohort correlations (Robinson et al., this volume), suggesting larger diagnostic heterogeneity. Both polygenicity and genetic heterogeneity will likely impact progress for these disorders. This indicates the necessity for even larger samples with additional (deep) phenotypes, including information on environmental risk (Nivard, this volume) available for further discovery.

Heterogeneity within a diagnosis is only one part of the complex story that genetic risk is telling us about mental illnesses. Another important finding that has emerged from both rare and common variant associations is pleiotropism of genetic disease risk (Lee et al. 2021). There is a large proportion of shared genetic risk across psychiatric disorders, as well as neurological and some medical disorders and traits (Brainstorm Consortium et al. 2018). In large-scale healthcare data sets, the polygenic risk score for schizophrenia, for example, has been found to associate not only with schizophrenia and psychotic disorders, but also with other psychiatric and medical disorders, often with confidence intervals of odds ratios mostly overlapping with those of odds ratios for schizophrenia and psychosis (Zheutlin et al. 2019). Such pleiotropy is also seen with rare variants of large risk for neuropsychiatric disorders. To date, no genes have been identified that exclusively confer risk for ASD and not also for ID or other neurodevelopmental disorders. This pleiotropy has impacted our progress in understanding genotype to phenotype correlation, and thus biological understanding of diagnoses, as well as our progress in utilizing genotype data to guide clinical diagnostic and treatment algorithms. The pleiotropy across multiple brain disorders raises the question whether more specific genotype to phenotype relationships should be evaluated specifically for individual diagnoses, or whether these diagnoses should be thought of as manifestations of underlying developmental brain dysfunction and thus investigated together. Indeed, cross-disorder approaches have already been taken for common psychiatric disorders (Cross-Disorder Group of the Psychiatric Genomics Consortium 2019).

Despite the issues of heterogeneity and pleiotropy, risk variants are indeed beginning to tell us more than just the structure of genetic risk; the identity of these risk variants is beginning to inform us about relevant neurobiology. Deleterious genetic variants in genes related to neurogenesis and nervous system development have been associated with increased risk for ASD, neurodevelopmental disorders but also schizophrenia (Iakoucheva et al. 2019; Singh et al. 2022). Pathway analyses of genome-wide association studies often point to similar biological systems implicated in different psychiatric disorders, such as synapse function (schizophrenia, ASD, bipolar, ADHD), chromatin remodeling (schizophrenia, ASD, depression), or immune function (depression, schizophrenia, ASD)—again not providing strong evidence for disorder-specific disruptions (Lee et al. 2021; Network Pathway Analysis Subgroup of Psychiatric Genomics Consortium 2015). Such pleiotropy also impacts how to move from genetic risk variant to function and ultimately pathomechanisms. For rare, but mainly common variants, the generation of large-scale data sets—annotating genetic variants to gene expression (including non-coding RNAs and splicing) and epigenetic modifications and 3D chromatin structure, specifically in brain tissue—has hugely accelerated our understanding of the potential function of these variants through system biology approaches (Gandal, this volume), especially since most associated common variants lie within regulatory and not coding regions of the genome.

While these resources have hugely accelerated discovery, there are important gaps, especially in cell-type specific annotations, missing developmental timepoints, and molecular resolution, especially in the protein space. The next step in functional understanding is to test how these variants influence function, from altered protein levels to cellular function and system-level changes. For psychiatric disorders this involves often specific brain circuits and influences risk of disease. This can only be achieved by using model systems. Human-induced pluripotent stem cell (iPSC)-derived model systems coupled with the possibility to generate humanized rodent and primate models now allow unprecedented possibilities to investigate gene-function relationships, including polygenic risk, on multiple levels up to complex behavior over the course of development. How such models can be best used, their promises as well as current limitations, is discussed by Brennand and Kushner (this volume).

While we have in-depth understanding of gene-function relationships in some specific rare (but also a few common) risk variants (e.g., Pak et al. 2021; Yilmaz et al. 2021), this information is lacking for a vast majority of associated variants. For all variants, it is so far unclear how they ultimately alter human disease risk. Especially for polygenic disorders, it remains to be understood which are the points of convergence (molecular, cellular, or circuit level) that lead to similar symptom presentation despite heterogeneous individual genetic risk composition, including different subsets of polygenic risk, rare variants, as well as a combination of rare and common variants.

Clinical Applications

The second major issue that we addressed is whether current advances in psychiatric genetics have impacted clinical practice. As with biology, the field can claim at least one significant advance. Currently, use of exome or genome sequencing is recommended as first-line testing for neurodevelopmental disorders such as autism; something on the order of one-fifth of children will have an identifiable, large effect size rare variant that likely played a causative role in their diagnosis. While such knowledge in and of itself can be important for individuals with a neurodevelopmental disorder and their families, the specific rare risk variant an individual carries does not typically affect clinical decision making, nor does it inform disease course. Thus, the practical utility of genetic diagnostics, even in this case, has not yet been fully realized (Chawner et al. 2021; Douard et al. 2021; Raznahan et al. 2022). Moreover, while sequencing is now offered to children with these disorders, adults with brain disorders are still underserved (Finucane et al. 2020). In the common variant space, aggregated polygenic risk scores hold potential to influence diagnoses, but the many caveats attached, including nonspecificity and low predictive value, are even more limiting. Indeed, even for well-characterized disorders like schizophrenia, polygenic risk scores are not ready for clinical use (see Smoller, this volume).

The promise of identifying genetic risk factors lies in their ability to reveal direct treatment targets. Small molecules from drug repurposing that interfere with pathways affected by the disrupted genes have been tested for tuberous sclerosis complex disorders and Fragile X disease. In neurology, genetic investigation has already led to the first successful antisense oligonucleotides trials and an FDA-approved treatment for spinal muscular atrophy. There are promising results and ongoing trials for gene replacement therapy using viral vector delivery, mainly for metabolic disease (for an overview, see Sahin, this volume). However, several obstacles need to be overcome, including gene delivery to the specific organ/cell type and delivery of the right amount of gene product to the end target, at the right time. Timing and dosing are particularly important in neurodevelopmental disorders like Rett syndrome, where decreased (Rett syndrome) but also increased (MECP2 duplication syndrome) function of the affected gene MECP2 is pathogenic (Sandweiss et al. 2020).

The coincidence of tremendous progress and increased knowledge as well as the relative lack of actionable clinical consequences prompts new questions regarding genetic counseling, especially for polygenic disease risk (see Austin, this volume), as well as ethical questions related to polygenic prediction. Before rolling out these diagnostic tools to clinical application (e.g., for predictions of disease vulnerability, treatment response, and disease course), careful evaluation of the risks and benefits of such technologies is required, as adverse effects (including stigmatization, demoralization, therapeutic nihilism, and self-fulfilling prophecies) have not been sufficiently evaluated (see Appelbaum, this volume).

The Ernst Strüngmann Forum: Exploring and Exploiting Genetic Risk for Psychiatric Disorder

In the context of these advances and the need to make further progress, this Ernst Strüngmann Forum was convened to discuss how best to realize the tremendous opportunities afforded by genetic discoveries. The task was to identify areas in the translation of genomics to neurobiology where a systematic, consensus-based, and collaborative approach to experimental science could help reveal the key neurobiological mechanisms associated with genetic risk for mental illness and foster translation of this knowledge into clinically useful approaches.

As noted above, experts from a variety of related disciplines were invited to participate. To ensure all participants were equally informed regarding the current state-of-the-art, papers were commissioned in advance to cover aspects of optimal sample collection (Robinson et al., this volume) and the impact of environmental risk and gene–environment interactions to further gene discovery (Nivard, this volume). Other papers address how common variants create risk for psychiatric disorders (see chapters by Hu and Won as well as Wray, this volume), how systems biology approaches have helped to understand underlying biology (Gandal, this volume), and optimal model systems for follow-up functional analyses of common and rare variants (Brennand and Kushner, this volume). A further set considers how new knowledge can be best communicated and translated to patients, delineating future steps in psychiatric genetic counseling (Austin, this volume), debating promise and challenges of precision medicine in rare neurodevelopmental disorders (Sahin, this volume), reviewing how polygenic risk score can be used in clinical psychiatry (Smoller, this volume), and, importantly, the ethical challenges associated with advances in genetic prediction of neuropsychiatric disorders (Appelbaum, this volume). Collectively, these authors demonstrate the tremendous progress made to date, while also highlighting the gaps in knowledge and challenges ahead.

One collective takeaway, implied in the theme of the Forum, is that psychiatric genetics seems to be at a turning point, with expectations running high on a return for biological understanding and clinical application. Accordingly, the Forum participants sought a critical evaluation of the status of this field and current knowledge to project the path forward. To accomplish these tasks, participants were divided into four working groups, each of which was tasked with addressing major challenges faced by the field.

Ronald et al. (this volume) focused on how best to identify additional genetic risk factors since much of the risk for psychiatric disorders remains unexplained. They looked at the importance of discovering additional risk factors as well as approaches on how best this could be achieved and explored the following issues:

- The advantages and disadvantages of studying quantitative versus categorical phenotypes and developmental phenotypes versus diagnostic outcomes.
- How to exploit heterogeneity and co-occurrence to do better gene discovery and hypothesis testing.
- What the costs and benefits of capturing the entirety of the allelic frequency spectrum will be both translationally and biologically, and how this differs by condition.
- How best to increase diversity in samples, and how this contributes to discovery, translation, and justice and equity.
- How to explore the space of environmental risk and gene–environment relationships.

Bearden et al. (this volume) focused on variants of large effect and discussed how best to move from lists of genes to insight into cell type, circuit-level action, developmental time and, ultimately, novel therapeutics. They structured their discussion around key issues in the field, including prioritization, convergent neurobiology, models, and clinical trials, and asked:

- With the goal of improving therapeutics, what are the key dimensions to prioritize genes and loci for neurobiological investigation?
- Which strategies will permit us to test for convergence/divergence in mechanisms between genetic loci, and how can we determine meaningful convergence?
- Which models should be used to interrogate genetic loci, how should they be leveraged, and how can their predictions be validated in humans?
- What are key advances required in natural history, biomarkers, and clinical endpoints to optimize the probability of success in clinical trials?
- How do we establish infrastructure and incentives to generate rigorous reproducible findings?

Won et al. (this volume) investigated common variants and how to understand the collective impact of common alleles with small effect size. Most genetic risk for psychiatric disorders seems to come from common alleles with small effect sizes, likely numbering in the hundreds to thousands. These common alleles of small effect are challenging as a starting point for understanding neurobiology. Won et al. present recommendations on how to best move from associated locus to causal variant, then from causal variant to gene, and ultimately from gene to function and phenotype. An important consideration in all these steps is context dependence (cell type, developmental period, exposure to cellular stressors) as well as gene–environment interplay. They present a new experimental paradigm that can capture polygenicity and allow us to move forward in understanding the aggregated functional impact of polygenic disease risk.

Davis et al. (this volume) explored clinical applications that leverage genetic associations to psychiatric disorders, specifically on how to move forward for diagnosis, treatment, and patient stratification: What can we do now? What can we envision doing in the near foreseeable future? And how do we get there? Their discussion considered the impact of genetic counseling and testing on the clinical management of mental illness, as well the impact of genetic education on the public discourse focused on mental illness. Further, they delineate near-term opportunities and challenges for copy number variants and rare variants in ethical clinical mental health practice as well as the opportunities and challenges for polygenic scores in ethical clinical mental health practice. Finally, they posit possible next steps and recommendations to maximize near-term clinical opportunities.

In conclusion, the chapters in this volume aim to convey the extensive discussions and recommendations that emerged from this Forum. We hope they will inspire the field to move forward in a coordinated, expeditious way, building on the tremendous advances of the past decade. In addition, we hope they will prompt further conversation and consensus-building. All these steps are necessary if we are to realize the true promise of psychiatric genetics; namely, to clarify the pathophysiological mechanisms of mental illness and transform the clinical practice of psychiatry.

Gene Discovery

2

Delineating Additional Risk Factors

Angelica Ronald, Joshua A. Gordon, Till F. M. Andlauer, Lukoye Atwoli, Na Cai, Thomas Lehner, Michel G. Nivard, and Kathryn Roeder

Abstract

This chapter highlights paths, processes, and considerations that become important as we build on the initial success of large genome-wide association studies of psychiatric disorders. As such, it largely focuses on research on common genetic variation and human genetic research. It proposes directing research toward interrogating how genetic variation acts on the developing brain. For this reason, it discusses the potential value and pitfalls of using developmental, circuit-based, and quantitative symptom-based phenotypes in parallel to the traditional approach of reliance on binary diagnoses in genetic research designs. With respect to heterogeneity and co-occurrence present in psychiatric disorders, analytic approaches are outlined that can advance understanding, improve gene discovery, and potentially influence nosology. It argues that increasing cohort diversity is nonnegotiable: it is essential to improve gene discovery, translation, social justice, and research equity. Furthermore, a range of methods that interrogate the processes of environmental risk, gene–environment correlation, and gene–environment interaction enable a more accurate understanding of direct genetic effects and of how environments operate together with genetic risk for psychiatric disorders. Far from being a diversion, these environmentally informed methods are likely to catalyze biological insights. To this end, considerations for optimal future experimental study designs are discussed, outlining their characteristics and the prioritized approaches. The overarching goal is to deliver, through gene discovery research, translational benefits for individuals living with neurodevelopmental conditions and psychiatric disorders.

Background

Over the last two decades, remarkable progress has been made in psychiatric genetics,[1] yet huge knowledge gaps remain, and the delivery of therapeutic

[1] In this chapter, psychiatric genetics is used as an umbrella term to encompass genetic research on both psychiatric and neurodevelopmental conditions; our focus is solely on human genetics.

options created from biological insights is lacking. In this chapter, we contemplate how we can move forward into new scientific territory in our field through a discussion of the following questions:

- What are the advantages and disadvantages of studying (a) quantitative versus binary phenotypes and (b) developmental phenotypes versus diagnostic outcomes?
- How can we best exploit heterogeneity and co-occurrence to improve gene discovery and hypothesis testing?
- What are the costs and benefits of capturing the entirety of the allelic frequency spectrum translationally and biologically, and how does this differ by condition?
- How will increasing diversity in samples contribute to discovery, translation, justice, and equity, and what strategies are needed to pursue this?
- How do we explore the space of environmental risk and gene–environment relationships?

We end with a proposal for an optimal future study of genetic variation in psychiatric conditions. Throughout, the common concerns within our field are featured, including the heterogeneity within and across psychiatric disorders, a discussion of priorities given limited resources, and means to exploit available opportunities where they exist.

Alternative Phenotypes

What are the advantages and disadvantages of studying (a) quantitative versus binary phenotypes and (b) developmental phenotypes versus diagnostic outcomes? While this question pits approaches against each other, as if they are mutually exclusive, the conclusion we reached is that all phenotypic approaches have strengths.

Diagnostic phenotypes arguably offer the greatest specificity for directly studying the phenomena themselves (i.e., psychiatric disorders). Developmental phenotypes enable us to study the site and time of action in which genes, together with any environmental risk, have their etiological effect; this site and time of action being the developing brain. Quantitative trait measures offer a range of strengths and analytical flexibility with complementary confounds to diagnoses. Importantly, given the investments already made in diagnostic approaches and the complexities of measuring novel traits, the field needs to demonstrate that quantitative and developmental traits provide new or better biological information than diagnoses. As outlined in Tables 2.1 and 2.2, respectively, the potential for additional advances using quantitative and developmental phenotypes seems high.

Table 2.1 Advantages and disadvantages of quantitative and binary phenotypes.

	Advantages	Disadvantages
Quantitative phenotypes	Can be collected in nonclinical samples (e.g., general population samples, community samples, research cohort studies). Can be more specific than a compound diagnosis, e.g., by focusing on specific symptoms, age of onset, or progression. This may increase potential for biological discoveries that yield effective treatment targets. Potential for transdiagnostic relevance (e.g., inattentiveness, executive control, impulsivity). Flexibility of measurement and application: often not time- or resource-demanding; amenable to repeated assessments, parametric/hierarchical modeling, and factor analyses. No need for a separate "control" sample. Statistical power gains because no artificial dichotomization necessary.	Known biases inherent in nonclinical samples, including in patterns of participation and attrition (e.g., Martin et al. 2016). Measurement is not always standardized to the same degree as DSM and ICD, though see Strengths and Difficulties Questionnaire for an example of a standardized quantitative measure (Goodman 1997). Distributions can be skewed (often be handled by transformations) and parametric models can require removal of statistical outliers, possibly contradicting the focus in psychiatry on the most severely affected individuals. Rarely show 100% genetic overlap with psychiatric diagnoses; ADHD traits and ADHD are sample exceptions of high genetic overlap between diagnosis and symptoms) (Demontis et al. 2019). Individual phenotypes often studied separately (although multiple single scales are used to create a latent factor) whereas a diagnosis assesses multidimensional symptom data and reduces it to a single outcome or scale. Can be time-consuming and expensive to develop; a rapid, scalable phenotyping protocol requires, e.g., validation and reliability data, language translations, age-specific norms, etc.
Binary phenotypes	There is an established liability threshold model on which they can be modeled. Established statistics and effect measures (e.g., odds ratios, prevalence) enable direct comparisons across studies. Available as yes/no disease status in electronic health records data.	Require a control sample which can introduce ascertainment issues, population stratification, and other unknown confounds. The liability threshold model requires the assumption of an underlying latent liability which is not directly measured. Dichotomization of quantitative data leads to loss of information and statistical power. Because of cross-sectional assessments, binary phenotypes are prone to contain false-positive cases and false negative controls.

Quantitative Traits

As noted in Table 2.1, quantitative phenotypes offer both statistical and biological advantages over binary phenotypes as targets for gene discovery. The possibility that some dimensional phenotypes, if closer to the neurobiological pathways governed by genes than binary phenotypes, might reveal new or more specific genetic information is tantalizing. However, this excitement must be tempered by the need to focus on the most promising quantitative phenotypes and to address issues of measurement and sample biases.

Measurement

Standardized quantitative trait measures are important for integrating and maximally utilizing data from cohorts. For example, one of the most significant issues in research on clinical characteristics and symptom profiles in major depression lies in the vast numbers of scales on which depression can be measured, and the inconsistency in their usage between studies (Fried 2017). Measurement heterogeneity across cohorts has made inferences challenging; even principled approaches for symptom and patient classification give mixed results depending on assessment instruments (van Loo et al. 2012). Heterogeneity across different measurements of a phenotype can lead to deflated heritability estimates in genetic studies of quantitative traits (Kalman et al. 2021; Wray and Maier 2014; see discussion below on Heterogeneity and Co-occurrence). As such, work to standardize quantitative trait measures that are consistently employed across studies is vital.

Issues also exist for binary phenotypes. Defining cases and controls is not straightforward. Any case/control study implicitly conditions on the selection of controls; for example, whether controls are selected with or without screening may influence genetic findings (Peyrot et al. 2016). This is another reason to avoid a binary diagnosis phenotype as the phenotype of interest relates to what will most help the patient. Case/control studies identify genes associated with a binary disorder (i.e., the biology relevant for the entire diagnostic construct irrespective of individual symptoms, age of onset, or illness progression). There is no guarantee that any of these genes will be functionally relevant for clinical symptoms observed in a patient at the point of diagnosis or treatment. By contrast, understanding the genetics of specific elements of the impairment in patients, such as symptoms or disease progression, could offer more fruitful avenues for translating gene discoveries into targeted therapeutic options (Stein et al. 2021).

Circuit-Based Phenotypes

For quantitative phenotypes to identify novel biology and/or therapeutic targets, they must contribute in a novel way beyond the progress already being made in gene discovery based on binary diagnoses. This potential is maximized when the quantitative phenotypes used for gene discovery are closer to the underlying biological pathways that genes directly encode. An oft-repeated trope is that genes do not encode mental illnesses; they encode proteins, which form biological pathways governing the behavior of cells, neural circuits, and neural systems, which in turn produce the behaviors that underpin mental illnesses. Mental illnesses are heterogeneous collections of various complex behaviors, several layers removed from basic molecular pathways encoded by genes. A promising approach would be to develop and quantify behaviors that represent the direct output of neural circuits, which lie several steps closer to genes along this pathway.

There are several examples of promising circuit-dependent behaviors ripe for exploitation in this manner. Fear-related behaviors, for instance, are quantifiable and represent the output of well-defined pathways involving an extended circuit that includes the amygdala and midbrain structures. Reward learning and especially the computation of reward prediction error are established, computationally modeled behaviors that map onto circuits, including the dopamine neurons of the ventral tegmental area and their targets in the nucleus accumbens. In both cases, translatable, quantitative measures exist that have the potential for scalable implementation in genetic studies (Haaker et al. 2019; Vassena et al. 2017).

Key outstanding issues are designing and validating these and other measures of circuit-level function and their heritability. Furthermore, to prove the promise of the approach, it would be useful to pilot a handful of such behaviors on a large enough scale to verify their potential to identify novel or more specific genetic findings.

Sample Biases

Though sampling biases are widespread in cohorts collected for genetic studies of psychiatric disorders, the directions and types of biases vary by data collection approach. First, there is a well-established WEIRD bias (western, educated, industrialized, rich, and democratic) in cohorts collected for genetic studies, and in data collected through voluntary participation there is a bias for well-educated and healthy individuals. For example, genome-wide association studies (GWASs) on participation in the mental health questionnaire in the UK Biobank (Fry et al. 2017) showed that the polygenic risk score (PRS) for mental health questionnaire participation is positively correlated with educational attainment and better health, and negatively correlated with psychological distress and schizophrenia (Adams et al. 2020). Similarly, data obtained from paying customers of consumer genomics companies may not be representative of the general population in terms of socioeconomic status and educational attainment (Hyde et al. 2016). Conditional attrition is an additional bias that can create challenges in genetic exploration of longitudinal cohorts (e.g., Martin et al. 2016).

Improved statistical modeling of participation bias, however, can aid valid inference. Careful socioeconomic and demographic reweighting of UK Biobank data to counter participation or healthy volunteer bias reversed spurious participation associations (van Alten et al. 2022). In biobanks where participants are recruited in clinical settings and may be less healthy than the underlying population, comprehensive reweighting based on medical information has proven effective in countering bias in PRS-based health care (Lee et al. 2022).

Developmental Phenotypes

Another underexploited area for future focus in gene discovery is that of developmental phenotypes, which refer to measures capturing infant, child, and adolescent development relevant to psychiatry. Examples include infant temperament, childhood behavior, cognitive constructs such as joint attention or effortful control, developmental milestones, and adolescent-onset traits such as risk taking and emerging mental health traits. Existing cohorts collecting developmental phenotypes that contribute to the psychiatric genetics literature include the Norwegian Mother, Father and Child Cohort Study (Magnus et al. 2016), the Twins Early Development Study (Rimfeld et al. 2019), and the Adolescent Brain Cognitive Development Study (Saragosa-Harris et al. 2022). Existing literature has focused on childhood and adolescence (Pain et al. 2018); to date, no well-powered ($n > 10{,}000$) gene discovery research is available on behavioral phenotypes in the infant years (0–3 years).

The advantage and justification for studying developmental traits is to understand the changes in the brain that occur prior to the onset of a neurodevelopmental or psychiatric condition. A pervasive hypothesis in psychiatry is that many psychiatric conditions have a developmental origin. As such, a complementary approach to studying the genetics of established diagnoses is to conduct gene discovery on pertinent developmental traits that capture the atypical development at the site of action: the developing brain (see Table 2.2).

Longitudinal population samples with reliable phenotyping are essential for unbiased estimates of prevalence, co-occurrence, and the temporal order in which phenotypes present themselves. As with all quantitative traits, gene discovery research on developmental phenotypes needs to reveal new or more specific genetic information relevant to psychiatric disorders to be justified in our field.

Psychiatric Diagnoses

The advantages and disadvantages of psychiatric diagnoses are listed in Table 2.2. At present, psychiatric diagnoses lack objectively measurable diagnostic criteria such as biomarkers. To boost sample sizes, some studies have relied on broad diagnostic definitions, such as allowing self-reported diagnoses instead of requiring diagnostic validation by a trained professional (Hyde et al. 2016).

Some studies exclude participants who have specific co-occurring conditions; it is not until the recent increase in availability of data from electronic health records and medical registries that diagnostic sequences or switches have been studied and accounted for in genetic studies (Krebs et al. 2021). Going forward, developments in methods to incorporate disease trajectories into genetic studies would undoubtedly reshape the research landscape of psychiatric genetics. Despite the disadvantages of psychiatric diagnoses listed in Table 2.2, considerable success has been achieved in gene discovery, likely owing to the relative ease of assembling large cohorts of individuals by diagnosis.

Table 2.2 Advantages and disadvantages of developmental phenotypes and psychiatric diagnoses.

	Advantages	Disadvantages
Developmental phenotypes	Developmental change and continuity can be accounted for through repeated measures or trajectory phenotypes. Closer reflection of nature to the extent that all individuals continually develop over time. Capture the developing brain, at a time when early interventions or preventive strategies would be appropriate. Potential to offer insights into diagnostic subtypes based on age of onset, trajectory subtype or prodromal features. High potential for transdiagnostic relevance.	The genetic correlation between a developmental phenotype and a psychiatric diagnosis is not always known. No guaranteed specificity to disorder of interest. The time-lag involved in prospective studies between time of data collection and transition of affected individuals to illness can impact feasibility. There are, however, strategic solutions in terms of design and methods.
Psychiatric diagnoses	Measurement typically relies on standardized diagnostic systems, including DSM and ICD; decades of research, clinical use and reiterations have refined these systems. Structured clinical interviews designed to handle a multidimensional symptomatology space and to dichotomize information with maximum reliability. Studying the same phenotype that is intended to benefit from the research.	Diagnoses are arguably not as objective as a biomarker. Some studies mix clinician-based best-estimate diagnoses with self-reported diagnoses, potentially adding heterogeneity and increasing error of measurement. Clinical samples susceptible to a range of biases, including over-representation of more severe cases and help-seeking characteristics in individuals. Heterogeneity in diagnostic practice across sites. Heavy reliance on combining data across multiple sites due to low numbers of cases at any single site. Cross-sectional assessments are prone to contain false-positive cases and false negative controls.

Summary

To expand research on quantitative and developmental phenotypes, concerted effort is needed to identify standardized measures. A definition of common standards and benchmarking of diverse measures across different cohorts, biobanks, and electronic health records is important to facilitate harmonization and to reduce heterogeneity between them. In the meantime, a phenotypic reference panel is one solution to model phenotypic heterogeneity if meta-analyzing across cohorts that have relied on different quantitative trait measures (Luningham et al. 2020; Luningham et al. 2019). We further note that phenotypes should be assessed for specificity and relevance to psychiatric outcomes. Though no sample is free of all bias, careful consideration of the range of biases that are present in clinical and nonclinical samples as described can help to ensure maximal specificity and relevance. A range of neurodevelopmental conditions have benefited from genetic research that focuses on both quantitative traits alongside the more traditional case-control design (Demontis et al. 2019; Pain et al. 2018). The next decade will reveal whether the merits of developmental and quantitative phenotypes will pay off in terms of biological innovations that provide translational benefits.

Heterogeneity and Co-occurrence

Heterogeneity and co-occurrence are rife in psychiatric illness, and the genetic data suggest that these phenomena are important and could be useful in understanding the causes of mental illness and developing targets for new treatments. How do we best exploit heterogeneity and co-occurrence to improve gene discovery and hypothesis testing?

Heterogeneity

There is heterogeneity in psychiatric genetics; accepting this statement as universal in psychiatry will enable our field to be constructive about heterogeneity in ways that have so far not been achieved. Here, we discuss how heterogeneity manifests in psychiatric disorders and the methods that can be used to account for this heterogeneity.

Why is tackling heterogeneity so important in psychiatric genetics? In short, heterogeneity in samples will reduce genetic signal and impede gene discovery. In both empirical data and simulations (Cai et al. 2020b; Dahl et al. 2020), heritability estimates based on single nucleotide polymorphisms (SNPs) are reduced when two phenotypes with heterogeneous genetic architectures are analyzed as one. For instance, the estimate of SNP-based heritability is deflated when different definitions of major depressive disorder that have different genetic architectures are analyzed as a single entity; major depressive disorder with and without prior severe stress exposures are both found to have higher SNP heritabilities than when they were analyzed together (Peterson et al. 2018).

Given mounting evidence that many psychiatric disorders may be the common outcome of heterogeneous pathways, it is becoming clear that treating each disorder as an entity and studying it at the level of a binary diagnosis or quantitative symptom total score is not the only or best solution. We suggest two alternative ways forward:

1. Examine the biological mechanisms behind the putative subtypes of psychiatric disorders delineated by the diagnostic (e.g., DSM-5) specifiers. Using major depressive disorder as an example, these specifiers came from decades of clinical experience and patients' own accounts; specifiers for major depressive disorder such as atypical, melancholic, and anxious depression have been proposed in addition to those based on developmental timing (Harrington et al. 1996), treatment resistance (Fagiolini and Kupfer 2003), and recurrence (Merikangas et al. 1994). Furthermore, studies have found that typical and atypical major depressive disorder subtypes show different patterns of associations with other PRSs for other traits or diseases (Badini et al. 2022; Milaneschi et al. 2016, 2017, 2020).
2. Refocus genetic discovery efforts on more granular phenotypes with higher validity and reliability than binary diagnoses or sum scores, such as individual symptoms or clinical characteristics (Fried 2015; Persons 1986). Staying with the example of major depressive disorder, its symptoms are genetically correlated with each other in the range of 0.6–0.9 (Howard et al. 2020; Jermy et al. 2022). Further, although disorders are often defined through sum scores of symptoms, genetic effects captured through symptoms may not account for all genetic risks for their corresponding disorders; the average genetic correlation between a specific major depressive disorder symptom and the disorder is 0.6 (Jermy et al. 2022). Looking into the genetics of individual symptoms and other clinical characteristics is likely a complementary approach to studying binary diagnoses, with the potential to generate new hypotheses and discoveries.

Approaches to Handling Heterogeneity

Covariates. To perform a GWAS, we regress the phenotype on the genotype, often including additional covariates. Appropriate analysis, however, depends upon whether the covariates are confounders or colliders. Confounding occurs when the phenotype and the genotype have a shared common cause that is not controlled for, thereby inducing a false association (e.g., ancestry). In contrast, a collider is a third variable that is influenced by both the phenotype and the genotype. Including a collider induces a false association between genotype and phenotype, which is called collider bias. Collider bias is a major statistical challenge that prevents the inclusion of a third variable (which may be a source of heterogeneity) from being "controlled for" in GWASs via a covariate approach. There are covariate selection methods, however, that can be used to avoid collider bias (Aschard et al. 2017; Dahl et al. 2019). Such methods have been used in smaller omics data sets to increase power for discovery (Gallois et al. 2019). In a GWAS design, these methods need to be applied for each individual SNP and, as such, need to be made more tractable for use in large sample sizes in psychiatric genetics.

Polygenic risk scores can be used to differentiate genetically defined psychiatric subgroups. For example, bipolar disorder type II was found to be most strongly associated with major depressive disorder PRSs whereas bipolar disorder type I was most strongly associated with schizophrenia PRSs (Stahl et al. 2019). Conducting separate GWASs by subgroups inevitably reduces power in terms of sample size. Nevertheless, the definition of disorder subtypes using PRS profiles is promising. This approach does not require further phenotypic data and should work even in small samples given the high statistical power of PRS analyses.

Case by case genome-wide association studies. Pooling data across disorders is an effective strategy for increasing statistical power for the discovery of loci related to psychiatric disorders (Grotzinger et al. 2022). Where heterogeneity is the specific research interest, the opposite might be effective. To this end, case by case GWASs, performed for one disorder versus those for other disorders, can identify loci that specifically distinguish between disorders (Peyrot and Price 2021), providing tractable biological leads that may aid in understanding one specific form of heterogeneity: differences between highly comorbid disorders.

Use genomic structural equation modeling to combine two disorder genome-wide association studies. Genomic structural equation modeling, or other tools suited for further analysis based on GWAS summary data, can aid in delineating distinctions between different aspects of a single phenotype (Grotzinger et al. 2019). An example from sociogenetics is the effort to disentangle the cognitive and noncognitive contributions to success in school. Demange et al. (2021) used the genome-wide association studies of cognition and education and split the GWAS signal for education into a cognitive component and a component not related to cognition. The specific noncognitive component related genetically to conscientiousness and delay of gratification and negatively to psychiatric traits such as bipolar disorder and schizophrenia. The ability to model both shared and trait-specific signals could be applied to study the relationships between psychiatric disorder subtypes. This would allow for the study of traits that have not themselves been directly subjected to gene discovery studies.

Relevance for Nosology

Heterogeneity in manifestations and etiologies within current diagnostic categories is a result of our operationalization of neurodevelopmental conditions and psychiatric disorders (Cai et al. 2020a; Ronald et al. 2011). Without knowing the biological mechanisms underlying them, we have created diagnostic categories that do not necessarily line up with etiological pathways. As a result, it is not surprising that many such diagnostic categories contain heterogeneous etiologies, some of which may be indexed by heterogeneous manifestations (through symptoms and other clinical characteristics). The process of developing testable hypotheses on disorder subtypes, and the knowledge gained through this research might ultimately improve diagnostic category operationalization.

Summary

Heterogeneity is the norm in psychiatry and addressing it is likely to pay off from a gene discovery point of view. Heterogeneity can be studied in several ways. Two options are to investigate diagnostic specifiers and focus on specific symptom profiles. Here we considered a range of methodological options to address heterogeneity. This area of future research may also lead to clinical impact by influencing nosology via refined biological understanding.

Co-occurrence

Co-occurrence of conditions is high in psychiatry, both within psychiatric disorders and between psychiatric and nonpsychiatric conditions. Ignoring co-occurrence means ignoring a fundamental feature of psychiatric disorders, impacting genetic analyses. By embracing transdiagnostic features of related disorders, however, we can surpass traditional diagnostic categories. Indeed, high co-occurrence (Kessler et al. 2005) and pleiotropy (Brainstorm Consortium et al. 2018; Gandal et al. 2018; Lee et al. 2019) between psychiatric disorders have motivated attempts to identify common genetic factors and implicated molecular pathways shared by multiple psychiatric disorders (Maier et al. 2015; Schork et al. 2019). Here, we focus on three approaches for exploiting co-occurrence to improve gene discovery and hypothesis testing.

Longitudinal Co-occurrence

One aspect of co-occurences that has not received sufficient attention is the temporal relationships between the multiple conditions. Any cross-sectional assessment, whether obtained through research, electronic health records, or nonclinical cohort studies, may only capture concurrently occurring diagnoses at the time of the survey. However, co-occurring conditions may have different times of onset, exhibit different peaks of severity, or even show completely nonoverlapping phases of manifestation, with underlying genetic factors acting pleiotropically. Importantly, co-occurring disorders share a common etiology, and/or one of the disorders could increase the risk of another over time. Therefore, more nuanced approaches to co-occurrence that aim to capture co-occurrence longitudinally rather than cross-sectionally may yield additional insight. Alternatively, co-occurring disorders might constitute a different disease entity altogether. These and other scenarios can only be examined by determining the longitudinal sequence of occurrence, accounting for the relative time of onset of the co-occurring conditions. Gathering such longitudinal information would facilitate modeling disorders as longitudinal occurrences, testing such models for their explanatory power, and mapping them onto the underlying genetics. For example, there might be a different genetic etiology for individuals whose co-occurring mood and anxiety disorders begin with major depression and progress to panic disorder, compared to those whose begin with panic disorder and progress to major depression. Moreover, longitudinal modeling might enable personalized risk profiles for psychiatric disorders including better predictions of disease progression.

Exploiting Nonpsychiatric Disorder Biology via Co-occurrence

Many individuals with psychiatric disorders have co-occurring nonpsychiatric disorders with potentially partly shared underlying genetic risk factors. For example, depression is more frequent in patients diagnosed with some nonpsychiatric disorders than in the general population (Boeschoten et al. 2017; Garrido et al. 2017). Conducting genetic analyses in patients showing co-occurrence of psychiatric with nonpsychiatric disorders for which the biology is well known might facilitate unraveling the etiology of psychiatric disorders.

Concepts and Methods to Model Co-occurrence on a Latent Level

Various models have been proposed to categorize features of psychopathology in hierarchical models. For example, the p factor (Caspi et al. 2014), derived from bifactor models, represents an underlying general liability for psychiatric conditions. Preliminary evidence suggests a genetic basis of the p factor (Selzam et al. 2018), but the utility of this construct continues to be scrutinized (Grotzinger et al. 2022).

Genomic structural equation modeling (SEM) is a method to perform modeling and hypothesis testing on complex etiological models after genome-wide association studies that is well suited for modeling psychiatric co-occurrence. In a specific application of genomic SEM sharing features with Mendelian randomization, Grotzinger et al. (2022) evaluated various forms of the latent p factor using genome-wide association studies of eleven psychopathologies. Genomic SEM analyses indicated a model where pleiotropy or co-occurrence was best explained by a set of correlated factors, each influencing two to three traits, rather than an overarching p factor. It remains to be seen whether alternate taxonomies of psychopathology, such as HiTOP (Conway et al. 2022), are consistent with these results.

Summary

The field of psychiatric genetics has mainly studied individual conditions, with some exceptions (Smoller et al. 2013). Moving forward, co-occurrence could be exploited by considering longitudinal co-occurrence, the biology of co-occurring nonpsychiatric disorders, by modeling co-occurrence latently, and by applying methods like genomic SEM.

Allelic Frequency Spectrum

What are the costs and benefits of capturing the entirety of the allelic frequency spectrum translationally and biologically, and how does this differ by condition? After a brief description of previous work from the psychiatric genetics community, including the Psychiatric Genomics Consortium, our discussion focuses on ways to advance future research. We explain what we mean by the entirety of the allelic frequency spectrum and which parts are currently not well studied. Examples are provided of work that has achieved findings on the "missing" part of the allelic frequency spectrum from other fields. We conclude that a likely by-product of the initiation and prioritization of genetic studies in diverse populations will be greater knowledge regarding the missing parts of the allelic frequency spectrum.

Work from the Psychiatric Genomics Consortium

Founded in 2008, the explicit goal of the Psychiatric Genomics Consortium was to perform large genome-wide association studies on neuropsychiatric disorders and to delineate their genetic and phenotypic architecture. Organized around 14 working groups to study 11 psychiatric disorders and cross-disorder genetics, the consortium has published more than 320 articles, including papers on the common variant risk architecture of schizophrenia, bipolar disorder, major depressive disorder, and autism spectrum disorder, as well as their genetic sharing and phenotypic overlap. By integrating discovery cohorts and generating genotypes for meta-analysis involving over 40 countries, and more than 800 investigators from over 150 institutions, the Psychiatric Genomics Consortium has become the largest collaboration in psychiatric genetics.

To date, the Psychiatric Genomics Consortium is focused on array-based common variants and array-derived structural variant analysis. While these methods capture many common variants with small effects on liability to disease, the approaches seldom capture low-frequency variants due to lack of power (except for rare variants with large effects). As such, current efforts do not capture the full allelic frequency spectrum of disease. Furthermore, though the consortium is international in nature, until recently the integrated cohorts were almost exclusively European in genetic ancestry and offered little diversity and limited genetic admixture.

What Is the Allelic Frequency Spectrum and What Is Missing?

It is estimated that any given human genome is different from that of another by about four to five million loci, many of which are SNPs (1000 Genomes Project Consortium et al. 2015). Variants lie on an allelic frequency spectrum largely determined by forces of population history (population size bottle necks, drift, and natural selection), which tend to limit effect sizes of common variants. Allelic frequency refers to the frequency with which a given variant is found in the population; a minor allelic frequency of 5% means that 5% of chromosomes carry that particular allele. Common variants are typically defined as those with a minor allele frequency of greater than 1%. Many of these are located in the noncoding regions of the genome and other places where genetic variation can be tolerated without catastrophic effects. Each associated common variant by itself confers a very small increase in risk. A PRS is commonly estimated as the aggregate genomic risk from the total of such variants in an individual. Since power for detection of a risk allele is a function of the variance explained (i.e., $2p(1-p)b^2$, where p is allele frequency and b is effect size) and sample size, rare-variant associations (minor allele frequency under 0.5%) are potentially detectable when they have large effect sizes. Hence, very large cohorts, such as UK Biobank, are powered to extend discovery to a minor allele frequency of $\geq$ 0.01% and to find alleles with smaller effect sizes, but only for common diseases and quantitative traits (as case numbers for less common disorders are lower). Sequencing studies of large case-control cohorts have identified rare genetic variants associated with schizophrenia with bigger effects (Martin et al. 2022). Individual variants may have frequencies as low as 0.005% but their association is established through gene-level burden tests. Between these two extremes exists an area of the allele frequency spectrum where variants occur with minor allele frequencies between 0.005% and 0.01%. Current experimental designs do not typically have the power to detect alleles with minor allele frequencies in this range (in Singh et al. 2022, see Fig. 6.).

Three potential reasons for directing efforts to find this missing part of the allele frequency spectrum (and effect size) space are as follows:

1. New biological pathways may be uncovered.
2. New gene-gene, gene–environment, and gene–sex interactions may be discovered.

3. There might be a combination of allele frequency and effect size that enables novel paradigms of neurobiological inquiry.

Existing research outside of psychiatry shows that alleles in this "missing" spectrum can be identified, but only with extremely large sample sizes. For example, genome-wide association studies on height identified variants in this space (Marouli et al. 2017; Yengo et al. 2022) as well as studies on neurodevelopmental disorders (Stoll et al. 2013) and inflammatory bowel disease (Luo et al. 2017).

Capturing the Entire Allelic Frequency Spectrum versus Other Research Priorities

Assuming a finite budget for data collection, obtaining sufficient sample sizes to fill out the missing regions of the allelic frequency spectrum for each condition must be weighed against other priorities, including the competing goal of expanding samples to encompass full global representation. With the information we have at hand and considering the current research landscape, we emphasize the importance of research efforts and resources on diverse ancestry populations over attempting to capture the "missing" part of the allele frequency spectrum. The missing part of the frequency spectrum will fill organically with larger sample sizes as they accumulate.

Focusing on Diversity

Historically, most gene discoveries have been conducted in European ancestry individuals. How will increasing diversity in samples contribute to discovery, translation, justice, and equity, and what strategies are needed to pursue this?

The failure to recruit individuals from diverse ancestry into genetic samples has significant repercussions in at least three areas. First, without diversity, the knowledge gained from genetics will be inequitable. It is challenging or impossible to apply genetic knowledge from existing data sets to risk prediction in non-European populations, and therapeutics developed based on this knowledge might not be globally applicable (Martin et al. 2017, 2019). Second, in some ancestral populations, additional risk variants may be present, or the frequency of associated variants might differ from other populations. Including diverse ancestries may therefore identify a greater variety of biological or therapeutic pathways potentially applicable to all ancestries. Third, due to the larger linkage disequilibrium blocks present in more recently diverged ancestries compared to ancestrally older populations, fine mapping of risk loci will be improved through genetic research on diverse samples. Recently, there has been a marked shift toward broader global representation in existing and new consortia-based studies.

In this section, we discuss strategies employed in such diversification efforts, and the lessons that have emerged from them. Subsequently, we address how increasing cohort diversity will contribute to gene discovery, translation, social justice, and research equity and consider optimal strategies to pursue this goal.

Strategies and Lessons Learned

In all attempts to increase diversity in global mental health research, there are problems inherent in researchers from high-income countries conducting research in low- and middle-income countries. These are largely fueled by different resources in terms of finances, human resource capacity, equipment availability, and institutional support. Kumar et al. (2022) examined this problem and have proposed recommendations for consideration by high-income country institutions as they establish collaborations with low- and middle-income country institutions. These recommendations include (a) the need to devolve global health research centers to where the health challenges being addressed are located and (b) to invest more in researchers from low- and middle-income countries. It is imperative that funding proposals include capacity development to ensure that local scientists are able to continue with similar work past the funding cycle.

An example of an attempt to design collaborations based on equity can be found in the Academic Model Providing Access to Health (AMPATH) collaboration between a consortium of North American institutions and Moi University in western Kenya. This relationship might provide a framework for broad-based collaborations of this kind, cutting across research, education, and health service delivery. Figure 2.1 provides a summary of the practical strategies that have grown out of this collaboration, based on principles articulated by Melby et al. (2016) and described in detail by Turissini et al. (2020).

A specific example of the application of these principles in the same setting, from a broad research perspective, is the Neuropsychiatric Genetics of African Populations Psychosis (NeuroGAP Psychosis) study (Martin et al. 2022; Stevenson et al. 2019). This collaboration brings researchers from Kenya, Uganda, Ethiopia, and South Africa together with collaborators from the United States. To date, this study has collected over 37,000 samples and is developing the capacity of local scientists to continue with the work beyond the funding cycle. Lessons learned from this work reemphasize the need for including local collaborators right from the beginning, designing clear and detailed collaboration agreements that keep equity in mind, and creating flexible funding mechanisms that recognize the resource and capacity differentials and intentionally set out to address them.

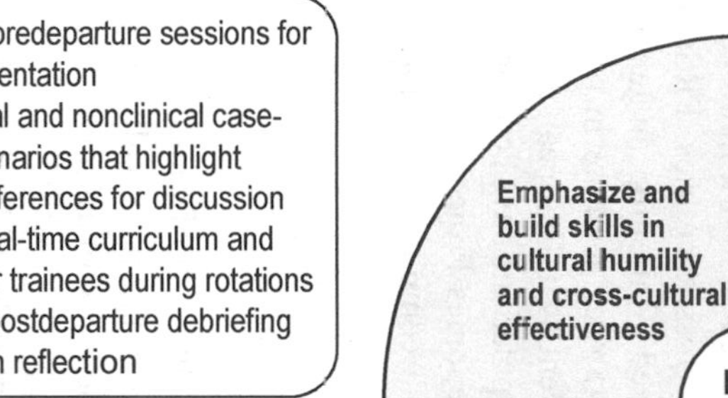

Figure 2.1 Practical strategies for implementation of Melby principles from the AMPATH experience. MOU: memorandum of understanding; LMIC: low- or middle-income country; HIC: high-income country.

Sample Diversity and Gene Discovery

Collection of diverse ancestry samples in psychiatric genetics will contribute to gene discovery and post-discovery follow-up. Due to migration patterns out of Africa, a substantial portion of allelic diversity was lost in ancestrally newer populations (1000 Genomes Project Consortium et al. 2015), and allelic diversity can only be determined by studying ancestrally older populations (Bentley et al. 2020). One example is the discovery of variants in *PCSK9*, which dramatically reduce low-density lipoprotein cholesterol concentrations. Discoveries such as this can identify key genes for drug therapy, which has implications for all populations.

Another advantage of studying diverse ancestries for gene discovery is that allelic frequencies vary by population, and power is greater when alleles are more common. Discovering specific alleles can thus be easier, due to higher allele frequencies, in some ancestries over others. For instance, the first two genome-wide significant loci for recurrent major depressive disorder in a Han Chinese population have high-risk allele frequencies (45% and 26%, respectively) in the Han Chinese population, but much lower allele frequencies in the European population (3% and 8%, respectively) (Converge Consortium 2015). Both have been replicated in an independent Han Chinese cohort, but not in European cohorts (Converge Consortium 2015).

Beyond gene discovery efforts, sample diversity will enable PRSs to be created that are optimized for all ancestries. It has been shown that even in examples where shared variants are discovered across ancestries, PRSs are not always portable across them. The PRSs generated from European genome-wide association studies on schizophrenia were 45% as accurate in predicting schizophrenia in samples with East Asian descent as in European ancestry samples (Lam et al. 2019). Ancestrally younger populations have considerably longer blocks of linkage disequilibrium (1000 Genomes Project Consortium et al. 2015). Long blocks of linkage disequilibrium complicate fine-mapping efforts and impair the portability of PRSs.

Sample Diversity and Fine Mapping

Statistical fine mapping is used to identify the credible set of causal variants at each GWAS-associated locus. Identifying these variants is typically the prerequisite for uncovering the associated gene and the mode of association (e.g., increased expression or alternate splicing).

When near one another, SNPs tend to be correlated due to linkage disequilibrium—a limiting factor for fine mapping. For example, when realizations of a "causal" SNP are perfectly correlated ($r = 1$) with one or more noncausal SNPs, no fine-mapping approach can distinguish between these variants. Fine-mapping intervals would be smaller if they were applied to a population with shorter correlated blocks (e.g., sub-Saharan African ancestry compared to

European ancestry). A large sample is required to detect each independent signal, and current samples of non-European populations are not large enough for this purpose. Clearly, increasing the sample sizes or incorporating information from both populations would yield tighter intervals for fine mapping.

Sample Diversity and Translation

Increasing diversity in samples is also essential for translation. Polygenic risk scores hold potential for clinical application to facilitate, for example, diagnosis and predict risk and progression. A PRS developed from samples of European ancestry, however, associates less strongly with the same phenotype in non-European samples (Curtis 2018; Yang and Zhou 2022). Notably, a PRS for schizophrenia was shown to be more strongly associated with ancestry than with schizophrenia (Curtis 2018). The challenge is largely expected to be due to linkage disequilibrium patterns and variant frequencies varying across ancestries, although differences in phenotyping also need careful consideration.

Phenotype differences between cohorts across ancestries further exacerbate the low portability of genetic findings. Phenotype differences can emerge as a result of study design, self-selection biases in participation, and other cultural differences in disease diagnosis. Concordance in phenotypes across ancestries also varies based on the specific psychiatric disorder. For example, while the genetic correlation for schizophrenia between East Asian and European populations is 0.98 (Lam et al. 2019) and the equivalent for bipolar disorder is 0.68, that of major depressive disorder between the same two populations is lower, at 0.33 (Bigdeli et al. 2017). In fact, just 11% of depression risk loci robustly identified in Europeans are associated with depression in East Asia (Giannakopoulou et al. 2021).

Moreover, efficacy of a treatment and risk of adverse effects may be dependent on genetic variants influencing drug metabolism or treatment-associated complications (e.g., neutralizing antibodies against biopharmaceuticals). The frequencies of these variants are ancestry dependent (Andlauer et al. 2020) and, hence, management of effective treatment and risk of adverse effects requires genetic analyses on diverse ancestries.

Increasing Diversity in Samples

The need for social justice and equity provides a strong argument for inclusion of diverse communities, both in the genetic samples we study and in the research workforce that conducts research on these samples. The social justice and equity arguments for diversifying our genetic samples derive from the need to ensure that all global citizens benefit from the advances that arise from gene discovery. Genetics provides opportunities for clinical advances in two independent ways. First, it is believed that genetic information about risk and resilience will be useful clinically at both the population and individual levels.

As theory predicts and empirical studies verify, the application of genetic information to risk prediction only works within a given genetic background. It is thus imperative for genetic studies to include diverse samples so that individuals from non-European ancestries can benefit from predictive knowledge. Second, the biological pathways elucidated from these studies can identify novel treatment targets. If we fail to study genetic risk in non-European populations, we may miss important clues to novel treatments that may be specific to, or especially important in, addressing mental illness in individuals from these populations.

Arguments for diversifying the genetic research workforce are equally compelling. We cannot hope to understand the nature and needs of global communities if those leading the research are not from those communities. Moreover, the benefits, both material and inspirational, of contributing to advances gained through genetics would be unfairly constrained without such participation. Our field of psychiatric genetics requires both sample and workforce diversity for it to reach its goals and contribute to better health across the globe.

Environmental Risk and Gene–Environment Relationships

How do we explore the space of environmental risk and gene–environment relationships? Environmental risk can impact disease development, without any contributing genetic factors. However, many environments are related to our genotypes. Only some rare, stochastic environments (e.g., experiencing a tsunami) do not correlate in any way with our genotype or the genotype of our close relatives. Most environmental influences are correlated with genetic influence (gene–environment correlation), or their effect is contingent on genetic influence (gene–environment interaction).

The classic twin design, the adoption design, and the monozygotic twin design have traditionally been used to parse out environmental variance from heritable effects. These remain powerful and well-tested designs. Still, new approaches in psychiatric genetics can be used to accelerate progress in understanding environmental risk and gene–environment relationships. These approaches measure and capture environmental variables known to have a large effect on psychiatric phenotypes—a key example being childhood trauma (Nelson et al. 2020)—and to incorporate them into genetic designs where possible. In particular, we need to strengthen the ability of psychiatric genetic studies to address and incorporate environmental risk by identifying environmental parameters that can be efficiently measured, are feasible to collect, and will generalize across studies.

Gene–Environment Correlation: Behavior Genetic Designs

Models using twin data can estimate the presence of gene–environment correlation by estimating the heritability of environmental measures and the degree of shared genetic influences between a measured "environmental" variable and a psychiatric phenotype (e.g., Shakoor et al. 2016). The advent of genome-wide complex trait analysis and genome-based restricted maximum likelihood (Yang et al. 2011) enables estimation of the SNP-based heritability of any environment measured in unrelated individuals (Plomin 2014).

Genome-Wide Association Studies of "Environments"

A natural next step from estimating the heritability of an environmental variable is to conduct gene discovery via GWAS to find genetic variants influencing measured environments. Early on, a GWAS of a measure of childhood family environment was conducted (Butcher and Plomin 2008); more recently, UK Biobank data have been used, for example, to identify SNPs associated with social deprivation and household income (Hill et al. 2016). This literature moves the field forward from hypothesizing about gene–environment correlation to identifying its underlying biology; that is, which genetic variants play a role in influencing the environments in which people live.

Polygenic Risk Score Associations with Environments

Another form of evidence for gene–environment correlation is through PRS associations. Polygenic risk scores should index a summed additive genetic signal of a phenotype. If a PRS is associated with a measured environment, it suggests some shared variance. For example, in a systematic review of all studies using the latest PRS for attention deficit hyperactivity disorder (ADHD) (Demontis et al. 2019), the ADHD PRS was consistently associated with lower socioeconomic status (Ronald et al. 2021).

Indeed, the signal in PRSs is thought to include direct genetic effects, but also to be inflated by a range of indirect effects including gene–environment correlations. Partitioning these indirect effects from the direct genetic effects, within-family analysis designs has been proposed (Selzam et al. 2019). Ultimately, this type of work helps to quantify the extent of genetic effects.

Within-Family versus Between-Family Genetic Association

Within-family designs, whether in GWASs or for PRS associations, enable direct genetic effects to be isolated from indirect effects. Indirect effects can include gene–environment correlation, population stratification, and assortative mating. For example, we can conduct analyses with PRSs using a within-family design (e.g., within sibling pairs) and compare effect sizes to those found for analyses with PRSs using a between-family design (i.e., unrelated individuals). This comparison enables us to gauge the extent of direct genetic effects relative to indirect effects (Selzam et al. 2019). When the within-family design involves comparing siblings, it controls for a wide range of environmental factors that are shared by the siblings.

Another within-family methodological development focuses on genes that are shared and not shared between parents and offspring. The traditional view is that within families, children's outcomes are influenced by the child's own genotype and the home environment shared with their parents. However, parents also have their own genotypes, some of which are shared with their offspring and some of which are not. Polygenic risk scores in parents can be partitioned into the alleles transmitted to their offspring and the parents' alleles that were not transmitted to their offspring but nevertheless may have influenced the child's environment. The latter process has been termed "genetic nurture" (Kong et al. 2018). These nontransmitted alleles may play a role in the offspring's outcome phenotypes through gene–environment correlation. This approach helps to unravel the causal pathways, both genetic and environmental, that contribute to risk for psychiatric disorders.

Gene–Environment Interaction

Twin Designs

Gene–environment interaction refers to the effect of environments being contingent on genetic influence, or vice versa. Twin models can test for gene–environment interaction (e.g., whether heritability varies as a function of environmental severity), while controlling for any gene–environment correlation. A recent example of gene–environment interaction in a twin design found that psychotic experiences are less heritable in individuals who have experienced greater environmental adversity and are more heritable for individuals who have experienced less environmental adversity, after controlling for any gene–environment correlation (Taylor et al. 2022).

Individual Loci and Polygenic Risk Scores

It is possible to identify interactions between multiple measured environments with specific genetic loci. First, iSet is a method based on linear mixed models that tests for interactions between sets of variants and environmental states or other contexts (Casale et al. 2017). It jointly tests for gene–environment interaction across multiple contexts and sets of adjacent variants in genomic loci across the genome and, as such, allows for characterizing the local architecture of gene–environment interactions. Second, the structured linear mixed model (StructLMM)—a variance component test to identify and characterize gene–environment interactions between individual SNPs and multiple environments—allows the identification of interactions that are simultaneously driven by multiple environments (Moore et al. 2019). Similarly, the linear environment mixed model analysis (LEMMA) uses a Bayesian approach and estimates a linear combination of environmental variables that interacts with genetic variants (Kerin and Marchini 2020).

Polygenic gene–environment interaction can be tested using extensions to genome-wide genomic restricted maximum likelihood (used to estimate SNP-based heritability from genome-wide data) under the mixed model for gene–environment interaction (GxEMM) framework, by allowing for environment-specific genetic variance and noise (Dahl et al. 2020). Importantly, GxEMM is further able to accommodate quantitative and multiple environments, an extension from previous models, and has already been used to show polygenic interactions with environmental stress indices for major depression (Dahl et al. 2020).

Using Results from Genome-Wide Association Studies to Test for Environmental Causality

Mendelian randomization is a form of instrumental variable analysis that uses genetic variants as instrumental variables (Davey Smith and Hemani 2014). It is now an established method for deriving a form of evidence of causality, which leverages genetic information (and yet does not focus on genetic influence itself) to estimate the causal effect of an exposure on an outcome. It has the potential to evaluate the causal effect of environments on psychiatric phenotypes more cheaply and in a complementary manner than randomized control trials. Mendelian randomization has a range of assumptions which, to some degree, are managed by a range of complementary methods (because different Mendelian randomization methods have differing assumptions). It is a method that exploits results from GWASs to study nongenetic processes; namely, the causality of environmental modifiers.

Summary

There is a range of methods that enable environmental risk and gene–environment correlation and gene–environment interaction to be tested empirically using the twin design, GWASs, and post-GWAS approaches. Far from being a diversion in our field, these methods are likely to catalyze biological insights because they enable a more accurate understanding of direct genetic effects and of how environments operate together with genetic risk. As such, the opportunities and benefits offered by these approaches should not be underestimated and very much add to the scoreboard of contributions made by psychiatric genetic genome-wide research in completing the picture of why psychiatric disorders develop.

Future Experimental Design

To integrate the various threads of our discussions, let us consider some key principles of experimental design that will optimize future discovery and advance our understanding of the genetic architecture of neurodevelopmental conditions and psychiatric disorders and their neurobiology, while accounting for equity and inclusion. Given finite time, resources, and consents, considering these principles will help guide future gene discovery studies to ensure maximum returns.

The most pertinent design features and the key approaches that offer the greatest potential for such advancements are summarized in Table 2.3. We consistently identified the need for well-powered global cohorts with a focus on diverse ancestral representation as the feature that should receive the highest priority. Appropriately designed studies that also account for local genetic variation will facilitate fine mapping, gene identification, and risk prediction.

Neurodevelopmental conditions and psychiatric disorders are developmental disorders and shedding light on developmental trajectories and their underlying genetic architecture will aid in defining the neurobiology of these disorders. Thus, study designs that allow for the collection of neurodevelopmental

Table 2.3 Key features of experimental design in psychiatric genetics.

Priorities	Approaches
Diversity	Aim for diverse ancestral samples on a global scale. Engage local researchers in sampling decisions. Enable diversity in the psychiatric genetics workforce where possible.
Development	Include collection of appropriate and feasible developmental data (e.g., birth records, milestones) collected through electronic health records.
Environment	Link by location (e.g., using the American Community Survey). Include siblings in a subset of the sampling frame to enable within-family designs. Measure known environmental influences for stratification (e.g., via birth records where available).
Heterogeneity	Incorporate heterogeneity into the study design and plan for subgroup analyses. Collect detailed information and make it available to analysts. Make future contact part of the consent.
Quantitative traits	Supplement diagnoses and symptom trackers with quantitative phenotypes and phenotypes closer to biology (e.g., circuit-based behaviors).
Co-occurrence	Be explicit about disorder exclusions. Collect detailed information and make it available to analysts. Consider the relative timing of onset of a co-occurring condition, beyond cross-sectional absence/presence.
Genetic platform	Aim to sequence at the highest practical coverage and resolution. Sequencing methods capture more diversity in the genome due to less reliance on imputation.

phenotypes (e.g., as a minimum standard, birth records and electronic health records data) are advantageous whenever possible.

Another crucial co-factor in the risk architecture of mental disorders is the environment. Study designs that allow for the collection of a minimum set of environmental exposure data (e.g., geolocation, trauma) would enable analytical tools to evaluate environmental factors and gene–environment interactions.

Historically, psychiatric genetics has relied on binary clinical diagnoses as outcome variables—an approach that has led to successes in gene discovery. There is, however, a vast distance between the different levels of analysis needed in psychiatry: from genes to molecules to cells to pathways to circuits and behavior (Figure 2.1). It is widely accepted that the binary phenotypes used in psychiatry are complex and heterogeneous and do not necessarily map well to their underlying biology. For this reason, heterogeneity is a core feature of neurodevelopmental conditions and psychiatric disorders and must be accounted for in study design and analysis. In addition to the collection of clinical diagnoses, it is thus important for heritable, disease-related, quantitative, and developmental phenotypes to be measured and analyzed.

Neurodevelopmental conditions and psychiatric disorders often do not occur in isolation and are frequently accompanied by the co-occurrence of other disorders of the brain or organ systems. The co-occurrence of other disorders reflects the underlying genetic and phenotypic heterogeneity and their complexity. Designs that permit all relevant phenotypes and enable analyses that include them are, therefore, advantageous. The co-occurrence of non-brain diseases should be leveraged as a possible pointer to the underlying biology and incorporated into the analysis.

Finally, it is important for genetic variation present in the cohort to be assessed on contemporary sequencing platforms, at the highest practical sequence coverage and resolution. The sequencing effort should be commensurate to the effort that goes into ascertainment, consent, exposure measurements, and collection of binary and quantitative phenotype data. Based on the continuing technological advancements in sequencing technologies, and the accompanying reduction in the cost of generating whole genomes, array-based technologies carry fewer advantages for most new studies. By using cost-effective sequencing methods, including low-pass whole-genome sequencing (Li et al. 2021; Martin et al. 2021), major shortcomings of microarrays, in particular poor imputation quality in diverse ancestries and a preselection of known variants, can be avoided.

In an era of limited resources, we realize that the strategies discussed in this chapter and summarized above may be difficult to implement concurrently in a single study. We believe, however, that through team-based national and international collaborations that are developed with community engagement and explicit emphasis on equity, these strategies are achievable and worthwhile. The study of non-European and older ancestral populations as well as study designs that we have outlined will assist in further delineating the genetic architecture of neurodevelopmental conditions and psychiatric disorders, dissect their phenotypic complexity, generate new discoveries of the underlying neurobiology, and ultimately achieve translational and clinical applications.

Acknowledgments

We thank Naomi Wray and Stephan Sanders for comments on earlier versions of this chapter. We also thank all the members of the Forum who contributed to the discussions in our group, in particular Jordan Smoller and Lea Davis. Views expressed herein do not necessarily represent the views of the NIH, HHS, or the United States Government.

3

Data Collection

Next Steps in Psychiatric Genetics

Elise B. Robinson, Heesu Kim, Daniel Weiner,
Alicia Ljungdahl, and Stephan J. Sanders

Abstract

Decades of twin and family studies have revealed the high heritability of neuropsychiatric disorders, suggesting an important causal role for genetic factors. Over the last decade, genetic studies have linked hundreds of genes and genetic loci to neuropsychiatric disorders as well as to behavior and cognition more broadly. Most large lists of genetic loci associated with disorders have been generated by consortia. These consortia aggregate data from similarly focused studies from around the globe, with historic emphasis on certain areas. This chapter explores what is necessary to deliver refined genetic insights rigorously and efficiently.

Identification of Genetic Variants in Neuropsychiatric Disorders

Any two unrelated individuals have about 3 million genetic variants (0.1% of the genome, 1 in a 1,000 bp) that differ between them. The majority of these are common single nucleotide polymorphisms (SNPs); that is, single base pairs of DNA that vary in at least 1% of the population. The remaining variation can be rare (<1% of the population) and/or larger (e.g., insertions, deletions, structural variants). Common variants can be detected using a genotyping array. The role of common variants in a disorder is assessed through genome-wide association studies (GWASs), which identify specific SNPs that are more common than expected in either cases or controls. Rare variants in protein-coding regions can be detected using whole-exome sequencing (WES). Due to their rarity, these variants typically must be grouped together (e.g., within the same gene) to assess whether their frequency differs from expectation between cases and controls. Whole-genome sequencing (WGS) enables the detection of variants across the frequency and size spectra, outperforming both genotyping arrays and WES, but it is expensive to conduct. Even with WGS data, moderately rare variants (0.1–2% population frequency) and rare noncoding variants associated with human disorders remain largely undetectable with current cohort sizes and methodologies (Sanders et al. 2017; Singh et al. 2022; Werling et al. 2018). Similarly, only the common variants and rare protein-coding variants with the highest effect sizes for neuropsychiatric disorders have been detected so far.

Natural Selection and Genomic Architecture

The choice of genetic characterization strategy often reflects the known or hypothesized genomic architecture of a disorder or trait, which is primarily influenced by natural selection. Strong selective pressure, as is present in early-onset neurodevelopmental disorders such as autism spectrum disorder (ASD) or intellectual disability (ID) (Power et al. 2013), imposes a limit on the effect size that a common variant can impart (Devlin et al. 2011), necessitating huge cohorts for GWAS discovery. Accordingly, genetic locus discovery for these disorders has focused on finding rare variants with high effect sizes, e.g., by the analysis of trios composed of both parents and an affected child to identify newly arising *de novo* mutations (Sebat et al. 2007). While each variant is individually rare, many different genes and many different disruptive variants within each gene can lead to symptoms. Combining all of these genes and variants, at least 30%–40% of ID cases and 10% of ASD cases can be explained by a single rare genetic event (Bishop et al. 2021). By comparison, it is rare for a single genetic variant to explain a meaningful fraction of individual risk for late-onset disorders, such as bipolar illness or major depressive disorder (MDD), and locus discovery for this type of disorder has accordingly focused on common variants discoverable through GWAS (Howard et al. 2019; Mullins et al. 2021).

In Table 3.1, we present a set of recent landmark psychiatric genetics studies of developmental (ASD, ID/NDD, and attention deficit hyperactivity disorder), mood (anxiety, MDD, bipolar disorder), and psychotic (schizophrenia) disorders. The studies listed reflect the largest collaborative efforts, in both genotyping and/or sequencing studies, for each outcome over the past five years.

In total, more than three million individuals participated in these studies, and more than 600 genes and genetic loci have been identified. Here, we discuss continuing data collection and association needs in neuropsychiatric statistical genetics, as gaps remain in both publicly available data collections and the published literature. We focus on three themes below: (a) completing discovery, (b) informing biology with genetic associations from across the frequency spectrum, and (c) improving global representation.

Table 3.1 Largest and most recent genomic studies across seven major psychiatric disorders: attention deficit hyperactivity disorder (ADHD), autism spectrum disorder (ASD), intellectual disability/neurodevelopmental delay (ID/NDD), anxiety (ANX), major depressive disorder (MDD), bipolar disorder (BD), and schizophrenia (SCZ). Single nucleotide polymorphisms (SNP), de novo (dn), ultrarare (ur), missense (mis), protein truncating variant (PTV), copy number variant (CNV), loss of function (LoF). N includes all samples from discovery and replications, where applicable.

Disorder	Study Design	Genetic Characterization	Variant	All cases (N)	All controls (N)	Total Subjects (N)	Significant loci/genes	Cohort	Reference
ADHD	Case-control	Genotyping	SNP	4,208	32,222	36,430	27	PGC, iPSYCH	Demontis et al. (2019)
		WGS	rare recurrent	205	670	875	1	iPSYCH	Satterstrom et al. (2019)
ASD	Case-control	Genotyping	SNP	18,381	27,969	46,350	5	Danish iPSYCH	Grove et al. (2019)
	Parent-child trios, case control	WES	dnPTV, dnCNV, mis	51,685	103,157	154,842	72	ASC, SSC, SPARK, iPSYCH	Fu et al. (2022)
ID/NDD	Case control, parent-child trios	Genotyping	SNP	7,715	10,726	18,441	0	DDD, ADD	Niemi et al. (2018)
	Parent-child trios	WES	dn	31,058	62,116	93,174	285	GeneDX, DDD, RUMC	Kaplanis et al. (2020)
ANX	Case control, continuous trait	Genotyping	SNP, eQTL	34,189	190,141	423,941	6	Million Veterans	Levey et al. (2020)
	Case control		SNP	44,465	58,113	102,578	5	UK Biobank	Purves et al. (2020)
MDD	Case control	Genotyping	SNP	660,418	1,453,489	2,113,907	87	UK Biobank, 23andMe, PGC	Howard et al. (2019)
			SNP	15,771	178,777	194,548	1	CONVERGE, TMDD, CKB	Giannakopoulou et al. (2021)
BD	Case control	Genotyping	CNV	23,979	383,095	407,074	53	UK Biobank	Kendall et al. (2019)
			SNP	41,917	371,549	413,466	64	PGC	Mullins et al. (2021)
			rare CNV	6,353	8,656	15,009	0	ICCBD	Charney et al. (2018)
		WES	urPTV	38,181	111,744	149,925	1	BipEx, SCHEMA	Palmer et al. (2022)
SCZ	Case control	Genotyping	SNP	69,369	236,642	306,011	270	PGC	Trubetskoy et al. (2022)
			CNV	21,094	20,227	41,321	8	PGC	Marshall et al. (2017)
	Case control, parent-child trios	WES	dnPTV, mis	24,248	97,322	121,570	10	CHEMA, gnomAD	Singh et al. (2022)

Completing Discovery

In our opinion, there is no objective point at which genetic discovery activities for neuropsychiatric disorders will be definitively complete, short of deploying the latest sequencing technology worldwide. Here we present some ideas relevant to the question of whether and how to emphasize future gene discovery.

There are several reasons to believe that identification of risk-conferring variation should continue. First, across the disorders listed in Table 3.1, we continue to identify new loci and do not see evidence of plateauing. Those loci provide new biological inferences and are furthering our understanding of the genetic architecture of neuropsychiatric disease. Schizophrenia provides a useful example, as it is the psychiatric outcome most comprehensively characterized with GWAS (about 70,000 cases have yielded over 250 common variant loci; Trubetskoy et al. 2022) and exome sequencing: about 24,000 cases by SCHEMA[1] have yielded 10 genes from rare variations (Singh et al. 2022). Combining these loci allows the relationship between effect size and population frequency of associated variants to be plotted. In Figure 3.1, we have adapted SCHEMA's figure (Singh et al. 2022) to highlight the search space in which discovery activities remain statistically underpowered. As an example, variants with 0.001 frequency and an odds ratio of 2 cannot be identified with current sample size and will require case samples of approximately 250,000 to be detectable (and at least an equal number of controls). At that same frequency, variants with an OR of 1.5 would be detectable with 900,000 cases.

For schizophrenia genetics, if we achieved a target sample of 250,000 cases, there would be several benefits. First, we would have access to the class of risk variation described above: variants of lower frequency and modest effect size. We do not know the degree to which the biology implicated by that class will overlap with either (a) very rare variants of large effect or (b) common variants of small effect. Second, by increasing schizophrenia case sample size further, we will identify more carriers of specific risk factors, which will permit better powered follow-up studies. For example, 15 SCHEMA individuals (out of 25,000 cases) carried a risk variant in SETD1A, the gene found to have the largest effect size. Expanding this total would enable detailed genotype-phenotype analysis (Sanders et al. 2018), comparison of developmental trajectories (Wickstrom et al. 2021), and the development of valuable cell line resources (Khan et al. 2020). Of course, such analyses and resource development necessitate studies in which the participants are contacted at different stages. Third, as we discuss in detail below, genetic studies of neuropsychiatric disease have, to this point, predominantly included individuals of European ancestry. Additional data collection in schizophrenia is necessary to progress toward equitable polygenic risk score (PRS) performance across ancestral groups, among other imperatives (for further discussion, see Ronald et al., this volume).

[1] The Schizophrenia Exome Sequencing Meta-Analysis

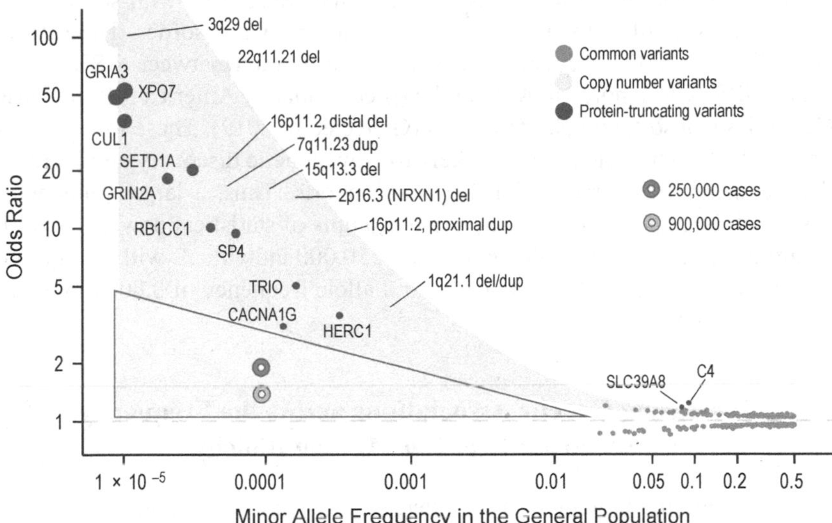

Figure 3.1 Effect size by allelic frequency for known genetic risk variants in schizophrenia. Updated from Singh et al. (2022).

While schizophrenia provides several useful points for consideration, it cannot be used as a model for all other psychiatric disorders. Schizophrenia has featured a relatively high rate of common variant discovery (as compared to MDD or ASD) and a relatively slow rate of rare variant discovery (as compared to ASD or ID). This pattern may predict average phenotypic differences between individuals with schizophrenia who carry strong-acting risk variants (e.g., in *SETD1A*) versus those who do not, as has been seen for other rare variant-mediated disorders (Ahn et al. 2014; Satterstrom et al. 2020). Such questions, however, can only be answered with larger schizophrenia case sample sizes.

Genetic data highlights other differences between schizophrenia and, for example, ASD and MDD. Schizophrenia has a very high "genetic correlation with itself," which we use to mean the estimated genetic correlation between one schizophrenia case-control data set and another. When one estimates this correlation between various schizophrenia cohorts that have contributed genetic data to the Psychiatric Genomics Consortium, those values almost uniformly exceed 0.9, and are typically close to 1. This can be interpreted to mean that the common variant influences on schizophrenia are extremely similar across different samples, regardless of where or how individuals with the diagnosis are being ascertained.

The same cannot be said for MDD or ASD. The average genetic correlation in MDD with itself is around 0.7. This is similar to the genetic correlation between schizophrenia and bipolar disorder. In other words, there is as much genetic heterogeneity between cohorts of individuals diagnosed with

MDD as there is between cohorts of individuals diagnosed with schizophrenia and cohorts of individuals diagnosed with bipolar disorder. The picture is similar for ASD. The estimated genetic correlation between ASD in the Danish iPSYCH cohort and ASD in the (predominantly American) Psychiatric Genomics Consortium cohorts is 0.74 (Grove et al. 2019). These low correlations reflect heterogeneity that is likely to slow genetic discovery and increase the frequency of nonreplication between cohorts. Thus, a larger number of cases will be required to reach equivalent points of statistical power. To put it quantitatively, we estimate that *more* than 250,000 individuals will be required to identify a risk variant with OR of 2 and allele frequency of 0.0001 in meta-analyses of MDD and ASD.

Increasing Genetic Associations across the Frequency Spectrum to Fill in Missing Biology

To understand the biology of a disorder, scientists must mechanistically connect causal factors to phenotypes. With the high heritabilities observed in neuropsychiatric disorders, genetic factors offer a critical causal starting point in this quest for biological understanding. Thus, a key motivation for genetic studies is as an entree into biology. All psychiatric disorders have elements of their genetic architecture that remain uncovered. For many, neither the common nor rare variant influences have been fleshed out. In this section, we link association goals to issues of biological understanding for both rare and common variation.

Rare variation underlies a substantial fraction of ID and ASD, early-onset disorders with high selective pressure. Rare variation is less prominent in late-onset disorders with weaker selective pressures. The majority of variation identified to date is from heterozygous protein-coding variation that disrupts one copy of a specific gene (e.g., *SCN2A*). These rare variants provide tractable targets for experimental model systems. However, the majority of genes associated with neuropsychiatric disorders perform myriad functions across development of the human brain (i.e., they are highly pleiotropic). While identifying a molecular, cellular, or behavioral consequence of disrupting the gene is relatively straightforward, showing that this consequence underlies the human phenotype is not, due to the absence of reliable endpoints in experimental model systems. This translational challenge limits the extent to which analysis of single genes can definitively inform biological understanding of the phenotype.

To overcome this challenge, convergent approaches aim to identify shared features or consequences across multiple genes as an indicator of relevant biology, demonstrating statistical enrichment of a biological measure across genes associated with a disorder compared to a relevant group of comparator genes (e.g., brain-expressed genes without evidence of statistical association).

This systems biology approach has provided key insights into ASD, including the enrichment of genes with a role in transcriptional regulation and neuronal communication (De Rubeis et al. 2014), prenatal onset (Parikshak et al. 2013; Willsey et al. 2013), and highlights the role of excitatory and inhibitory cortical neurons (Satterstrom et al. 2020). Convergent approaches, however, are very sensitive to the choice of background genes, which, in turn, rely on gene discovery efforts. While current analyses can reliably distinguish genes associated with ASD, they lack the sensitivity to exclude genes that are not associated with ASD. Larger discovery cohorts would improve our ability to distinguish genes associated with ASD versus those which are not, providing deeper insights into the underlying neurobiology.

Meanwhile, common polygenic variation contributes the majority of genetic liability for neuropsychiatric disease and is highly distributed across the genome. For example, more than 71% of 1 Mb blocks of the genome contain at least one schizophrenia-influencing variant (Loh et al. 2015). Significant loci are largely noncoding, which presents a formidable challenge to biological interpretation and identification of causal genes. Here, we consider three strategies for learning risk biology from common polygenic variation, each of which requires further characterization of the common variant signal to be employed effectively.

First, there is the classic approach of (a) fine mapping to identify the causal variant from the GWAS-identified variant and (b) using bioinformatic and experimental approaches to identify the manner in which the causal variant creates risk (e.g., through regulation of a nearby gene). This approach has achieved some notable successes, including identifying expression quantitative trait loci (eQTL), which co-localize with schizophrenia risk loci (Fromer et al. 2016), and the association of specific C4 haplotypes with schizophrenia (Sekar et al. 2016). However, with currently available data, the great majority of neuropsychiatric GWAS loci cannot be resolved to a single variant that alters gene expression or splicing behavior. Efforts to identify brain-related eQTLs and the eGenes that they regulate remain limited by sample size as well as the current state of knowledge of gene expression patterns in specific developmental stages, brain regions, and cell types (Table 3.2). Improved sample size would aid fine mapping of known loci and permit the discovery of new loci as would more specific and complete data regarding gene expression in the brain across the lifespan.

Second, new statistical approaches aim to use neuropsychiatric risk genes uncovered by rare variation to provide an interpretative scaffold for common variation. The degree to which these genes mediate the effects of common variation could be highly informative to questions of rare and common variant convergence. One recently developed approach, the Abstract Mediation Model (Weiner et al. 2022), estimates the fraction of common variant heritability mediated by a set of genes without relying on measured gene expression levels or eQTLs. Most strikingly, more than 90% of heritability for schizophrenia and

Table 3.2 Representative quantitative trait locus (QTL) discovery in the human brain. DLPFC: dorsolateral prefrontal cortex.

QTL Type	Brain Region	Developmental Stage	Total Subjects (N)	eGenes / loci	Cohort	Reference
Expression	DLPFC	Prenatal, postnatal	176	5,728	BrainVar	Werling et al. (2020)
Expression	Cortex	Prenatal	201	6,546	UCLA	Walker et al. (2019)
Expression	Cortex	Adult	1,433	18,433	AMP-AD (ROSMAP) Mayo TCX	Sieberts et al. (2020)
Expression	10 regions	Adult	72–103	853–3,454	GTEx	GTEx Consortium (2020)
Splicing	13 regions	Adult	63–124	1,590	GTEx	Zhang et al. (2020b)
Expression	DLPFC	Adult	1,866	32,944	PsychENCODE, CMC, GTEx	Wang et al. (2018)
Chromatin	DLPFC	Adult	292	8,464	PsychENCODE, CMC, GTEx	Wang et al. (2018)
Protein	DLPFC	Adult	380	32	NA	Yang et al. (2021)

ASD are mediated by genes other than those implicated in neurodevelopmental disorders through rare coding variation (n = 373 genes; Figure 3.2). In contrast, 21 genes implicated in Mendelian forms of lipid dysregulation are massively enriched for lipid heritability (> 100x), mediating about 25% of overall heritability. These results reflect the differential effect of negative selection on common variation, where negative selection against neuropsychiatric traits limits the allelic effect size of common variants, "flattening" the distribution of heritability across the genome (O'Connor et al. 2019). In contrast, selective pressures act much less strongly on lipid phenotypes, permitting common variants of large effect to co-localize at physiologically important genes.

These observations provide a critical look into the prospects for deriving biological insight from neuropsychiatric polygenicity. First, genome-wide observations such as these do not preclude instances of common and rare overlap; for instance, in schizophrenia, both common and rare associations implicate glutamatergic dysfunction in disease pathogenesis (Singh et al. 2022; Trubetskoy et al. 2022). However, they do suggest that rare variant-implicated genes mediate only a small fraction of polygenic heritability and, consequently, that a very large number of genes mediate heritability for these traits. Sophisticated approaches and biological assays are needed to derive these insights that extend beyond canonical gene set enrichment methods.

A third option is to develop methods to learn risk biology directly from a common polygenic signal. This is a new area of inquiry, becoming more possible through the growth of human or human-derived cell line resources, specifically those paired with genome-wide genetic data. A recent analysis

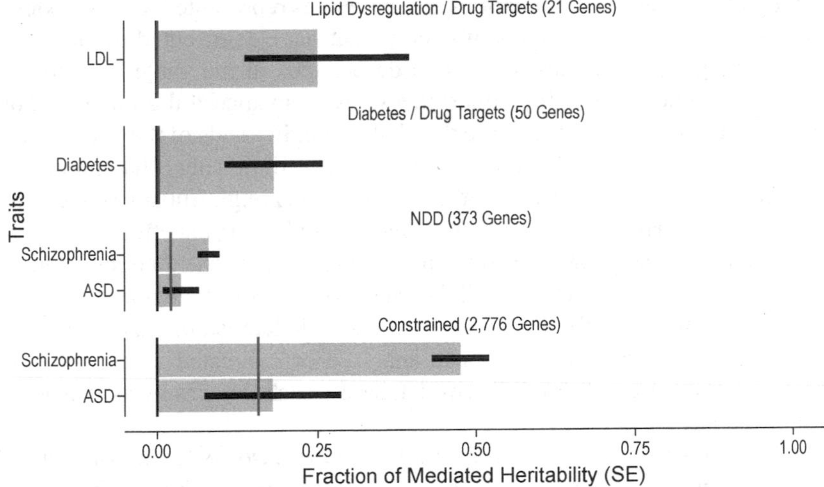

Figure 3.2 Fraction of common variant heritability explained by specific gene lists (LDL: low-density lipoprotein).

of common variant risk for ASD exemplifies such an approach (Weiner et al. 2022). In their study, Weiner et al. uncovered an unexpected concentration of common variant signal distributed across the 30 Mb p arm of chromosome 16. The region includes one of the best-established neuropsychiatric risk copy number variations (CNVs), deletions, and duplications at 16p11.2. Using human cell line resources, they found that both common polygenic influences on ASD and isogenic deletion of the 16p11.2 CNVs were associated with decreased gene expression across the full 30 Mb p arm. The per gene effects of the deletion and the PRS of ASD were correlated, suggesting convergent functional impact. The region also exhibited an unusually high degree of chromatin contact with itself, potentially explaining the convergent effects of common and rare variation in the region. These findings suggest that biological insight can emerge from highly distributed polygenic liability, though cell line and other omics resources will need to grow substantially to be most successfully used for this purpose.

Improving Global Representation

Genomic studies have historically relied on data from nations with the resources to fund large-scale research. Reflecting disparities in these resources, Fatumo et al. (2022) estimate that 86% of all genomics studies have been conducted in populations of European descent.

Psychiatric genetics studies are no exception to this trend. Among all studies listed in Table 3.1, only one focuses centrally on a non-European population, although other ancestral populations are sometimes represented to some extent. To dissect the ancestral origins of cohorts that have contributed to landmark psychiatric genetics studies, we took a deeper look at the Table 3.1 cohorts. First, we assigned each major cohort in a study to an ancestral group based on the majority of that cohort: if more than half the individuals of the cohort were of European ancestry, we assigned it to European; if the cohort had no majority group, it was assigned to "other"). In some cases (e.g., Autism Sequencing Consortium, SCHEMA, or Psychiatric Genomics Consortium efforts), the goal was to develop a large data set from an aggregate of very small cohorts. Under these scenarios, we counted the full data set as one cohort, particularly because the consortium-led databases continue to be used in later studies as one cohort. Consistent with this, if a study meta-analyzed or replicated across different large cohorts sourced from different databases, each database was deemed a distinct cohort.

In addition to the studies from Table 3.1, we also added non-European GWAS cohorts with more than 50,000 total samples within the past five years, if such studies existed. We found two such papers, both of which studied East Asian cohorts: Lam et al. (2019) conducted a study of schizophrenia and Giannakopoulou et al. (2021) studied MDD. We summarize these results in Figure 3.3.

It will be very difficult to achieve numerically equal ancestral representation in neuropsychiatric genetics collections, particularly in light of the need to drastically increase sample size for many disorders. However, it is possible to achieve parity in the performance of genetic data across populations. Parity has been widely discussed in terms of PRS performance, as PRSs are now being incorporated into clinical care in a number of settings. Should PRS become clinically useful in psychiatry (see Davis et al., this volume), the use of current PRS would exacerbate health disparities (Doan et al. 2019; Martin et al. 2019b). PRS perform best when deployed in the same ancestral populations that provided data for the GWAS activity used to develop the PRS. For example, the schizophrenia PRSs, derived from predominantly European ancestry samples, becomes less associated to schizophrenia liability and less predictive of correlated behavioral outcomes in ancestral groups that are genetically distant from Europeans.

Problems of parity also extend to rare variation. Rates of *de novo* variation do not differ markedly by ancestry, leading to the expectation that similar genes will be associated with neuropsychiatric disorders worldwide through heterozygous rare variation (unless ancestry-specific protective factors exist). Interpreting rare variation for clinical diagnostics, however, relies on using population cohorts, such as gnomAD, to distinguish rare-standing variation from disease-causing new variation. The marked underrepresentation of people of African ancestry extends to gnomAD, in which only 14% of individuals have some African ancestry and these are predominantly from African Americans with a mixture of West African and European ancestry (Gudmundsson et al.

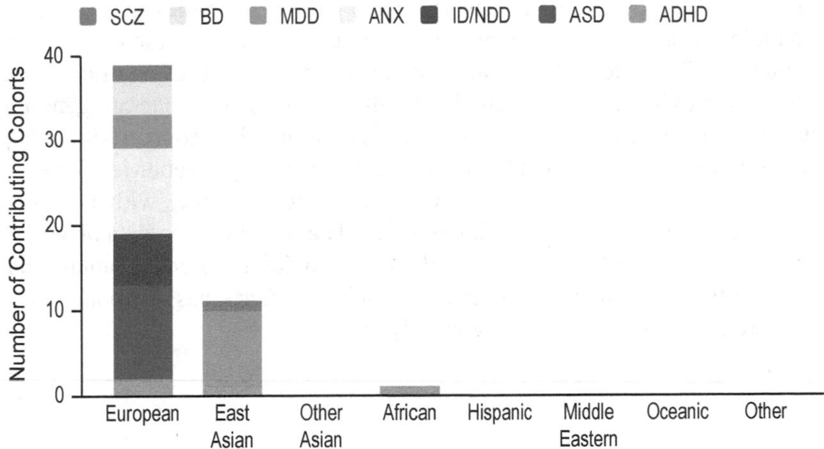

Figure 3.3 Distribution of majority ancestries of cohorts contributing to major and most recent psychiatric genetic studies.

2022; Karczewski et al. 2020). Measures are underway to improve this, including the NeuroDev Kenya collection, which aims to identify genetic diagnoses in hundreds of East African individuals and families, and improve medical, genetic, and diagnostic pipelines for individuals of all types of African ancestry. Because people of African ancestry carry more genetic variation than people of European or Asian ancestry (groups better represented in genetic studies), they are more likely to carry variants of unknown significance and receive ambiguous results from genetic testing (Popejoy et al. 2018). They are also more likely to receive false positive and false negative genetic diagnoses (Caswell-Jin et al. 2018; Lek et al. 2016; Popejoy et al. 2018). Biallelic rare variation also plays a role in neuropsychiatric disorders (Lim et al. 2013). Since these rely on rare standing variation, we would expect dramatic differences across ancestries, as are seen with disorders such as cystic fibrosis or mucopolysaccharidosis.

Conclusion

Increasing sample size is critical to further progress in delineating genetic risk for neuropsychiatric disorders; however, advances in assays (e.g., WGS), statistical methodologies, and functional biology will also contribute. Although immense progress has been made, substantial gaps remain, including many psychiatric diagnoses, most major ancestral populations, variants of moderate effect size and/or population frequency, and rare noncoding variation. Further progress will continue to refine our understanding of existing rare and common loci, extend neurobiological insights from these loci, and potentially uncover entirely new biological insights.

Neuropsychiatric disorder consortia have led the genomics field in terms of building international collaborations to share data across researchers. The Psychiatric Genomics Consortium, Autism Sequencing Consortium, and SCHEMA provide active models. While these groups still generate genomic data, they have increasingly integrated data from other sources, including nonprofit (e.g., Simons Foundation) and for-profit (e.g., 23andMe, GeneDx, Regeneron) organizations. This trend is likely to continue, with consortia increasingly focusing on integrating external data or generating data on ancestrally or phenotypically diverse populations. Providing an environment conducive to these ongoing large-scale international efforts has the potential to deliver refined genetic insights rigorously and efficiently.

4

Environmental Risk and Gene–Environment Relationships in Psychiatric Disorders

Michel G. Nivard

Abstract

Insisting on a distinction between "environmental" and "genetic" risks for psychiatric disorders is imprecise and can be counterproductive. The effect of a genetic variant on a psychiatric outcome may act through environmental pathways. Environmental exposures encountered in life are partly a consequence of how our own heritable traits and predispositions, or those of our parents, interact with our surroundings. This chapter reviews key methods to establish whether an environmental exposure causes an increase in the risk to develop psychopathology or whether it causes psychopathology to relapse. A set of widely studied environmental risks are reviewed for their impact on psychopathology: bereavement, loss, family strife, childhood maltreatment, childhood sexual abuse, trauma, migration and minority stress, exposure to (substance) abuse, sleep, education, and income.

Introduction

The "environment" is a general term and when viewed to be a cause of psychopathology, it evokes different interpretations across disciplines. Sociologists might view racism, sexism, ageism, government policy, or social conventions as possible structural, environmental causes of psychopathology. Health economists might find economic inequality, differences in access to (preventive) care, and market failure in health insurance or health provider markets to be possible environmental causes of psychopathology. Psychologists and psychiatrists might consider parenting, family structure, attachment, stress, and trauma as environmental causes of psychopathology. Developmental biologists and brain scientists might consider hormone levels, vitamins, nutrients, toxins absorbed through exposure or diet to underpin environmental causes of psychopathology. None of these perspectives or levels of analysis are wrong; causes at one level (e.g., lead exposure) may mediate causes at another level (e.g., access to safe housing) and require interventions at yet another (e.g., policy changes). It is natural for scientists or practitioners trained in a particular discipline to gravitate to what they have frequently observed or where they feel they can intervene, but an interdisciplinary perspective is necessary to provide clarity and generate valuable avenues for intervention. In fact, innovations in one area (e.g., better preventive psychotherapy) often requires change in another (e.g., policy or funding reform) for those in need to receive effective treatment.

Genetic Risk and Environmental Risk Are Not Mutually Exclusive

It is crucial to recognize that genetic and environmental risk factors are deeply intertwined. If we were to perform a large enough genome-wide association study (GWAS) of the effectiveness of clozapine treatment for schizophrenia, we would almost surely recover an effect of loci in the *CHRNA3/5* (nicotinic receptor) gene cluster. Certain genetic variants in that region predispose people to smoke (more), and because smoking reduces serum levels of clozapine (Tsuda et al. 2014), any allele that predisposes people to smoke will, on average, reduce clozapine treatment success. Whether the effect of variants in the nicotinic receptor gene on clozapine response would be considered a genetic or environmental effect depends on one's perspective. Finding the effect would be highly illuminating if we had no prior knowledge on the role of smoking in clozapine metabolism. If this example is too hypothetical because we do not have very big clozapine GWAS yet, consider that the most significantly associated genetic variant in any lung cancer GWAS that does not control for smoking is in the region of the *CHRNA3/5* gene (nicotinic receptor), clearly the consequence of a causal genetic pathway that acts through the environment.

Even if the mechanisms uncovered by a GWAS reflect a direct biological causal path that plays out entirely within the body or brain, the most direct intervention might be entirely environmental. The most strongly associated genetic variant in the largest clozapine GWAS to date (Pardiñas et al. 2019) is also a lead hit for the coffee consumption GWAS (Coffee and Caffeine Genetics Consortium et al. 2015)—an association that is a likely consequence of the shared metabolism of caffeine and clozapine by the *CYP1A1* and/or *CYP1A2* genes. Regardless of mechanism, the easiest way to improve patient lives directly, given what we have learned from this clozapine GWAS, might involve tighter regulation or monitoring of caffeine (and based on prior evidence nicotine) intake in patient populations (Rajkumar et al. 2013; Tsuda et al. 2014). Genetic associations might reflect environmental associations or highlight paths for environmental interventions. Based on a GWAS of a psychiatric outcome alone, we cannot adjudicate whether a specific significant locus or pathway implies a genetic, biological, psychological, or environmental risk for psychiatric disorders or symptoms. In many cases, a pathway involves "all of the above."

It is important to note that genetic associations are not studies of mechanism or etiology; they are a prerequisite for the study of disease mechanism or etiology. GWAS associations allow us to link psychopathology to other complex traits: brain traits, metabolic traits, and molecular traits that confirm or reject specific associations and hypothesized causal relations. While GWAS can help further our understanding of the causes of psychiatric disorders, regardless of whether those causes are understood to be environmental, psychological, or biological, there are certain exogenous (understood to be environmental) risks for psychopathology for which genetic analysis is not the best or obvious answer. As genetic risk and environmental risk are deeply intertwined, it almost always helps to try and account for genetic effects when studying environmental risk of psychopathology.

Risk of *What* Exactly?

A critical nuance that muddles the discourse on the (relative) contribution of environmental and heritable risk for psychopathology is that one must clearly define risk for *what*. Schizophrenia and bipolar disorder are among the most heritable psychiatric disorders, a fact that has been confirmed through multiple orthogonal methods (Golan et al. 2014; Lichtenstein et al. 2009). In the lives of most people diagnosed with schizophrenia or bipolar disorder, they may experience periods of remission as well as relapse, including periods of hospitalization, incarceration, and other adverse outcomes (Jørgensen et al. 2021). The psychological, social, and structural triggers of relapse, hospitalization, or incarceration could be environmentally influenced, even if individual differences in lifetime risk of these occurrences are highly heritable or biological.

The causes of developing schizophrenia need not be the same as the causes of being (un)able to participate in social, economic, and family life with a psychiatric disorder. While these two processes may be correlated and more severely affected patients may generally have significant levels of functional impairment, it would be a categorical mistake to assume that environmental or genetic influence on the disease itself, as well as on its functional consequences, is entirely the same.

Establishing Whether Environmental Risk Factors Are Causal

To determine whether an association with environmental risk is causal (i.e., the environmental factor plays a role in the etiology of the associated outcome rather than simply being correlated with other causal factors) can be challenging. Ideally, we would study the effects of environmental risk factors experimentally in randomized controlled trials, but in many cases, ethical and practical considerations prevent experimental manipulation of environmental risks. In the absence of experimental control over environmental risk factors, alternative strategies are needed to ensure that the risk factors are indeed causal and not simply correlated to other causes of psychopathology. It is tempting to fall back on the worn-out meme: "correlation is not causation." Still, it is important to emphasize that not all observational or correlational studies are equal in terms of the evidence they offer for a specific causal relation. We can systematically assess which types of observational study will offer the greatest certainty about the effects of environmental exposures on psychopathology. Here I highlight three specific designs: natural experiments, instrumental variable analyses, and family control analyses. As each of these has potential pitfalls and biases, it is prudent to consider any specific effect of interest across multiple designs when possible. It is also worth noting that all three techniques are sometimes held up as being very close to or fundamentally the same as experimental studies. They are not truly causal experiments, but despite their correlational nature, they enable a more rigorous evaluation of the nature of the exposure and the threats to validity that can offer evidence exceeding a mere correlation.

Natural Experiments

A natural experiment relies on a natural exposure that randomly affects some but not all people in a cohort or study. One critical aspect of a natural experiment that authors need to argue or readers need to be able to confirm is that people randomly encountered the natural exposure. That is, the exposure being studied is uncorrelated to possible other causes of the specific outcome or form of psychopathology of interest. Put in counterfactual terms: by comparing the two groups, we are comparing people that are *interchangeable*; that is, they could have been placed in either group but chance determined their placement in a group. If the exposed group is truly randomly exposed, then measuring the rate of psychopathology in the exposed and unexposed groups after the exposure is sufficient to test whether the exposure effects the risk of psychopathology. If, however, the exposed group is for some reason meaningfully different from the unexposed group, then ideally we would have measures of the rate of psychopathology prior to the exposure and would not need to assume that the exposed and control group are interchangeable, other than their exposure status. Instead, we could assume that *had the exposure not occurred, any prior difference between the exposed and unexposed group would have remained constant*. This assumption is known as the "parallel trends assumption." What does this mean in practice for psychiatric epidemiology?

Consider a fictional experiment that compares a group of Dutch divers on a Pacific diving holiday, who experience a traumatic claustrophobic accident, to the rest of the Dutch population. When analyzing rates of psychopathology and use of psycho-pharmaceuticals, pre-exposure risk must be assumed to be identical in both groups. However, people who go on an expensive and somewhat adventurous diving holiday are likely to be wealthier and might have a higher risk tolerance—qualities that could contribute to differences between the divers and other members of the Dutch population. When designing a study or evaluating the work of others, there are two ways to improve this natural experiment. The first involves better matching. One could sample divers who took the same holiday trip the year before as controls; these divers would be well matched for income, risk tolerance, and other unmeasurable or unforeseen confounders. The second concerns the inclusion of pre-exposure measures in both the experimental and control groups. If we have access to pre-exposure measurement of the outcome, we do not need to assume the groups had identical risk prior to exposure but rather that the difference in the groups would have remained constant had the exposure not occurred. Often, researchers cannot access or measure outcomes prior to the natural exposure. In other cases, the parallel trends assumption might fail: even with careful controls in place and a well-selected comparison group, there may be other differences in the groups, had the exposure not occurred. The probability of the parallel trends assumption holding becomes more plausible as the exposed group is better matched to the unexposed group, in terms of known confounders such as age, sex, and prior psychiatric history.

When performed with care, natural experiments provide a powerful way of evaluating the impact of exposures that cannot be ethically or practically manipulated experimentally. Nonetheless, they are limited, because it is difficult to know with certainty whether a natural experiment occurs randomly with respect to all kinds of potential confounders. These confounders may result in differences between the exposed and unexposed group in unknown ways and may bias results.

Instrumental Variables

The use of instrumental variables is another way to examine the causal nature of environmental risk associations. In evaluating treatments or exposures outside the confines of a randomized control study, we are blind to any and all unmeasured influences or processes that could correlate the exposure or risk factor to the outcome. For example, there is concern that the use of selective serotonin reuptake inhibitors (SSRIs) predisposes a person to self-harm or suicide compared to the use of placebo, tricyclic, or other antidepressants (Fergusson et al. 2005; Gunnell et al. 2005). Yet other than through direct comparison in clinical trials (which has been done, but due to the relative rarity of these outcomes require very large sample sizes to offer precise estimates), the relation between being prescribed an antidepressant and self-harm or suicide attempt is deeply confounded by disease severity and numerous other confounders. If there is a source of variation in SSRI prescription (relative to other antidepressants) that is unrelated to disease severity or outcome, we could use this as an *instrumental variable*. In instrumental variable regression, we first predict SSRI prescription with the instrumental variable and then regress the outcome of interest (self-harm/suicide) on the *predicted* SSRI use. Key assumptions inherent in this approach include:

1. The instrument influences the outcome *only* through the exposure and not through other related processes.
2. There is no correlation between the instrumental variable and any confounder of the relation between exposure and outcome.
3. The instrument must have a substantial impact on the exposure (SSRI prescription).

Provided these assumptions hold, using an instrumental variable approach can provide unbiased estimates of the causal effects of environmental associations, such as the association of SSRI prescription and self-harm or suicide.

How can this be done in practice? One potential instrument for medication use is found in idiosyncratic personal preferences in the prescription practices of physicians. A British study of approximately 880,000 tricyclic antidepressants (TCA) and SSRI prescriptions (Davies et al. 2013) showed that physicians who in the past were more likely to prescribe an SSRI (relative to TCAs in this study) were more likely to do so in the future, and that while the prescription of an SSRI or a TCA strongly related to the patient characteristics (age, BMI, smoking, prior depression), the long-term prescription preferences of physicians did not relate to these patient characteristics. Thus, physician prescription preference reliably influences whether a person gets prescribed an SSRI or a TCA but appears unrelated to obvious potential confounders of the relation between medication and suicidal behavior. Physician drug preference, therefore, could serve as an instrumental variable that would enable the discernment of drug-specific risks while reducing the confounds induced by patient-specific factors.

While there are numerous other processes that give rise to potential instrumental variables, it is impossible to guarantee or empirically test that an instrumental variable will meet all assumptions and yield unbiased estimates. A specific class of instrumental variables well known to geneticists will be "Mendelian randomization," where a genetic variant serves as an instrumental variable (Sanderson et al. 2022). Critical caveats around the exact interpretation of the effect size arise for instrumental variable analysis, where the instrument, exposure, or outcome is binary—a situation that is fairly common in psychiatric epidemiology.

Family/Sibling Designs

Family designs enable close matching between exposed and unexposed individuals for a range of additional risk factors. The sibling differences model, also known as the sibling control model or the family fixed-effect model, is an intuitive model used to study causes of mental illness when unknown or unmeasured confounders are thought to be shared between siblings. By comparing the within-sibling relations between exposure and outcome, we automatically match closely (but not perfectly) the exposed and unexposed groups for parental socioeconomic status, genetic influences, and childhood environment. When twins are used, the exposed and unexposed groups are also matched for prenatal exposures as well as cohort and age effects; monozygotic twins are perfectly matched for genetic risk. We use sibling differences to reframe a research question from "are those who experienced trauma more likely to become depressed" to "are those who experienced *more* trauma than their siblings more likely to become depressed" (Kendler et al. 1999)? In the case of a causal relation between stressful life events and depression, we expect their relationship to persist, even when controlling for anything shared between siblings, as demonstrated by (Kendler et al. 1999).

There are certain limitations in the use of sibling differences models. These models predate modern causal thinking, and interpretation of specific sibling differences models (e.g., stratified Cox proportional hazard models) defy straightforward causal interpretation (Petersen and Lange 2020). The model trades perfect control of shared confounders for risk of bias due to measurement error and confounders specific to a sibling (Frisell 2021). Most applications of sibling difference models consider only linear effects, whereas there are various examples of nonlinear relations in psychiatric epidemiology. I propose that several nonlinear extensions of the sibling model be tested to determine the conditions under which resulting estimates can be interpreted as causal, in a manner consistent with modern causal thinking. Bias due to measurement error or unshared confounders is unavoidable, and other designs have different sources of bias. Thus, triangulation of results across different methods is recommended to safeguard against method-specific biases.

Historically Emphasized and Plausible Environmental Risk Exposures

Several studies have linked environmental factors to mental illness risk. In this section, I review some of these results, both for exposures that plausibly increase the risk of onset of psychiatric disorders and that modify outcomes for people with a history of psychiatric diagnosis. There is a certain risk of bias involved in surveying the scientific literature (whether systematically or casually). Due to limits on what we can measure or the structure of scientific funding, certain topics have historically received more attention and therefore may be overemphasized in a survey or review. Environmental risk for psychopathology is no exception. The survey here inherits these biases, as they are embedded in the underlying literature and thus reflected through the risk factors that

I have selected. Nonetheless, these risk factors, along with the way in which they were studied, can offer a guide to study further environmental risk factors.

Acute Traumatic Events

The literature on exposure to acute traumatic events as a cause of psychopathology is vast and robust. One notable natural experiment concerns Swedish survivors of the 2004 South East Asian (Christmas Day) tsunami. The nature of this traumatic event was entirely unpredictable. Owing to Sweden's excellent national registries, researchers could link all Swedes that arrived from selected Asian airports into Sweden during the three-week period that followed the tsunami to socioeconomic status and age-matched controls and compare their psychiatric outcomes (Arnberg et al. 2015). Posttraumatic stress disorder and other stress-related diagnoses were strongly elevated among the exposed Swedes (highest aHR = 7.51 for PTSD), and exposure severity was related to outcome severity. The effect was strongest in the first three months after they returned but persisted throughout the entire five-year follow-up period. It is important to note, however, that the researchers did not study differences between exposed and unexposed groups in the change in disease prevalence from before to after exposure (so-called difference in differences analysis), but only considered psychiatric outcomes after exposure.

Bereavement

In the DSM-III and DSM-IV, bereavement was specifically excluded as a cause of major depressive disorder. If a depressive episode resulted from the loss of a loved one, it was implicitly considered a passing state, qualitatively different from other stresses. The situation changed with the publication of the DSM-5. This was a controversial decision. Some argued there was a risk of medicalizing mourning (Frances 2013), while others felt that bereavement should not prevent people with serious morbidity from getting treatment and that obtaining a diagnosis could facilitate proper treatment (Iglewicz et al. 2013). Furthermore, there is evidence that the bereavement period is associated with serious morbidity. For example, the severity of depression symptoms after bereavement is predictive of physical illness in a five-year period following bereavement (Domingue et al. 2021a).

Considering bereavement as a risk factor brings us back to the question: A risk factor for *what*? Some data suggest that manifestations of depression after bereavement do not differ from depression after other stressful life events (e.g., divorce, illness, and job loss as reported by Kendler et al. 2008). However, in a sample of older adults, bereavement raises some but not all symptoms of depression, a finding seemingly consistent with the consequences of grief being different from other forms of depression. It is possible that grief may cause symptoms of depression in a manner inconsistent with depression in many or most bereaved individuals, while those who do suffer depression after bereavement are not dissimilar from patients who suffer depression due to other trauma.

Bereavement is also linked to other psychopathologies. For example, in a population-wide study of Danish and Swedish registry data, childhood bereavement (death of a parent) has been associated with a 39% increased risk for schizophrenia (Liang et al. 2016). Some of this risk, however, may be due to a confound of unrecognized parental psychopathology and consequent familial risk factors; if death due to suicide or accident are excluded, the risk increase is only 21% (95% CI13-30%). Others have found children suffering sudden childhood bereavement—due to loss of a father or sibling (N = 6136) compared to loss of a father or sibling due to illness (N = 5719)—is associated with an elevated risk of bipolar disorder and schizophrenia (Clarke et al. 2013), even when excluding suicide as a cause of sudden bereavement.

Finally, a population register-based study in Sweden found that parental bereavement and other trigger events (e.g., traumatic brain injury, self-harm, exposure to violence, unintentional injury, and substance intoxication) are related to an elevated risk of violent crime in the week after the event. For schizophrenia patients, the risk of violent crime is particularly elevated after parental bereavement. Parental loss may affect schizophrenia patients specifically as they may still be socially, emotionally, and economically dependent on the parent (Sariaslan et al. 2020).

Childhood Maltreatment and Sexual Abuse

Various forms of abuse and maltreatment have been linked to psychopathology. A co-twin-controlled study of 1,411 female twins, (Kendler et al. 2000) found that twins who were sexually abused (measured with self and co-twin report) in childhood were at elevated risk for major depressive disorder, generalized anxiety disorder, panic disorder, bulimia, as well as alcohol and drug dependence. The risk of psychopathology was more steeply elevated for those who experienced genital childhood sexual abuse or for whom the abuse involved forced intercourse. Replication in Australian twins discordant for self-reported sexual abuse confirmed elevated depression risk, substance abuse risk, and other adverse outcomes, and generalized the effect to men exposed to sexual abuse in childhood (Nelson et al. 2002). Others have found similar effects of childhood traumatic events (including, but not exclusively, sexual abuse) on the risk for depression, anxiety, somatization, and eating disorders (Brown et al. 2014).

Exposure to Substance Abuse

A large study of high-risk siblings and half-siblings—where one child was adopted out of a family and at least one parent had an alcohol use disorder

(AUD)—elegantly established the influence of the rearing environment beyond the influence of genetics (Kendler et al. 2021). For siblings from high-risk families, the overall risk of developing AUD was almost fourfold that of the general population, a fact that could be attributed to either genetic or environmental influences. However, siblings adopted out of a family with a parent with AUD had a significantly lower risk of developing AUD [HR sibs = 0.76 (0.65–0.89) and HR half-sibs = 0.77 (0.70–0.84)] than siblings who remained in the birth family, thus establishing a role of the rearing environment on AUD. Risk was reduced less for those adopted into a family with an adoptive parent with AUD than for those adopted into a family without a parent with AUD, further confirming the influence of the rearing environment and extending the finding to include the adoptive environment.

Poverty, Income, and Unemployment

Numerous findings demonstrate associations and causal relationships between economic factors and mental illness. Experimental work in lower- and middle-income countries has demonstrated that when one alleviates monetary poverty in caregivers (or in some cases to youth directly) through cash transfers, the internalization of problems in their children—a strong indicator of causality—is reduced (Zaneva et al. 2022). Importantly, in extreme high-risk situations, the effect of modest cash transfers is insufficient, and the imposition of strict conditions can have negative effects. A quasi-experimental study in the United States showed a benefit of parental income supplementation on offspring mental health in an American Indian population (Costello et al. 2010). Recent register-based studies in Norway, which link parental income to (adopted) childhood outcome, show a modest effect of parental income (Kinge et al. 2021), whereas a Finnish study that leverages sibling discordance for parental income did not find an effect on children's mental health (Sariaslan et al. 2021b). These results suggest a modest or no-effect of income (not poverty) in Scandinavian countries with a well-functioning welfare state. Analysis of Slovenian register data of the entire Slovenian workforce over at least the past decade finds that unemployment is correlated to a steeply heightened risk of suicide and treatment with psychiatric medication. Risk of suicide, but not psychiatric medication use, remained when unemployment was restricted to those cases that had a probable cause unrelated to the individual (i.e., unemployment was caused by a mass lay-off event) (Vodopivec et al. 2021).

For several reasons, the absence of average effects of income on mental health in high income countries with strong social policies should not be considered evidence for the absence of effects of poverty on the individual level in these countries, or the absence of effects in other Western countries with less adequate social policies. First, average effect estimates of income consider the effects of income across the entire distribution and fail to capture nonlinear effects, such as the likelihood that the risk/resource relationship might vary at different ends of the income continuum. Relatedly, job loss is buffered by social programs and private savings, which can obscure the relationship between income and risk. Finally, some segments of the population evade adequate capture even in data registers (e.g., the homeless, those with informal or unregistered debts, and those financially deprived by a spouse or parent).

Overall, there is inconclusive evidence on the value of an asset transfer program in middle- and lower-income countries, yet some conditional asset transfer intervention studies register mental health benefits (Lund et al. 2011). In countries that lack a social safety net, there may be a causal relation between poverty and mental health. Finally, the effect of income, employment, and poverty could be mediated by various psychological processes that require additional attention.

Placement in Out-of-Home Care

There are situations where the state needs to step in and help parents or help protect children from their parents. Approximately 5% of children in Western countries are in foster care at some point in their childhood (Fallesen et al. 2014). Placing children in the care of the state has the potential for significant consequences and is so common that it should be the target of sustained empirical study. The long-term consequences of removing a child out of their family home are impossible to study through controlled experiments, because randomly placing children in or out of state care is unethical. Equally, the consequences of foster care cannot be studied through observational studies by simply comparing the outcomes of foster children to the general population, because the causes of family dysfunction that contribute to the risk of placement outside the home are also likely to impact long-term outcomes for the child.

Pioneering work by the economist John Doyle used the fact that case workers in Illinois were assigned to families in an essentially random fashion to examine the effects of foster care. These studies were made possible because these case workers differed substantially in their rate of placing children in foster care as an instrumental variable (Doyle Jr. 2008). Doyle showed that children at the margin of placement who remained at home—those who might have been put in foster care if they had been evaluated by a different case worker—were less likely to be arrested as an adult. Consistent with these findings, nationwide register data analysis of 855,622 children born in Finland between 1986 and 2000 show that children placed in out-of-home care had worse outcomes than their siblings who remained in the home, in terms severe mental illness, anxiety disorder, depression, and personality disorder (Sariaslan et al. 2021a). Further contrasting the type of care for siblings who were both placed in out-of-home care (N = 11,092) revealed that within-sibling pairs, and controlling for a wide array of pre-placement behavioral indicators and risks, the highest risk for depression and serious mental illness occurred in children who received institutional care (vs. foster care) as well as those with the highest number of episodes in out-of-home care (Sariaslan et al. 2021a). These studies point to the importance of evaluating the risk of out-of-home-care placement and features of that care (institutional vs. foster care) which can potentially impact adult mental health.

Migration and Minority Stress

Both migration and minority stress contribute environmental risk for mental illness. A widely cited early empirical work by Odegard in 1932 (cited in Cantor-Graae und Selten 2005) established elevated rates of schizophrenia in Norwegian migrants to Minnesota. Similarly, Maltzberg (1936) established that white migrants (controlled for age and urbanicity) to New York state were at 1.4-fold higher risk of being diagnosed with dementia praecox and a 1.2-fold elevated risk for manic depressive psychosis; they were not, however, at elevated risk for alcoholic psychosis. Later work by Maltzberg (1962) established a similar elevated rate of dementia praecox admissions in Black migrants compared to Black native-born New Yorkers. A later meta-analysis (Cantor-Graae and Selten 2005) and Danish population-wide studies (Cantor-Graae et al. 2003) revealed that migrants from a wide variety of countries of origin and with a wide variety of destinations are more frequently diagnosed with schizophrenia. The Danish study also tested but rejected differences in rates of schizophrenia across age upon first residence in Denmark. For those who were born in Denmark to mothers born in Denmark, the study found that those who resided abroad before age 15 had an elevated risk of schizophrenia diagnosis (RR = 1.6, 95% CI 1.25–2.05). In addition, a more steeply elevated risk was observed in migrants from ethnic minority communities compared to migrants from what might be perceived as ethnically the same (evident in higher relative risk for schizophrenia for African, Asian, and Greenlandic migrants than for migrants from other Scandinavian countries). Further evidence of elevated rates for schizophrenia were found in Afro-Caribbean migrants to the U.K. (Van Os et al. 1996), in migrants from Suriname and the Antilles to the Netherlands (Selten et al. 1997), and in migrants to Sweden, with a particularly high-risk in East African and Middle Eastern migrants (Zolkowska et al. 2001). Collectively, these findings suggest that minority stress may further increase the risk conferred by migration.

The leading alternate model to explain the elevated rates of schizophrenia in immigrant communities is selective migration. Those at elevated but subclinical risk for schizophrenia may be more likely to migrate, which would elevate rates of schizophrenia in migrant populations. To test the selective migration hypothesis, Selten et al. (2002) studied Surinamese immigrants to the Netherlands. After Suriname gained independence, over one-third of its population migrated to the Netherlands, which allowed Selten et al. to compare the rate of schizophrenia in Surinamese born immigrants in the Netherlands, using the total Surinamese population prior to migration as a denominator. The data showed that the rate of schizophrenia among Surinamese immigrants was higher than among native-born Dutch. A smaller orthogonal test of the selective migration hypothesis compared rates of migration among adopted children who had a biological parent with schizophrenia with adopted children who did not; it found lower migration rates in those with an affected biological parent (Rosenthal et al. 1974). Selective migration does not appear to account for the elevated risk for schizophrenia in migrants and their children.

Prenatal Exposure to Famine

Several studies suggest prenatal exposure to famine as a risk factor for serious mental illness. Two key long-running studies have looked at severe caloric restriction during pregnancy:

- Dutch hunger winter studies, which contrasted women who were exposed to famine in the winter of 1944–1945, when allied offensive and German export embargoes to occupied territories caused severe food shortages in cities in the west portion of the Netherlands.
- Studies of the Chinese Famine from 1959–1961, which was associated with the "great leap forward" set of policies intended to industrialize China.

Contrasting those born in places hardest hit by the famine during the first trimester of pregnancy to those born elsewhere in the Netherlands or immediately before or after this period, researchers identified an elevated risk for schizophrenia in the Dutch national psychiatry register (RR = 2.0, 95% CI = 1.2–3.4) (Hoek et al. 1998). Exposure to the Chinese famine in the first trimester of pregnancy was also associated with an elevated risk for schizophrenia (Xu et al. 2009). A recent comprehensive review also implicates famine as a risk factor for affective and personality disorders as well as for psychotic disorders (Dana et al. 2019).

In the developed world, it is questionable whether famine is still severe or frequent enough to be considered a common or even rare cause of psychopathology. However, most people do not live in the developed world. Even in developed countries, specific vulnerable groups, such as mothers with eating disorders, are observed to give birth to babies with a lower birthweight (Micali et al. 2007). Studying the consequences of malnourishment during pregnancy in the developed world may require nonlinear analysis so that the effects of extreme deprivation can be isolated from other risk factors, as other physical or psychophysical stresses may affect the health of a child. It may also be useful to evaluate the effects of deeply stressful events, such as war (e.g., the London Blitz), in the absence of famine, or stressful personal life events (sudden or violent bereavement during pregnancy) on the risk of psychopathology in the offspring of those affected.

Sleep

A natural experiment that recurs yearly is the switch to daylight savings time, which moves the sleep midpoint by one hour. Danish registry data shows an 11% (95% CI = 7%–15%) increase in episodes of unipolar depression after wintertime goes into effect (Hansen et al. 2017). This result is corroborated by Mendelian randomization analysis, which reveals that an hour change in sleep midpoint changes depression risk by 23% (95% CI = 6%–33%) (Daghlas et al. 2021). The two studies rely on different designs and different data sets yet reach very similar conclusions. Their consistency illustrates how a fully independent natural experiment and instrumental variable analyses can be leveraged to corroborate a plausible causal relation. Unlike some of the other environmental exposures discussed, sleep can and has been the subject of experimental manipulations. An example is a small, targeted experiment with a more extreme (and qualitatively different) exposure. Researchers compared 25 healthy adults rested at baseline and, after 56 hours of continuous wakefulness, found increased symptoms of anxiety, depression, somatic complaints, and paranoia (Kahn-Greene et al. 2007). Between these extremes and the natural experiments discussed here, there is a wide literature of sleep, restlessness, and insomnia treatment studies. For example, a review of daily diary and momentary assessment studies found that within-person aspects of sleep quality correlate with affect the following day; note also that affect associates with later sleep (Konjarski et al. 2018). These findings point to the widely recognized need to adjust the type of measurement and measurement frequency and interval in studying psychopathology to the timeframe in which the relation between environment and psychopathology occurs.

What About Gene–Environment Interactions?

There is broad interest in the effects of interactions between genes and the environment on psychiatric risk. The study of gene–environment interaction requires both the environmental and genetic risk to be well established (i.e., to be a convincing cause and not just an incidental correlate of psychopathology). Reliably estimating the effects of a gene–environment interaction faces several unique methodological challenges. First, analytic issues (e.g., improper modeling of the distribution of outcome variables) can induce false-positive interactions, even if they do not cause a false-positive main effect (Domingue et al. 2021b). Second, omitting interactions between the environment and the covariates may induce false-positive gene–environment interactions (Keller 2014). Finally, for an interaction to be convincing, we would ideally have tight control over any correlation between genotype and confounders (using, e.g., sibling genetic analysis.), In addition, the environmental exposure would have to be exogenous to ensure it is not potentially correlated with other environments that either confound the analysis or are the true source of interaction (Biroli et al. 2022). A rigorous program to study gene–environment interactions would have to contend with these methodological challenges. One study which finds gene by traumatic experience interaction effects on depression risk (Coleman et al. 2020) addresses some but not all of these methodological challenges to validity, and can be viewed as a starting point for future improvements.

Conclusion

This chapter has detailed some experimental design issues inherent in efforts to delineate environmental risk for mental illnesses, reviewed some of the more widely demonstrated examples of environmental risk factors, and briefly considered approaches to gene–environment interactions. There is a massive literature full of carefully performed studies that find specific environmental exposures that relate to risk for psychopathology; some of these (reviewed above) represent a somewhat arbitrary set for which evidence exists from quasi-experimental, instrumental variable, or within-sibling designs. These have been supplemented with experimental designs or intense longitudinal assessments if the nature of the particular environmental exposure was amenable to such studies. Notably, the literature focuses predominantly on mean effects, and one could imagine that the risk of psychopathology increases nonlinearly at the extremes of an exposure. Nonlinear regression and causal inference techniques could help establish whether an exposure has a linear or nonlinear effect on risk and better identify who is at risk. One should avoid confusing effect sizes and estimates of population average causes based on empirical work with the causes and effect sizes of psychopathology in a certain individual. For example, while the magnitude of effect of sleep on psychopathology as assessed in various studies is small, those studies (and their findings) are not necessarily ecologically valid for a mother who has not had an uninterrupted night's sleep for months, due to night feeding and care responsibilities. Future studies aimed at a mechanistic understanding of psychiatric disease risk would do well to consider approaches that take these complexities into account, to move the field forward in a way that is relevant to real-world clinical scenarios.

Understanding Rare Variation

5

Rare Variants

Shared Paths for Therapeutic Development and Neurobiological Investigation

Carrie E. Bearden, Sumantra Chattarji, Ricardo Dolmetsch, Lilia M. Iakoucheva, Steven A. Kushner, Mustafa Sahin, Nenad Sestan, Tomomi Shimogori, and Stephan J. Sanders

Abstract

The revolution in human genetics has led to the identification of hundreds of rare genetic variants that underlie neuropsychiatric disorders. This technological leap presents both an opportunity and a dilemma for developing new therapies. Monogenic diseases are simpler to study and can be used to develop a road map for progressing from a genetic cause to both an understanding of neurobiology and a disease-modifying therapy. This trajectory involves the development of cellular and animal models, the understanding of the natural history of a disease, and the identification of biomarkers and clinical endpoints. However, the large number of mutations and the rarity of the diseases requires criteria for prioritization and strategies for connecting these diseases to more common causes of neuropsychiatric disorders. The goal of this chapter is to provide a road map to help prioritize investments that will improve our understanding of rare neuropsychiatric diseases, connect these diseases to common disorders, and help to catalyze the development of new therapies.

Introduction

Therapeutic development relies either on serendipity or on understanding the pathophysiology of a disease sufficiently to design a rational intervention. For most of history, the development of therapies for diseases of the central nervous system has been based on serendipity combined with astute clinical observation. However, over the past decade, advances in genetics and neurobiology combined with new therapeutic modalities have led to some successes based on rational drug design, including:

- Nucleic acid therapies: Nusinersen (Spinraza™), Onasemnogene abeparvovec (Zolgensma™), and Risdiplam (Evrysdi™) in spinal muscular atrophy (Vignette 5.1) (Finkel et al. 2017; Gidaro and Servais 2019; Keinath et al. 2021; Kim et al. 2019; Messina and Sframeli 2020),
- Selective immune-modulating antibodies: Ocrelizumab in multiple sclerosis (Juanatey et al. 2018), and
- A GABA-receptor modulating neurosteroid: Brexanolone in postpartum depression (Faden and Citrome 2020; Leader et al. 2019).

Our goal is to leverage the tremendous progress in understanding the genetics of neuropsychiatric disorders to extend these successes to other rare diseases and, ultimately, to common psychiatric disorders such as depression.

Rare variants with large effect sizes at well-defined genomic loci represent a highly tractable starting point for both investigating neurobiology and developing therapeutics. These quests are highly synergistic. Many of the characteristics that make a specific rare variant suitable for neurobiological inquiry also make it suitable for therapeutic discovery. Furthermore, many of the investigative steps are also shared, including understanding genotype-phenotype relationships and natural history, delineating the direction of effect, assessing whether mechanisms are preserved across species, and identifying endpoints and biomarkers. However, we also face substantial challenges, including a limited understanding of how the brain functions or develops, highly pleiotropic effects as well as incomplete penetrance from the rare variants, the inaccessibility of the human brain, and the absence of clearly defined equivalents of

Vignette 5.1 Spinal muscular atrophy (Bonanno et al. 2022).

Symptoms	• Early-onset, lower motor neuron atrophy. • Resulting paralysis leads to respiratory failure. • Severe forms are usually fatal by two years of age.
Genetics	• Recessive loss-of-function variants in the *SMN1* gene (often deletions of exon 7) lead to loss of the SMN protein, which leads to progressive lower motor neuron degeneration. • The neighboring *SMN2* gene encodes an identical protein but with substantially reduced efficiency due to a cryptic splice site in exon 7. • Copy number of *SMN2* varies substantially across the population and modifies the severity of spinal muscular atrophy symptoms (type 0–IV).
Incidence	• 10 in 100,000 in Europeans. • Carrier frequency of 1 in 35 in Europeans but penetrance modified by *SMN2* copy number. • Lower incidence in other ancestral groups.
Endpoints	• Mortality, respiratory support, motor milestones
Therapies	• AAV gene replacement (Zolgensma™) • Splice modifying ASOs to increase *SMN2* translation efficiency (Spinraza™) • *SMN2* splice modifying small molecule (Evrysdi™).

neuropsychiatric phenotypes in experimental model systems. To overcome these challenges, we need large-scale concerted efforts to better define the impact of rare variants across multiple dimensions of neurobiology in humans and multiple experimental model systems.

This chapter summarizes our discussions at the Forum, which were guided by the following key questions:

- With the goal of improving therapeutics, what are the key dimensions to prioritizing genes and loci for neurobiological investigation?
- What are strategies for testing for convergence/divergence in mechanisms between genetic loci? How do we determine meaningful convergence?
- Which models should be used to interrogate genetic loci and how should they be leveraged? How do we validate their predictions in humans?
- What are key advances required in natural history, biomarkers, and clinical endpoints to optimize the probability of success in clinical trials?
- How do we establish infrastructure and incentives to generate rigorous reproducible findings?

As each topic is considered in turn, we propose an optimal study design for achieving testable hypotheses regarding the neurobiology of rare, highly penetrant variants, across multiple models, and levels of analysis.

Prioritizing Genes and Loci for Neurobiological Investigation

What are the key dimensions to prioritizing genes and loci for neurobiological investigation?

To improve therapeutics, we need to explore the multiple dimensions necessary to prioritize genes and loci for neurobiological investigation. Prioritization strategies vary based on the characteristics of the genes and loci. Recognizing that all neuropsychiatric disorders are polygenic, but that the genomic architecture varies between them (see Robinson et al., this volume), we considered three levels of complexity: single gene disorders, structural variants with multiple risk genes, and common variants.

Single Gene Disorders

To date, most single gene disorders are in childhood-onset phenotypes, including neurodevelopmental delay and autism spectrum disorder (ASD). Recent, large-scale cohorts have demonstrated that single gene disorders also play a role in schizophrenia and bipolar disorder, albeit in a very small number of individuals (see Robinson et al., this volume). As a consequence of natural selection, the effect sizes of rare variants associated with neuropsychiatric disorders on neurobehavioral phenotypes are estimated to be high, with odds ratios over 10, and several variants with odds ratios in excess of 50 (Fu et al. 2022; Marshall et al. 2008; Sanders et al. 2017; Satterstrom et al. 2020; Singh et al. 2022). These effect sizes are substantially larger than the odds ratios below 1.05 observed for the majority of common variants associated with neuropsychiatric disorders (Robinson et al., this volume), but smaller than those observed in Mendelian disorders (e.g., ≥ 500), in keeping with a substantial contribution from genomic background, environmental factors, and stochastic effects, even in individuals with a rare variant. These large effect sizes provide two major opportunities:

1. Human cellular and animal model experimental systems with the genetic variant are likely to provide an opportunity to acquire knowledge about the pathophysiology of the disorder.
2. Rescuing the genetic variant, or restoring the relevant gene's function, within the right neurodevelopmental window is likely to improve symptoms.

Modeling a genetic variant whose impact is sufficient to cause the phenotype in a suitable genetic background simplifies subsequent investigation. In theory, each disorder has only one therapeutic target and needs only one experimental model system. This, however, makes the assumption that a gene is the appropriate level of resolution, which may not always be the case. For example, numerous genes have multiple transcription start sites and variable splicing isoforms, and these can impact protein function (Araki et al. 2020; Chau et al. 2021; Dai et al. 2019; Liang et al. 2021). Alternatively, if a gene is a transcription factor, it may impact multiple other genes, and in this case, rescuing downstream targets may be more effective. Similarly, functional and phenotypic consequences can vary between missense variants in the same gene (Sanders et al. 2018). Attention to genotype-phenotype relationships in human populations is key to ensuring that research insights represent the observed disorder.

Gene Prioritization

In considering criteria for rare variant prioritization, we drew inspiration from the successes and obstacles encountered in developing therapies for rare neurodevelopmental disorders, reviewed by Sahin (this volume), and the implications of these on understanding neurobiology. We identified numerous factors (detailed below) to consider in gene prioritization and were struck by how similar the weighting of these factors was between the two goals of therapeutic development and understanding neurobiology (Figure 5.1).

Phenotypic Association. In an era in which there are hundreds of genes associated with neurodevelopmental phenotypes at genome-wide significance, crossing this threshold is a requirement for a gene to be prioritized (unless

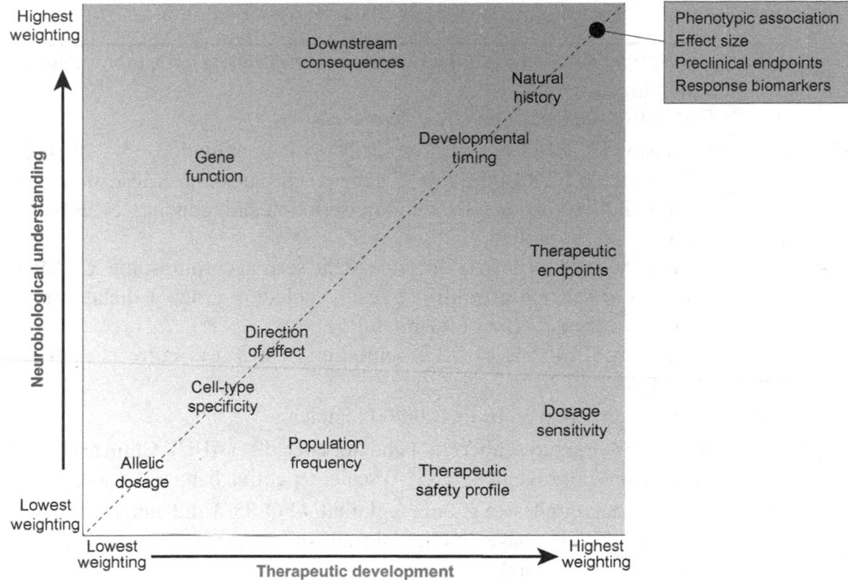

Figure 5.1 Gene prioritization in single gene disorders. The relative weighting for 15 factors in determining gene priority is shown qualitatively for therapeutic development (X-axis) and neurobiological understanding (Y-axis).

hundreds of genes are being assayed, and a more liberal threshold is appropriate). Statistical techniques exist for integrating multiple modalities of genetic data (e.g., *de novo* and inherited variation; Fu et al. 2022; He et al. 2013), but exceptions requiring human curation remain (e.g., triplet repeats in Fragile X syndrome undetected by exome sequencing; see Vignette 5.2). Further ranking by evidence of association is driven largely by population frequency and effect size, which we will consider separately.

Population Frequency. High population frequency simplifies natural history studies, genotype-phenotype analysis, clinical trial design, and commercialization of therapies and offers an opportunity to help more individuals. While a higher population frequency is useful for understanding neurobiology, it is a more important consideration for developing therapeutics. From a therapeutic perspective, the *prevalence of diagnosed individuals* matters more than the incidence; for example, there are larger cohorts of individuals with tuberous sclerosis (*TSC1*, *TSC2*) due to the longstanding clinical awareness of these disorders than there are with *CHD8* mutations, despite the predicted incidence of *CHD8* mutations being higher than *TSC1/2* due to the larger gene length. However, even N-of-one studies can be informative if there is clear natural history and a large effect size of the therapy (Gupta et al. 2020), so this criterion may carry less weight than others in specific cases.

Vignette 5.2 Fragile X syndrome (Bear et al. 2004; Berry-Kravis et al. 2016).

Symptoms	• Developmental delay, intellectual disability, ASD, ADHD, motor coordination impairment. • Distinctive physical signs may be present.
Genetics	• Expansion of CGG repeats (typically ≤44, premutation 55–200, FXS >200) in the 5′UTR of the *FMR1* gene on chromosome X leads to methylation of the promoter, silencing transcription and reducing levels of the FMRP-encoded protein. • Females have milder symptoms due to the second chromosome X. FMRP regulates translation of multiple genes, including group 1 metabotropic glutamate receptors (mGluR1/mGluR5). • In preclinical models of FXS, inhibition of mGluR5 corrects multiple phenotypes.
Incidence	• 20 in 100,000 males; 10 in 100,000 females.
Endpoints	• Behavioral measures: aberrant behavior checklist (ABC), Clinical Global Impression–Improvement (CGI-I) scale, repetitive behavior scale.
Therapies	• mGluR5 antagonists (e.g., mavoglurant/AFQ-056) did not modify the ABC endpoint in phase 2b clinical trials of adults (18–45 years) or adolescents (12–17 years). • Preclinical trials are also focusing on reactivation or replacement of the *FMR1* gene.

Effect size. With larger effect size of the variant, we would expect greater benefit from therapy and more dramatic downstream consequences for understanding neurobiology. Accurate estimates of effect size are often challenging due to the absence of sufficient numbers of unaffected carriers with phenotype data. For haploinsufficient genes (i.e., when the loss of one allele leads to clinically relevant functional impairments, often leading to monoallelic or dominant inheritance patterns), the "loss-of-function observed/expected upper bound fraction" (LOEUF) score—an estimate of constraint based on the extent to which loss-of-function mutations in genes are under purifying selection in large population cohorts (Karczewski et al. 2020)—may help quantify this.

Natural history. Detailed natural history studies are critical to defining prognosis, phenotypic endpoints, therapeutic requirements of the affected individuals, genotype-phenotype correlations, and potential biomarkers (Gupta et al. 2020; Zerres and Rudnik-Schöneborn 1995). The availability of these data is highly beneficial and often essential for therapeutic development since the data helps select appropriate age ranges and therapeutic endpoints specific to the disorder. They are equally important for neurobiology, where understanding genotype-phenotype relationships and relating data from experimental model systems to human phenotypes are key.

Dosage sensitivity. Haploinsufficiency (i.e., sensitivity to low gene expression) underlies the majority of neurodevelopmental disorders (Fu et al. 2022).

In a subset, overexpression can also lead to symptoms; for example, insufficient MeCP2 protein leads to Rett syndrome but duplications of the *MECP2* gene also cause neurodevelopmental delay. Similarly, both deletions and duplications at the 16p11.2 locus are associated with neurodevelopmental sequelae. In contrast, moderate overexpression (in contrast to gain-of-function) of *SCN2A* does not appear to have functional consequences (Tamura et al. 2022). For neurobiological inquiries, this can be controlled (or may even aid experimental design) so it plays little role in prioritization. For therapeutic development, genes with bidirectional dosage sensitivity (e.g., the "Goldilocks effect") might be expected to have a narrow therapeutic window, and techniques to exert fine control over expression are in their infancy. For now, genes with unidirectional dosage sensitivity should be prioritized over bidirectional dosage sensitivity for therapeutic development.

Allelic dosage. Since effect size and dosage sensitivity are considered separately, we felt that both biallelic (autosomal recessive) and monoallelic (dominant or X-linked) disorders were appropriate starting points for both therapeutic development and understanding neurobiology, giving this factor a lower weight.

Functional understanding. To date, progress in therapeutics and neurobiology has followed a detailed understanding of gene/protein function, direction of effect, cell-type specificity, and downstream consequences. These factors are essential steps in leveraging the gene to understand neurobiology, while only "sufficient" detail is required to aid therapeutic development; for example, the mechanisms by which survival motor neuron (SMN) protein deficiency leads to lower motor neuron death are still not clear. Consequently, the following factors were weighted slightly higher in prioritizing genes for understanding neurobiology:

- *Gene/protein function*: Genes with specific downstream functions (e.g., ion channels) or clearly annotated functions in well-known pathways (e.g., *CUL3*) may be more tractable for understanding neurobiology and defining the direction of effect than others (e.g., transcription factors).
- *Direction of effect*: The effects of rare variants can be loss-of-function, gain-of-function, dominant negative, or increased-function, either alone or in combination (Sanders et al. 2018). Once these effects are defined (which relies on defining and assaying gene function), they can be factored into experimental design or therapeutic development. Gain-of-function effects may require allele-specific or DNA/RNA-editing therapies. In theory, DNA and RNA editing could succeed without prior knowledge of the direction of effect.
- *Downstream consequences*: Defining the impact of the rare variant on brain function and development is critical to understanding neurobiology. For therapeutic design, it can help identify preclinical and

therapeutic endpoints. Of note, if a therapy is directed at downstream consequences rather than the underlying genetic variant (e.g., mGluR5 in Fragile X), then the evidence base underlying these consequences should be a major consideration in gene prioritization.

- *Cell-type specificity*: Like direction of effect, it is important to characterize the cell types in which the gene/protein is expressed, and this needs to be factored into experimental and therapeutic design.
- *Developmental timing*: Like cell-type specificity, it is critical to define the developmental timing; however, this is often more challenging and harder to control experimentally. Disorders with substantial prenatal pathology may be especially challenging to treat (Herzeg et al. 2022; Zylka 2020); however, without validated preclinical endpoints, only successful therapies in humans would truly resolve the developmental critical window.

Preclinical endpoints. A robust preclinical endpoint relevant to the human disorder greatly benefits both neurobiological understanding and therapeutic development. The efficacy of such endpoints is not always immediately obvious. For example, SMN levels and tail necrosis in the mouse model of spinal muscular atrophy successfully predicted the benefits of antisense oligonucleotide (ASO) therapy in humans with spinal muscular atrophy (Finkel et al. 2017; Hua et al. 2010), while it is less clear that behavioral assays in rodents with particular genetic mutations (e.g., Fragile X syndrome) reflect intellectual disability or ASD in humans (Berry-Kravis et al. 2016).

Therapeutic safety profile. The field of nucleic acid therapies in the human central nervous system is in its infancy (Kuzmin et al. 2021) and may be associated with substantial risk, which must be balanced against potential benefit. In contrast, repurposing existing drugs with known safety profiles carries substantially lower risk. These considerations are critical for therapeutic development but matter less for understanding neurobiology.

Therapeutic endpoints. Clinical trials must predefine a single primary endpoint by which they are assessed; thus, the choice of endpoint is critical. Quantitative and "clean" endpoints, such as seizure frequency, are likely to be better powered than qualitative and "noisy" endpoints, such as behavioral symptoms. At the same time, given the urgent need to develop therapies for neurobehavioral manifestations of these conditions, the development of improved quantitative behavioral endpoints is a high priority. Precedence that the endpoint can be modified at a specific developmental stage is also an advantage. Like the safety profile, this is a critical consideration for therapeutic development and may also impact neurobiological inquiry, by demonstrating the relevance of findings to the human disorder.

Response biomarkers. The availability of objective evidence that a therapy is engaging with the target and having the desired effect (such as a response biomarker) enables critical insight into dosing, duration of therapy, and patient stratification. At best, a response biomarker can act as a surrogate endpoint (e.g., HbA1c in diabetes) and be translated between experimental model systems and humans to act as a preclinical endpoint. Effective biomarkers for spinal muscular atrophy are emerging (Pino et al. 2021). For other neurodevelopmental and neuropsychiatric disorders, we are unaware of any robust biomarkers (Parellada et al. 2023; Sahin et al. 2018).

Application to Spinal Muscular Atrophy, Fragile X Syndrome, and Angelman Syndrome

Comparing these prioritization categories for (a) spinal muscular atrophy (Vignette 5.1), where there are widely adopted therapies, (b) Fragile X syndrome (Vignette 5.2), where phase 2 clinical trials failed to meet the endpoint, and (c) Angelman syndrome (Vignette 5.3), with promising interim data in phase 1 and 2 trials, many similarities can be identified (Table 5.1). In Fragile X syndrome, the relatively wide age ranges in developmental timing of disease onset, the lack of certainty that mGluR underlies symptoms in humans (downstream neurobiology), and the challenging nature of identifying robust

Vignette 5.3 Angelman syndrome (Judson et al. 2021; Noor et al. 2015; Wolter et al. 2020; Ultragenyx Pharmaceutical Inc. n.d.).

Symptoms	• Neurodevelopmental delay, often with ataxia, seizures, and microcephaly.
Genetics	• Loss-of-function of the maternal copy of *UBE3A*, which is imprinted in neurons. • Can be caused by *de novo* deletions, *de novo* small disruptive mutations in *UBE3A*, or uni-parental disomy. • *UBE3A* encodes an E3 ubiquitin ligase, which impacts the levels of multiple proteins. Overexpression of *UBE3A* has also been implicated in neurodevelopmental disorders.
Incidence	• 6 in 100,000 across ancestry groups. Deletion is the most common mechanism (70%).
Endpoints	• Developmental milestones, Clinical Global Impression–Improvement (CGI-I) scale.
Therapies	• Antisense oligonucleotides directed at the *UBE3A* antisense transcript (*UBE3A-AS*) that mediates imprinting can reactivate the paternal copy of *UBE3A*. • Several such therapies are under development, including GTX-102 that shows promise in a phase 1/2 open label clinical trial (NCT04259281). • CRISPR and gene replacement approaches are in preclinical development.

Table 5.1 Comparison of therapeutic development in spinal muscular atrophy, Fragile X syndrome, and Angelman syndrome.

	Spinal Muscular Atrophy	Fragile X Syndrome	Angelman Syndrome
Phenotypic association	Robust	Robust	Robust
Population frequency	10 in 100,000	20 in 100,000	6 in 100,000
Effect size	Very high	Very high	Very high
Dosage sensitivity	Unidirectional	Unidirectional	Bidirectional
Allelic dosage	Biallelic (recessive)	X-linked	Monoallelic (dominant), but imprinted
Functional understanding	Low SMN protein and lower motor neuron death but the mechanism is unclear	Low FMRP affects translation of multiple proteins; preclinical evidence for mGluR5 being key	Low *UBE3A* in neurons impacts the levels of numerous proteins; unclear how this leads to symptoms
Preclinical endpoints	Mortality, SMN levels and tail necrosis in rodents	Behavioral measures in rodents	Motor performance, seizure susceptibility, and behavioral measures in rodents
Therapeutic action	Genetic rescue of causal gene or paralogue (*SMN1/2*)	Antagonist of downstream protein (mGluR5)	Genetic reactivation of imprinted causal gene (*UBE3A*)
Therapeutic safety profile	High risk: first ASO in human central nervous system	Low risk: repurposed drug	High risk: ASO in human central nervous system
Therapeutic age	After birth	12–45 years	4–17 years
Therapeutic endpoints	Mortality, respiratory support	Behavioral measures	Clinical impression
Response biomarkers	None	None	None
Natural history	Well-characterized	Well-characterized	Well-characterized

preclinical and therapeutic endpoints in neurodevelopmental delay probably contributed to failure (Berry-Kravis et al. 2016; Grabb and Potter 2022). These lessons helped refine subsequent studies, including for Angelman syndrome, which used younger ages, alternative endpoints, and gene-directed therapy. However, it is easy to draw such conclusions in retrospect. We can imagine a version of events where we are drawing inspiration from Fragile X syndrome and critiquing the early developmental onset and the high risk of ASOs in both spinal muscular atrophy and Angelman syndrome. Selecting the most tractable disorders for therapeutic development now helps pave the way for other disorders in the future.

Structural Variants

Structural variants (SVs) include copy number variants (CNVs, e.g., deletions and duplications), inversions, translocations, and aneuploidies, either alone or in combination. Due to hypermutability, some SVs have population frequencies that are substantially higher than expected (e.g., non-allelic homologous recombination leading to 16p11.2 CNVs or meiotic nondisjunction leading to Trisomy 21). In addition to the factors already listed, we considered the impact of known "causal genes" when prioritizing SVs:

Causal genes. In some SVs, most of the phenotypic risk is mediated by a single gene (e.g., *NRXN1* in 2p16.3 deletions, *SHANK3* in 22q13 deletions, *UBE3A* in 15q11-13 maternal deletions). In these SVs, exome-sequencing data of cohorts with neurodevelopmental delay independently identify the single gene but not others within the SV (Fu et al. 2022; Sanders et al. 2015; Satterstrom et al. 2020). For these SVs, our prioritization schema for single gene disorders, above, applies.

In contrast, other SVs, such as CNVs at 16p11.2 and 22q11.2, appear to have a more complex risk architecture. Exome-sequencing data do not suggest a single gene is mediating risk or may implicate multiple genes (Sanders et al. 2015; Satterstrom et al. 2020). Systematic knockouts of each gene in experimental model systems have claimed to identify individual genes; for example, *KCTD13* at the 16p11.2 locus (Golzio et al. 2012) or *FZD9* at the 7q11.23 Williams syndrome locus (Chailangkarn et al. 2018). However, these results are not easily reconciled with the absence of gene association in human exome-sequencing data (Fu et al. 2022; Sanders et al. 2015; Satterstrom et al. 2020) or other similar analyses (Escamilla et al. 2017; Qiu et al. 2019). A polygenic or oligogenic model is a parsimonious explanation. However, it is possible that the genes within these SVs have combinatorial effects (i.e., interactions; Corominas et al. 2014; Lin et al. 2015) that individual gene knockouts miss or that risk is mediated by noncoding regions or surrounding loci. We considered how rare variant prioritization should be weighted by a polygenic SV locus.

Therapeutic development. Without a single gene target, nucleic acid therapies are challenging to apply, therefore we felt that SVs currently should not be prioritized for therapeutic development. We saw three possibilities for future therapeutics in polygenic SVs:

1. identifying and targeting the gene mediating the most risk,
2. targeting multiple genes, and
3. identifying downstream targets that might be amenable to repurposed drugs or small molecule screens.

Neurobiological understanding. Several SVs mediate high effect sizes with high population frequencies (e.g., 16p11.2, 22q11.2), providing unparalleled opportunities to study genotype-phenotype relationships and natural history in rarer variant disorders in human populations (Cable et al. 2021; Jacquemont et al. 2022). However, with current techniques it is challenging to induce, rescue, or manipulate large mutations, complicating many lines of inquiry. Similarly, questions of cell-type specificity, gene function, and development timing are complicated by the numerous genes involved; combinatorial effects may also be present.

In summary, due to the complexities of multiple genes within SV loci, we think that SVs without a clear single gene locus should be down-weighted for both therapeutic development and neurobiological understanding. Across SVs with multiple genes, the factors and weights we described for single gene disorders (Figure 5.1) can be used to prioritize them, though we note that the inclusion of more than one causal gene complicates several of these.

Common Variants

The majority of trait liability in neuropsychiatric disorders is thought to arise from numerous common variants, each mediating small effects (Corvin and Sullivan 2016; Gaugler et al. 2014; Owen et al. 2009; Sullivan 2005). The utility of these variants *en masse* to investigate neurobiology is considered by Won et al. (this volume). Below, we focus on which individual common variant loci, if at all, should be prioritized for therapeutic development or understanding neurobiology (cf. Won et al., this volume).

Fine mapping. As described above, the absence of a single gene target complicates experimentation. With sufficient genomic or functional genomic data, many common variants can be fine-mapped to individual genes (Sekar et al. 2016) with a specific mechanism (e.g., decreased expression), direction of effect, effect size, or causal variant (see Ronald et al. and Won et al., this volume). In prioritizing individual common variant loci, we would want to include a factor relating to whether the locus has been resolved to a single gene or variant in this manner and carries a high weight (Trubetskoy et al. 2022).

Overlapping loci. We observe substantial overlap in the genes from rare variant analyses of ASD and schizophrenia (Fu et al. 2022; Singh et al. 2022) and loci from common variant analyses of schizophrenia (Trubetskoy et al. 2022). Where such overlap exists for a given disorder between individual genes or loci arising from both common and rare variant studies, this adds to the prioritization of both the gene and locus.

Therapeutic development. There was consensus in our group that individual common variants should not be prioritized for therapeutic development due to the small effect sizes. We acknowledge, however, that a therapy with a large impact on a gene identified by a common variant with a small effect size might be beneficial, especially if there was overlapping rare variation. Further, in the presence of a rare variant, polygenic risk scores might be beneficial to consider for patient stratification (Davies et al. 2020).

Neurobiological understanding. The small effect sizes of individual common variants also pose a challenge for exploring neurobiology, compounded by the lack of conservation between species of noncoding regions, where most common variants are found. Investigating the gene targeted by a common variant provides a simpler starting point and may lead to larger effect sizes (Sekar et al. 2016). This strategy would add the additional requirement of demonstrating that the observed effects were relevant to the human disorder. As such, we felt that individual common variants should not be prioritized for investigating neurobiology, but this should be reevaluated as more data becomes available.

Gene Prioritization

While we qualitatively defined weights for the prioritization factors (Figure 5.1), we did not apply these to rank single gene disorders. We note that this ranking would vary based on requirements (e.g., a specific phenotype) and therefore be somewhat subjective. As such, the ranking would best be performed by a group of domain experts guided by these factors rather than by applying an algorithm based on the qualitative weights. We also note that these factors are dynamic. For example, the discovery of a response biomarker or changes in the perceived safety profile of a therapeutic modality could change the ranking of a gene radically.

Convergent Neurobiology

What are the strategies for testing for convergence/divergence in mechanisms between genetic loci? How do we determine meaningful convergence?

Therapy aimed at a specific gene offers hope for the minority of patients with a single gene disorder. For the majority of patients that lack such a clear target, therapies will need to focus on the neurobiological pathways that causally mediate phenotype. Single gene disorders can be used to illuminate these neurobiological pathways, leveraging the large effect sizes to identify causal pathways from genotype to phenotype (Figure 5.2a). In neuropsychiatric disorders, this process is complicated by pleiotropy (Figure 5.2b)—many functional consequences for each genetic variant—and the genetic heterogeneity (Figure 5.2c)—many genetic loci associated with each neuropsychiatric disorder.

In the absence of a clear endpoint (e.g., face-valid behavior such as seizures or pain response) or biomarker (e.g., cholesterol), the identification of convergent consequences across multiple genetic variants offers a mechanism to distinguish the biological processes by which genetic information influences

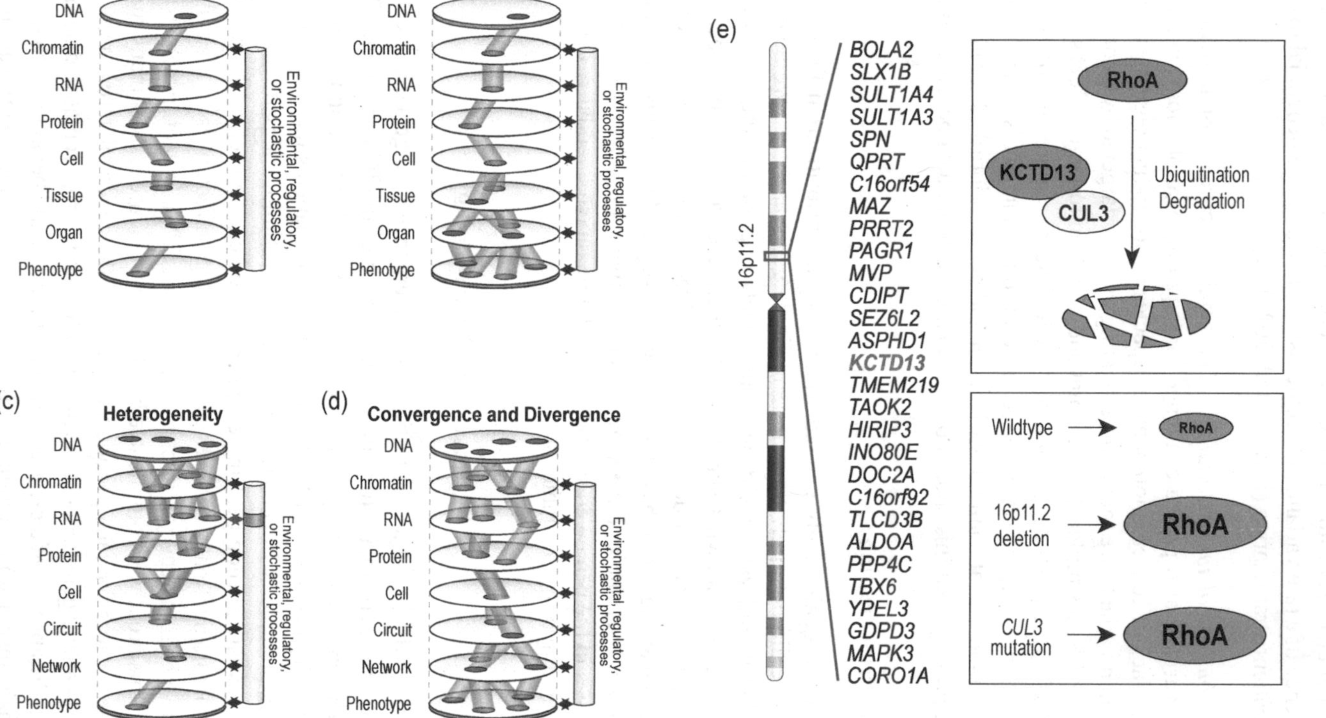
(a)
Causal Pathway
DNA
Chromatin
RNA
Protein
Cell
Tissue
Organ
Phenotype
Environmental, regulatory, or stochastic processes
(b)
Pleiotrophy
DNA
Chromatin
RNA
Protein
Cell
Tissue
Organ
Phenotype
Environmental, regulatory, or stochastic processes
(c)
Heterogeneity
DNA
Chromatin
RNA
Protein
Cell
Circuit
Network
Phenotype
Environmental, regulatory, or stochastic processes
(d)
Convergence and Divergence
DNA
Chromatin
RNA
Protein
Cell
Circuit
Network
Phenotype
Environmental, regulatory, or stochastic processes
(e)
16p11.2
BOLA2
SLX1B
SULT1A4
SULT1A3
SPN
QPRT
C16orf54
MAZ
PRRT2
PAGR1
MVP
CDIPT
SEZ6L2
ASPHD1
KCTD13
TMEM219
TAOK2
HIRIP3
INO80E
DOC2A
C16orf92
TLCD3B
ALDOA
PPP4C
TBX6
YPEL3
GDPD3
MAPK3
CORO1A
RhoA
KCTD13
CUL3
Ubiquitination Degradation
Wildtype
RhoA
16p11.2 deletion
RhoA
CUL3 mutation
RhoA

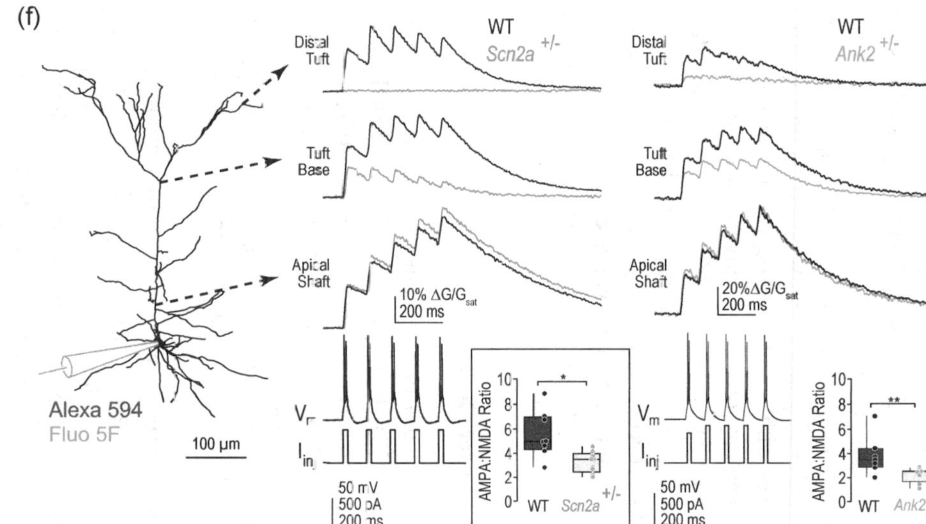

Figure 5.2 Causal pathways and convergence across causal factors in neuropsychiatric disorders. (a) We hypothesize that the mechanisms underlying genotype-phenotype associations act via different levels of biology that are discoverable. (b) Due to the complexity of the brain, each causal factor is likely to be pleiotropic (i.e., it can contribute to numerous phenotypes and multiple intervening biological processes). (c) Similarly, neuropsychiatric phenotypes are heterogeneous with multiple causal factors (both genetic and environmental). (d) We expect that a large number of causal factors might converge on a smaller number of intervening biological processes such that convergence might help guide the discovery of the causal pathway; see (a). However, divergence might be observable at other levels of analysis. (e) The gene *KCTD13* in the ASD-associated 16p11.2 microdeletion/duplication region has been implicated as a contributor to phenotype. The KCTD13 protein interacts with CUL3, encoded by the *CUL3* ASD-associated gene, and both proteins regulate the degradation of RhoA. This is an example of experimental "micro-convergence" providing a shared mechanism between two ASD-associated loci. (f) A second example of micro-convergence: heterozygous knockouts of both *Scn2a* and *Ank2* in mice lead to reduced backpropagation, with action potentials unable to reach the distal end of the dendritic tree. In both knockouts, the AMPA:NMDA ratio is reduced, suggesting immature synapses and a deficit in synaptic plasticity.

phenotype (Figure 5.2). This concept rests on the assumption that shared phenotype reflects some degree of shared neurobiology and that a large number of genetic loci act via a smaller number of biological processes, necessitating similarities in downstream processes between some genetic variants. Such convergence may be detectable at one or more levels of analysis (e.g., RNA, protein, subcellular location, pathway, cell type, circuit, brain region, developmental stage) but may not be readily detectable at others (Figure 5.2d). A biological process (e.g., excitatory neuron function) that truly mediates risk arising from combined effects across multiple loci might be expected to show convergence across experimental models of these loci. However, a closely related biological process (e.g., serotonergic neuron function) might also show a degree of convergence due to this similarity. Convergence is thus relative: we are searching for the processes with the greatest degree of convergence at each level of analysis, rather than any degree of convergence. Furthermore, convergence may be dynamic; for example, observable only at a specific stage in development or under specific conditions. This suggests the need for systematic analysis across multiple levels of analysis (e.g., cell types) to detect the biological process with the strongest convergent evidence based on a measure of effect size (e.g., correlation or enrichment) or variance (e.g., degree of phenotypic variance explained).

Multiple Autism Spectrum Disorder Genes

To date, 72 genes have been associated with ASD at genome-wide significance (Fu et al. 2022; Satterstrom et al. 2020); the majority act via haploinsufficiency (i.e., pathogenic for ASD when one of the two alleles does not produce a functional protein). While analysis of each gene independently can provide insight into the downstream neurobiological consequences, pleiotropy (Figure 5.2c) makes it hard to distinguish which of these consequences are relevant to neuropsychiatric symptoms. Again, the absence of a clear endpoint or biomarker prevents definitive experiments.

An alternative approach is to assess convergence across multiple ASD genes, and there is some evidence that this concept can provide insights. Many of the genes associated with ASD are enriched for *de novo* protein-truncating variants in genes that have been shown to be intolerant of such variants in the general population; this suggests convergence in a loss-of-function effect in haploinsufficient genes (Fu et al. 2022; Satterstrom et al. 2020). At the level of protein function, we observe the majority of genes associated with ASD-encoding proteins with a role in gene regulation (e.g., transcription factors, chromatin modifiers) or neuronal communication (e.g., synaptic proteins, ion channels; De Rubeis et al. 2014; Sanders et al. 2015; Satterstrom et al. 2020). Integrating these results with gene expression data from the developing human cortex shows that ASD-associated genes are enriched during mid-fetal gestation (Chang et al. 2015; Parikshak et al. 2013; Willsey et al. 2013), though the majority of genes continue to be highly expressed in the postnatal cortex. Single-cell transcriptomic data from the human brain shows strong convergence across ASD-associated genes in cortical excitatory and inhibitory neurons in the developing brain (Fu et al. 2022; Satterstrom et al. 2020).

These data provide some initial insights into key questions of function, cell type, and developmental period—questions critical to consider for the development of therapeutics (Dominguez et al. 2016; Hua et al. 2007; Liang et al. 2017; Muntoni and Wood 2011; Qi et al. 2013; Rinaldi and Wood 2018). The predominant heterozygous loss-of-function effects suggest that overexpression of the wildtype allele (e.g., CRIPSRa or knockdown of a repressor of the ASD-associated gene using antisense oligonucleotides) could be beneficial in many single gene disorders associated with ASD and neurodevelopmental delay. Animal models already show promise for several causes of neurodevelopmental delay (Colasante et al. 2020; Luoni et al. 2020; Schmid et al. 2021; Valassina et al. 2022); however, therapies for haploinsufficient genes may fail without sufficient knowledge of the disease-relevant biology (Hill and Meisler 2021).

While the assessment of convergent patterns has provided some insights, we must be mindful of the limitations of this approach. For example, cell-type enrichment strongly implicates cortical neurons. The developing brain is enriched for neurons compared with the mature brain: Is the prenatal enrichment of ASD-associated genes due to the high proportion of neurons, or is the neuron enrichment a reflection of the prenatal onset, or does ASD act through neurons in the prenatal cortex? Such questions are now being addressed with newer single-cell RNA-sequencing methods (e.g., Velmeshev et al. 2019). Transcription-based enrichment studies act on the assumption that high gene expression correlates with "cause," but there is no guarantee that this is true. If we were to study neurons in a different brain region (e.g., postnatal striatum), would we observe a higher degree of convergence that might change our conclusions? At present, we do not have a clear experimental or mathematical framework to address these issues.

Micro-Convergence across Autism Spectrum Disorder Loci

16p11.2 and CUL3. The concept of convergence can also be applied to experimental data from small numbers of loci associated with neuropsychiatric disorders (Figure 5.2e). Deletions and duplications at the 16p11.2 locus are associated with multiple neuropsychiatric disorders (see Vignette 5.4). A recent study using patient-derived induced pluripotent stem cells and brain organoids identified dysregulation of the neuronal cytoskeleton, neuronal migration, and RhoA signaling as potential biological processes underlying the 16p11.2-associated brain phenotypes (Urresti et al. 2021). Interestingly, one of the 16p11.2-encoded proteins, KCTD13, is a direct interacting partner of Cullin 3 (CUL3) ubiquitin ligase encoded by the *CUL3* gene (Lin et al. 2015), which has been associated with neurodevelopmental delay at genome-wide

Vignette 5.4 16p11.2 deletion and duplication syndromes (D'Angelo et al. 2016; Martin-Brevet et al. 2018; McCarthy et al. 2009; Weiss et al. 2008).

Symptoms	• Both deletions and duplications are associated primarily with developmental delay, intellectual disability, and ASD. • Deletion is associated with increased head circumference and body mass index. • Duplication is associated with reduced head circumference, reduced BMI, and schizophrenia risk.
Genetics	• Loss (deletion) or gain (duplication) of ~600 kb in the short (p) arm at the 11.2 position on chromosome 16. • Surrounding segmental duplications create a locus susceptible to non-allelic homologous recombination, leading to the high population frequency. • Unlikely that any single gene underlies all the symptoms (e.g., exome sequencing has not identified a risk locus). • Risk mediated by two or more genes remains possible.
Incidence	• 60 in 100,000, split equally between deletion (30 in 100,000) and duplication (30 in 100,000).
Endpoints	• Language, social communication, motor milestones.
Therapies	• Behavioral focused (symptom-based) interventions (at present).

significance (Fu et al. 2022). Of note, the haploinsufficient *Cul3* mouse model also has defects in neuronal cytoskeleton and RhoA signaling, similar to those observed in 16p11.2 organoids (Amar et al. 2021). Furthermore, the resulting complex between KCTD13 and CUL3 regulates RhoA levels by ubiquitination and degradation: RhoA is known to be involved in neuronal migration, axon growth, dendrite formation, and cytoskeleton remodeling during brain development (Govek et al. 2011). RhoA activation has also been observed as a consequence of *CACNA1C* disruption (encoding the $Ca_V1.2$ calcium channel) in Timothy syndrome (Krey et al. 2013), which is associated with ASD. Some of the 16p11.2-related neuron migration phenotypes observed in organoids were rescued using a small molecule inhibitor of RhoA activity Rhosin (Urresti et al. 2021); this approach is currently being tested in the *Cul3* mouse model. This "micro-convergence" provides a complementary experimental approach to complement the larger-scale convergent patterns observed across many genes.

SCN2A and ANK2. A second example of micro-convergence has recently been described between two other ASD-associated genes. Heterozygous loss-of-function mutations in *SCN2A* (encoding the voltage-gated sodium channel $Na_V1.2$) are a major cause of ASD (see Vignette 5.5). Characterization of the *Scn2a* heterozygous knockout mouse (*Scn2a*$^{+/-}$) has demonstrated a persistent deficit in action potential backpropagation by which action potentials reach the dendrites of the cell that generated the action potential, in contrast to forward propagation down the axon to other neurons (Figure 5.2f) (Spratt et al.

Vignette 5.5 *SCN2A* mutations (Li et al. 2021c; Sanders et al. 2018; Tamura et al. 2022).

Symptoms	• Seizures, ranging from severe epileptic encephalopathy to late-onset seizures. • Developmental delay, ASD, movement disorders, ataxia.
Genetics	• *De novo* mutations in the *SCN2A* gene that encodes the $Na_V1.2$ voltage-gated sodium channel. • Protein-truncating variants and loss-of-function missense variants lead to developmental delay, ASD, ±late-onset (≥ 3 years) seizures. • Gain-of-function missense variants lead to early-onset (≤ 6 months) epileptic encephalopathy. • Mixed gain/loss-of-function missense variants lead to seizures with an onset of 6 months to 3 years and developmental delay ± movement disorders. • Inherited mild gain-of-function missense variants lead to benign infantile seizures.
Incidence	• 9 in 100,000 across populations • 7.5 in 100,000 with loss-of-function • 1.5 in 100,000 with gain-of-function or gain or loss-of-function
Endpoints	• Mortality (epileptic encephalopathy), seizure frequency, developmental milestones
Therapies	• Sodium channel blocking antiepileptics for early onset seizures. • Non-sodium channel blocking antiepileptics for late-onset seizures. • PRAX-222 ASO nonselectively decreases *SCN2A* expression for gain-of-function therapy and is beginning clinical trials. • CRISPRa therapy upregulates *SCN*2A expression for loss-of-function therapy and is in preclinical development.

2019). This reduction in backpropagation leads to a reduced AMPA:NMDA ratio, suggesting immature synapses and a deficit in plasticity. In the *Scn2a*$^{+/-}$ mice, this synaptic phenotype can be rescued by a single *in vivo* CRISPRa injection via the tail vein (Tamura et al. 2022). The gene *ANK2* encodes the protein ankyrin-B, which has recently been shown to be essential for scaffolding $Na_V1.2$ to the dendritic membrane. Like *SCN2A*, *ANK2* is associated with ASD and neurodevelopmental delay at genome-wide significance (Fu et al. 2022). Analysis of the *Ank2* heterozygous knockout mouse (*Ank2*$^{+/-}$) reveals the same deficit in backpropagation and synaptic plasticity (Figure 5.2f) (Nelson et al. 2022).

Neurexins and neuroligins. Mutations in neurexins (*NRXN1*, *NRXN3*) and neuroligins (*NLGN2*, *NLGN3*, *NLGN4*) are associated with ASD and neurodevelopmental disorders. *NRXN1* is also associated with schizophrenia (Pak et al. 2015; Tromp et al. 2021). All these genes encode proteins that form transsynaptic signaling complexes anchored on the pre- and postsynaptic membrane that shape the properties of synapses (Eichmüller et al. 2022; Südhof 2008, 2017b).

Divergence across Levels of Analysis

Fragile X syndrome provides a counterexample, in which functional "divergence" emerges across levels of neural organization despite "convergence" at the molecular level (see Figure 5.2d, Vignette 5.3, and Sahin, this volume). Our current understanding of the pathogenesis of Fragile X syndrome and the role of group I metabotropic glutamate receptors (including mGluR5) is based primarily on studies in the hippocampus and neocortex in rodents (Bear et al. 2004). In these regions, Fragile X syndrome leads to increased signaling through mGluR5, which leads to elevated synaptic plasticity as evidenced by an enhancement of long-term depression (LTD) (Fitzjohn et al. 2001; Hou et al. 2006; Huber et al. 2002; Nakamoto et al. 2007; Palmer et al. 1997). As predicted, downregulating mGluR signaling in mice corrects multiple abnormalities induced in Fragile X syndrome in these regions, including the LTD phenotype, impaired inhibitory avoidance extinction, audiogenic seizures, and enhanced cortical spine density (Dölen et al. 2007). However, the opposite effect occurs in the lateral amygdala, where mGluR5 mediates reduced synaptic plasticity via long-term potentiation (LTP) (Rodrigues et al. 2002; Suvrathan et al. 2010). Accordingly, an mGluR antagonist failed to reverse deficient amygdalar LTP in *Fmr1*$^{-/y}$ mice (Suvrathan et al. 2010).

In a more recent study using a rat model of Fragile X syndrome, activation of mGluRs reversed LTP impairment in the lateral amygdala as well as its behavioral correlate: impaired recall of conditioned fear (Fernandes et al. 2021). Interestingly, this study also revealed the presence of presynaptic mGluR5 at the same thalamic inputs that mediate LTP in the lateral amygdala. In contrast, much of the earlier work on synaptic deficits associated with Fragile X syndrome and their reversal in the hippocampus focused primarily on postsynaptic mechanisms. In other words, while mGluR-dependent synaptic signaling mechanisms in Fragile X syndrome pathophysiology are a point of convergence in the hippocampus and amygdala, the pharmacological correction of synaptic defects serves as an example of divergence: mGluR-inactivation is effective in the hippocampus, whereas mGluR-activation has been shown to *reverse* synaptic and behavioral deficits in the amygdala of Fragile X syndrome rats. Further, while we observe molecular convergence across brain regions at the level of mGluR, we observe subsequent divergence at the level of synaptic plasticity and behavioral outcomes (Figure 5.2d). Notably, this also highlights the importance of modifying the prevailing mGluR-based framework for therapeutic strategies to include circuit-specific differences in Fragile X syndrome pathophysiology.

Summary

The identification of convergent functional consequences across multiple genetic loci associated with a disorder increases the likelihood that the specific functional consequence is on the causal pathway between genotype and phenotype (Figure 5.2). However, convergence is relative and, if demonstrated, a greater degree of convergence in a related process might dramatically change interpretation. Identifying convergent effects requires systematic analyses across genes at multiple levels of analysis and across development. There is considerable scope to improve the analytical framework of convergent analyses to facilitate better comparisons and aid causal inference.

Models to Interrogate Genetic Loci

Brain development is extremely sensitive and complex. This process is crucial to future brain function, and investigating it is key to understanding how neurodevelopmental disorders alter brain function. Given the uniqueness of the human brain across species, the best tissue for enquiries to illuminate these developmental processes is from humans. There is a critical need for more molecular, structural, functional, and clinical information on typical and atypical human brain function across development as the primary source of information on these processes and as a comparator to validate experimental model systems. However, we cannot experimentally manipulate human subjects or gain access to living tissue with sufficient resolution. As such, we advocate for a systematic analysis of human-induced pluripotent stem cells (hiPSCs) as well as rodent and nonhuman primate (e.g., marmoset) models of single gene disorders in tandem with human studies. While there are concerns about the predictive efficacy of rodent studies for therapies of neuropsychiatric disorders in humans (see Vignette 5.2), there is limited data on how nonhuman primate models will fare. Here, we consider how data from experiment model systems can be used to make and validate predictions of human phenotypes (see also Brennand and Kushner, this volume).

Rodent Models

Since the publication of the first knockout mouse in 1987 (Thomas and Capecchi 1987), mice have been the mainstay for modeling most rare genetic disorders. More than 99% of mouse genes have human homologs; thus, genetically engineered mouse models have construct validity (or etiologic validity), which refers to how closely the molecular underpinnings of a disease in an animal model mirror those in humans. Whether those models have face validity as well, such that the phenotype in an animal model has significant overlap with the phenotype in humans, is still open to investigation. There is substantial skepticism about the behavioral traits observed in neuropsychiatric disorders. Finally, predictive validity (predicting successful therapy in humans) of these models does not yet exist for the most part because there are no FDA-approved treatments for most neuropsychiatric symptoms associated with rare genetic disorders; there is also an absence of validated preclinical endpoints and biomarkers. Nonetheless, mouse models can be extremely helpful in providing insights at the level of cellular function. They may be less useful, however, at the level of circuits or behavior. Additionally, genetic background effects play a substantial role in many phenotypes, consequently demonstrating consistent findings across mouse strains is critical.

Rats have been used extensively for pharmacological modeling but less so in the genetic modeling of brain disorders. Extension of CRISPR editing and advances in embryonic stem cell methods now allow for the efficient generation of rat models of single gene disorders. Rat models have the advantage that they display more complex behaviors and communications than mice (Ellenbroek and Youn 2016). Comparison of mouse and rat models of genetic diseases is starting to reveal that while cellular functions may be conserved, behavioral manifestations may differ across species in response to genetic manipulations (Till et al. 2015). Whether rat models will have improved face and/or predictive validity compared to mice in terms of developing new treatments for rare genetic disorders is not yet known.

Prairie voles have also been proposed as a suitable model for neuropsychiatric disorders because of the long-term social attachments formed between mating partners (Berendzen et al. 2023). Again, face and/or predictive validity remains to be demonstrated.

When modeling disorders with rodents, several steps can be taken to increase rigor and reproducibility (Gulinello et al. 2019). The issue of strain-specificity can be overcome by using multiple background strains, outbred mouse models, and multiple genetic models for the same disease. Issues related to statistical power can be addressed by preregistering behavioral assays and metrics (similar to clinical trials), increasing sample sizes, and replicating significant positive findings independently before moving to clinical trials (Howe et al. 2018). Finally, translational biomarkers shared by humans and rodents are needed to assess the therapeutic efficacy of an intervention (Modi and Sahin 2017).

Human-Induced Pluripotent Stem Cell Models

To investigate the molecular mechanisms of neurodevelopmental disorders, hiPSC-based models are now widely used. Given the limited opportunity for studying fetal brain tissue from individuals with neurodevelopmental disorders, hiPSC technology provides a unique opportunity to study developmental processes in a human context. Somatic cells derived from individuals are reprogrammed and differentiated into two-dimensional neuronal cultures, three-dimensional models (organoids), or more complex models, such as assembloids (Kelley and Paşca 2022; Paşca et al. 2022). Alternatively, specific genetic variants can be engineered into existing hiPSCs lines. It has been demonstrated that organoids are particularly well-suited for studies of prenatal neurodevelopmental disorder studies because their transcriptional profiles, cellular composition, and even electrophysiological properties largely capture those of the human early- to mid-fetal brain, despite certain noted limitations (Amiri et al. 2018; Bhaduri et al. 2020; Camp et al. 2015; Luo et al. 2016; Trujillo et al. 2019; Velasco et al. 2019). Many studies to date have used 3D cortical organoids to model neurodevelopmental disorders, such as lissencephaly (Bershteyn et al. 2017), idiopathic ASD (Mariani et al. 2015), microcephaly (Lancaster et al. 2013), Timothy syndrome (Birey et al. 2017), and 16p11.2-associated ASD (Urresti et al. 2021). These models may enable high- and medium-throughput drug screening for preclinical endpoints that emerge early in neurodevelopment. In addition, recent technological developments allow transplantation of organoids and assembloids into animal brains to create grafted "chimera" models that could provide further insights into diseases within more physiological conditions, including later stages of neurodevelopment, vascularization, and integration of more diverse cell types (Daviaud et al. 2018; Mansour et al. 2018).

Despite their many advantages, hiPSCs have some substantial limitations. It is hard to differentiate the cells beyond the equivalent of mid-fetal development, limiting insights into postnatal development, let alone the adolescent, adult, or elderly brain. For organoid models, there is substantial variability in cellular composition between organoids from the same hiPSC line, adding heterogeneity to assays. The use of hiPSC-derived models is further limited by patient availability or the heterogeneous genetic backgrounds of the patients, which can complicate the investigation of genetic variants of small effect (e.g., common variants from genome-wide association studies), and the prohibitive cost of producing such models on a large scale (e.g., hundreds to thousands of patients). Some of these limitations (e.g., accessibility to relevant patient populations) could be overcome, for example, by generating isogenic models by CRISPR engineering the desired mutation(s) into control iPSC lines (Ben Jehuda et al. 2018) or correcting the mutation from patient lines to independently assess the role of genetic background. Further avenues to pursue include lowering the cost of hiPSC reprogramming and organoid production and adapting the technology to a high-throughput low-volume format. Overall, despite many interesting insights into neurodevelopmental disorders achieved with hiPSC-derived models, the current state of the field still suffers from small sample sizes and variability in protocols that are used to generate these models, which makes cross-comparison difficult (Anderson et al. 2021). The application of appropriate statistical models that account for technical and biological replicates from different iPSC clones, and mixed models that treat the individual as a random-effect variable should be used in the analyses (Hoffman et al. 2019). As with rodent models, predictive validity remains to be demonstrated, though there are examples of treatments that have gone directly from hiPSC models to clinical trials without testing in an animal model (Wainger et al. 2014). These potential pitfalls notwithstanding, hiPSC-derived models clearly serve as an essential asset for future studies and therapeutic interventions for neurodevelopmental disorders.

Nonhuman Primate Models

Currently, most animal work is conducted in rodents, primarily because there is an extensive range of genetic tools with which to investigate these models and infrastructure to support these efforts. However, the human brain is quite distinct from that of rodents (Marshall and Mason 2019). To fill the gap, it is crucial to have a model animal that is closer to humans, and nonhuman primates represent the closest species. The common marmoset (*Callithrix jacchus*), a small New World monkey, has recently emerged as a new animal model for studies of neurological and neuropsychiatric disorders, basic and behavioral neuroscience, neuroimaging, stem cell research, and drug toxicology (Hikishima et al. 2011; Iwanami et al. 2005; Kishi et al. 2014; Leuner et al. 2007; Mansfield 2003; Mashiko et al. 2012; Poswillo et al. 1972; Sasaki et al. 2009; Tomioka et al. 2010; Yamazaki et al. 2011). Similar to humans, but unlike rodents, wild marmosets live in stable extended families. Group members support infant care by the breeding mother with strong parental and familial relationships. These and other human-like characteristics of marmosets are likely to be advantageous for cognitive behavioral research.

In addition, the recent generation of transgenic marmosets will enable researchers to investigate the molecular genetic basis of higher cognition and complex brain disorders that contain endophenotypes related to human-like conditions (Kishi et al. 2014; Okano et al. 2012; Sasaki et al. 2009). Moreover, comparisons revealed substantial similarities in cell types and gene expression patterns within prefrontal and visual cortices between marmosets, humans, and other species (Kita et al. 2021; Onishi et al. 2022; Ma et al. 2022). The above results suggest that the marmoset is likely to be a good animal model for human developmental brain disorders, and there is a reasonable expectation of face and predictive validity not achieved in other experimental model systems of neuropsychiatric disorders.

Using nonhuman primates for all experimental goals, however, raises ethical and economic issues. It is important to consider what is the best model animal for a given experiment. For example, if a rodent or cellular model recapitulates the human condition, then it is hard to justify a nonhuman primate model. Thus, failure to identify such a feature in other model systems may be a prerequisite for beginning to generate a nonhuman primate model. Currently, there are also practical considerations, as there are few marmoset colonies available for experimentation, limiting the number of conditions that can be modeled.

Nonhuman primates are not a panacea, since humans have capacities not found in marmosets or other nonhuman primates, and their brains differ in important ways. Key to understanding the extent to which marmosets can model human conditions is developing large-scale data sets that can be directly compared between species in typical and atypical brains. Such data sets would include whole-genome sequencing, epigenetic (e.g., ATAC-sequencing method), transcriptomic (e.g., single nuclei RNA sequencing and *in situ* hybridization), high-resolution structural and functional imaging, and deep phenotyping. Most of these assays will need to include the developmental axis. As an initial step in this direction, the marmoset ISH database provides an invaluable reference tool that helps translate knowledge from rodents to primates and advance primate molecular neurobiology research.

Summary

It remains unclear whether neuropsychiatric disorders are human-specific (necessitating hiPSC models), brain region-specific (necessitating animal models), or circuit- and behavior-specific (potentially necessitating nonhuman primate models). Until a clear consensus emerges driven by robust predictive validity in neuropsychiatric disorders, there is a role for all experimental models. We identified three advances that are required:

1. Reduced reliance on single strains of inbred animals.
2. Increased use of large mammalian models, especially the marmoset nonhuman primate model including single gene disorder models.
3. Systematic data generation in parallel across multiple models at multiple levels of analysis to provide clear data to judge which processes are conserved across models, which are not, and whether there are biomarkers or endpoints in common between models.

Requirements for Clinical Trials

What key advances are required, in terms of natural history, biomarkers, and clinical endpoints, to optimize the probability of success in clinical trials?

Natural History

Natural history studies define the natural course of a disease, providing critical insights into the needs of the patient population, potential therapeutic endpoints, and potential biomarkers. Obtaining this data requires the collection of standardized prospective longitudinal information, ideally across multiple developmental points in time. Since individuals affected with rare genetic disorders are likely to be geographically distributed, it is essential to have a platform to perform standardized assessments of such individuals across the distributed sites. Such a multisite platform requires tight standardization of neuropsychological assessments and biomarkers (e.g., EEG and MRI). Standardization of protocols is often achieved by using human controls or artificial "human phantoms," who travel from site to site at regular intervals (Prohl et al. 2019; Saby et al. 2021). Although such efforts are time- and labor-consuming, they are essential to obtain meaningful and reproducible data from multisite observational or interventional studies.

Biomarkers

Reliable, quantifiable, and translatable biomarkers of disease are needed to transform the investigation, diagnosis, and management of neuropsychiatric disorders. Multiple types of biomarkers have been defined by the BEST (Biomarkers, EndpointS, and other Tools) Resource from the FDA–NIH Biomarker Working Group (see Table 5.2). All of these are valuable (Califf 2018); however, response biomarkers that could assay target engagement of an intervention are especially important from the perspective of drug discovery (Parellada et al. 2023). Having reliable biomarkers and related mechanistic biological understanding is key for establishing target engagement and making "go/no-go" decisions, even in the absence of a clinical effect. With this framework, every failure informs the next study; a single success has the potential to transform the field due to the knowledge gained regarding therapeutic development.

The discovery of biomarkers that translate between species, including humans, would transform the utility of animal models. The utility of rodent behavior varies by phenotype, but measures of pain or seizures have predictive validity as preclinical endpoints in humans (Howe et al. 2018). Nonetheless, behavioral assays are complicated, and response biomarkers that correlate with these endpoints (e.g., neuronal excitability, EEG, or autonomic activation) could lead to more efficient comprehensive therapeutic screens. Other potential response biomarkers include myelination (as measured by MRI) or motor response (as measured by wearable technologies). Since demyelination is a hallmark of several neurological conditions (e.g., multiple sclerosis), validation of *in vivo* biomarkers of myelin is a particularly active area of investigation. A recent systematic review of published quantitative validation studies found that magnetization transfer and relaxometry-based measures showed the strongest correlations with myelin content (Mancini et al. 2020). Currently, however, there is no MRI-based measure of myelin that is true to histology, and more reproducibility studies are needed in the field. Likewise, noninvasive, wearable sensor technologies hold great potential for quantifying and continuously tracking real-world motor function, both in relation to disease progression and treatment response (Ganesalingam and Bowser 2010; Tyler et al. 2020). Greater collaboration across multiple disciplines (clinicians, bioengineers, data scientists, and software developers) from both academia and industry is needed, however, to fulfill their promise.

Developing response biomarkers that could provide reliable and valid measures of cognitive and behavioral phenotypes is of paramount importance for

Table 5.2 Definitions of biomarker types, adapted from the FDA–NIH Biomarker Working Group (2016).

Susceptibility/risk	Biomarker that indicates one's potential for developing a disease/condition of interest.
Diagnostic	Biomarker used to detect or confirm the presence of a disease/condition or to identify individuals with a disease subtype.
Monitoring	Biomarker that is measured repeatedly to assess the status of a disease/condition or for evidence of exposure to (or effect of) an intervention.
Prognostic	Biomarker used to indicate the likelihood of a clinical event, disease recurrence, or progression in individuals with disease/condition of interest.
Predictive	Biomarker used to identify individual(s) more likely to experience a particular effect from exposure to an intervention.
Response	Biomarker used to show that a biological response (potentially beneficial or harmful) has occurred from exposure or intervention, with the following subcategories: • Pharmacodynamic: reflects the biological activity of an intervention without necessarily indicating efficacy or a particular mechanism of action; could be used to establish proof of concept, dose selection, or to measure treatment response. • Surrogate endpoint: can be used as an endpoint in clinical trials as a substitute for a direct measure of patient response; is expected to predict the clinical benefit or harm.
Safety	Biomarker measure before/after exposure to an intervention to indicate possible toxicity as an adverse effect.

neuropsychiatric and developmental disorders. To date, no response biomarkers have been validated in ASD (Parellada et al. 2022). The majority of studies are underpowered and few studies aim to systematically screen multiple biomarkers with robust statistical thresholds and replication. As challenging as it is to find such biomarkers, their importance merits the large-scale collaborative efforts that will be required to find them.

Importance of Developmental Timing

Interventions for phenylketonuria and amblyopia have identified critical periods for cognitive and visual development, respectively. Whether there are critical periods for the treatment of behavioral symptoms in neurodevelopmental or psychiatric disorders remains unknown; similarly, the extent to which cognitive impairments can be rescued later in development has not been determined. There are specific time periods in which the brain undergoes dramatic shifts in neural organization; specific circuits are likely differentially affected based on developmental timing. This suggests that focusing on time periods involving dramatic shifts in synaptic organization, as well as the early postnatal period (in rodents as well as nonhuman primate models), is essential for gaining insight into how specific mutations affect brain development. However, neurodevelopmental periods of the most rapid change (gliogenesis/synaptic organization) may not necessarily correspond directly to the optimal window for treatment (Guy et al. 2007; Koene et al. 2021; Milazzo et al. 2021; Rotaru et al. 2018; Silva-Santos et al. 2015; Tsai et al. 2018; Ure et al. 2016).

There may be points in development where correcting gene function no longer benefits the patient. Thus, pinpointing critical periods for therapeutic intervention for specific outcomes is essential: What is the recoverable fraction of the target outcome at a given time in neurodevelopment? Even for traits like binocular plasticity, there is a gradient of response (Wang et al. 2010). Some circuits are dynamic and continuously remodeled, such as adult mouse hippocampus (Attardo et al. 2015).

The best answers to these questions may come directly from attempting to treat these disorders in humans, as has been done in spinal muscular atrophy. Therefore, the ability of genetic therapies to pinpoint the extent to which neuropsychiatric symptoms can be modified across developmental stages and degrees of severity may inform the potential of future therapies aimed at idiopathic cases lacking a simple single gene target.

The Rocky Road to Treatment Success

There are many potential pitfalls on the path to therapeutic success (see Sahin, this volume). The cumulative impact of all these pitfalls leads to a low probability of success, even when the probability of making a correct decision at each stage is relatively high (Table 5.3). For example, if there were nine major decisions to be made and each had an 80% probability of being correct, the overall chance of success is only 13%.

In the face of these challenges, it is clear that we need to attempt more "shots on goal" to maximize chances of successful treatment; we also need to optimize decision making at each stage. More attempts should be made in the context of repurposed (i.e., safe) drugs, where prior experience may help increase the probabilities of success at several stages. Genetic therapies have the advantage of near certainty on the choice of "target," marginally increasing the overall chance of success as well as the confidence that even an unsuccessful trial has lessons to refine future trials. Accordingly, the sharing of data for negative outcomes is essential. A successful trial of even a single neurodevelopmental disorder would provide critical insights that could increase the probability of success at multiple stages of future trials. There is also an urgent need to improve efficiency in clinical trial design to reduce resource needs. A closer relationship with industry would be mutually beneficial, creating a precompetitive space for characterizing disorders in model systems and humans, and helping train the next generation of researchers for clinical translation.

Table 5.3 Hypothetical probability of success at each stage of therapeutic development and overall.

Decision	Probability of Correct Decision				
Target	95%	90%	80%	70%	60%
Therapy	95%	90%	80%	70%	60%
Dose	95%	90%	80%	70%	60%
Duration	95%	90%	80%	70%	60%
Population	95%	90%	80%	70%	60%
Age range	95%	90%	80%	70%	60%
Sample size	95%	90%	80%	70%	60%
Endpoints	95%	90%	80%	70%	60%
Side effects	95%	90%	80%	70%	60%
Total:	63%	39%	13%	4%	1%

Implementation

How do we establish infrastructure and incentives to generate rigorous reproducible findings?

Better alignment of incentive structures between academia and industry is key (see Figure 5.3). There is a precompetitive need for understanding biology, and establishing training programs with a translational focus (e.g., T32 training grants to gain experience in clinical trial implementation) will benefit both. This approach should meet the synergistic goals of research findings with higher clinical impact, more successful therapies for industry, and better treatments for people who need them. In addition, as a global effort, implementation is key to the success of the field, as it is critical to increase

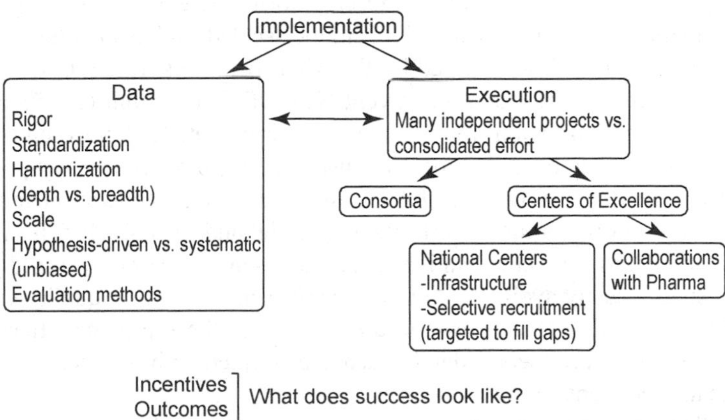

Figure 5.3 A model for implementation. Incentive structures between industry and academia must be better aligned to optimize chances of successful therapeutics.

the representativeness and diversity of the workforce, as well as to ensure widespread access throughout the world to innovative therapies. Training programs that better integrate trainees and mentors from industry and academia are needed to establish greater synergy. For example, industry could provide funding for internships in academic centers with a translational focus.

Rigor and Reproducibility

Presently, across science, the novelty of experimental proposals and methodologies may be prioritized ahead of investigative rigor. In practice, this leads to a paucity of studies that are able to confirm or refine new findings, even in cases when this may be most warranted. In concept, this may continue to support the phenomenon that "new" is assumed to be equal to "true." Yet the penalties for potential errors that could arise under this mantra are nontrivial, and they could be especially costly for large-scale studies or consortia charged with creating resources to be used broadly across diverse scientific disciplines. Fortunately, there are standout examples where truth by replication and revision is appreciated (e.g., the Human Genome Project). Still, there remains a strong need for journals and funding bodies to incentivize programs for multiple labs to create, check, and replicate crucial data iteratively and collaboratively.

In a similar example from translational studies, a recent comprehensive review of potential biomarkers for evaluating ASD diagnosis and treatment found that no current candidate biomolecule has sufficient evidence to inform clinical decisions in trials related to symptom reduction (Parellada et al. 2022). This review highlighted a major problem in the field; namely that, of the nearly 1,000 candidate biomarkers evaluated, 80% were unique to a single publication. This points to the urgent need for greater standardization and collaboration to solve these challenges for achieving treatment success.

Large-scale examples of collaborations prioritizing experimental rigor and reliability that may provide a model for smaller-scaled studies include the brain structure and gene atlases created by the Allen Brain Institute (Hawrylycz et al. 2012; Li et al. 2018), and the PsychENCODE Consortium (2015) among others. These collaborations are notable for their operating plan which coordinated, organized, and enabled identical usage of the best technology possible in concert with the best labs possible. In these cases, data generation and validation occur through multiple streams, in parallel and recursively. This model also requires that data, code, and other resources are made public rapidly and from a single, easily available point of access. Since stringent quality control and data availability are intrinsic to the mission of these projects, their track record of creating products widely valued and credited with advancing the field may be a direct consequence.

Another collaborative framework that provides a model for other studies of practical and translatable scientific rigor is the Rare Diseases Clinical Research Network—an NIH-supported consortium of 20 research groups that are specified to include scientists, patients/community members, and clinicians, each focused on a group of rare disorders. Since such groups and the diseases of interest are extremely unique and heterogeneous by definition, care is taken by the network to assure that methods are validated in all cases and unified whenever possible. Furthermore, when singular findings are encountered that may hold great scientific interest but cannot meet statistical significance owing to rare diagnoses and current sample availability, oversight by the network assures that expanded studies have a higher likelihood of definitive results.

Studies within the network of nonhuman primate research centers may also exemplify policies, ideals, and incentive structures that could promote scientific reproducibility and increase overall productivity. In these settings, research ethics and relative resource limitations predetermine that experiments are planned and carefully coordinated within groups so that each part of the model system (the animal, its exposures, and/or behavior) is used optimally. This process is organized both within and between national primate research centers to assure that such models and methods are standardized and that integration with preclinical and clinical studies is consistent. Thoughtful translation of these principles to other experimental platforms can assure that rigor and reproducibility, as well as the speed, simplicity, and lower costs inherent in other models, all can be maximized.

An Experimental Model for Investigating Rare Variants

Across the five questions that we addressed in our discussions, we identified multiple opportunities to refine the analysis of rare variants and inform the study of neurodevelopmental and psychiatric disorders. Here, we combine these insights to propose an optimal experimental model to advance the field (Figure 5.4).

As we considered the prioritization of genes, we appreciated that the dual goals of neurobiological insight and therapeutic discovery share many synergies and lead to similar rankings of genes for investigation. In our discussion of the search for convergent biology, we observed utility from both large-scale systematic analysis of many genes as well as "micro-convergence" from in-depth systematic analyses of small numbers of genes. Regarding the utility and validation of models and recognizing our ignorance about how neurodevelopmental and psychiatric symptoms emerge, we saw value in both human cellular and animal models. We felt there was an urgent need to embrace nonhuman primate models, such as marmosets, in the hope that they might yield the necessary preclinical endpoints that are essential to demonstrate causal relationships and effective therapies. As we considered how to optimize the probability of success in clinical trials, we described the need to perform natural history studies, search for biomarkers, and define therapeutically actionable windows of development. Finally, to improve the rigor and reliability of experiments,

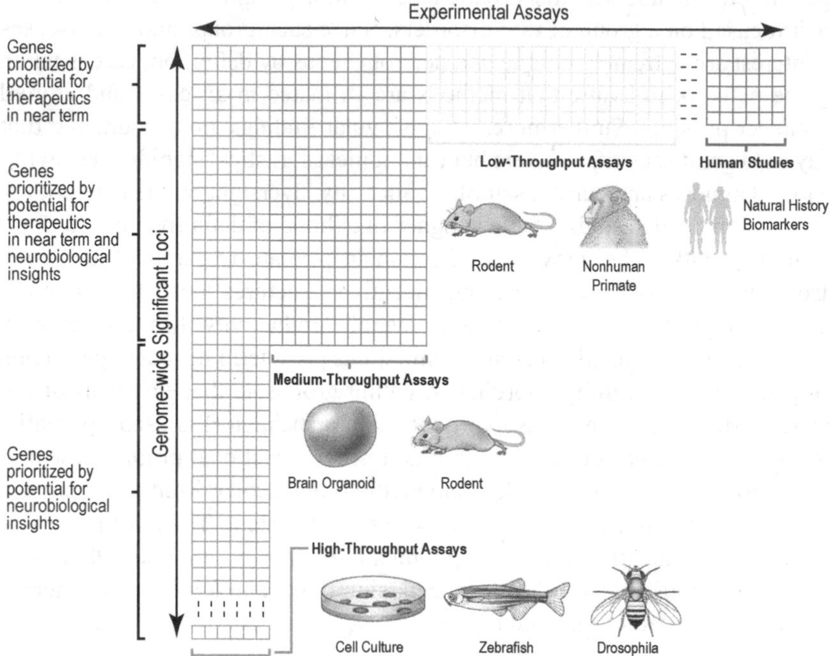

Figure 5.4 A proposed model for collaborative investigations of rare variants.

we stress the contributions that large-scale collaborative endeavors can contribute to help achieve this.

We envision our proposed framework as a large-scale collaborative endeavor, one that aims to generate systematic data across multiple levels of analysis. We start by prioritizing all genome-wide significant loci from rare variant discovery efforts according to the schema described earlier (see section, Prioritizing Genes and Loci for Neurobiological Investigation). We aim to define three groups:

- Group 1: a small number of single gene disorders with the greatest short-term therapeutic potential,
- Group 2: a medium number of genes prioritized for therapeutic and neurobiological potential, and
- Group 3: a large number of genes prioritized for neurobiological potential (Figure 5.4).

Next, we identify experimental assays to help understand these single gene disorders and split these into three groups:

- High-throughput assays that can be applied to groups 1, 2, and 3 for large-scale convergent analyses,

- Medium-throughput assays to be applied to groups 1 and 2 for in-depth convergent analyses,
- Low-throughput assays and preclinical translational assays to be applied to group 1 for therapeutic development, biomarker discovery, assessment of predictive validity of model systems, and examination of micro-convergence across multiple levels of analysis.

It is important to note that this experimental design is modular. For example, if a technological advance enabled a medium-throughput assay to be deployed at higher throughput, or if an assay showed such clear potential in group 1 or 2 that it should be deployed in a larger group, it would be clear which genes remained to be assayed. Furthermore, the resulting data would still be systematic, allowing convergent analyses across multiple genes. Similarly, if a preclinical therapy was developed for a gene in group 2, there would be a clear roadmap of how to perform the additional group 1 assays for clinical translation. The experimental design also lends itself to generating comparable data across model systems and humans, allowing the model systems to be validated.

For low-throughput assays in group 1, human and nonhuman primate studies are essential. These activities would include natural history studies (standardized across multiple genes to allow comparisons) and assays across multiple brain regions and developmental stages in cellular and animal studies with a particular emphasis on nonhuman primates.

To utilize these data to assess convergent patterns, it is essential that we do not rely on shared controls. If all assays are compared to the same set of pooled controls, it is inevitable that similar patterns will be seen across the genes assayed, leading to false convergent signals. Therefore, substantial resources will need to be devoted to data generation in wildtype models and healthy human control subjects. This, however, will create a data set that provides critical insights into the typical distribution of values in the assay. It also offers a chance to create reference data across brain regions and developmental stages in typically developing animals and cells that can be compared directly with equivalent data from typically developing humans. Thus, the extensive control data are critical to both validating experimental model systems and systematically quantifying convergence patterns across the entire experimental framework.

Conclusions and Major Outcomes

At present, variants with large effect sizes represent the most tangible starting point for both investigating neurobiology and developing therapeutics. The dual quests for treating single gene disorders and understanding neurobiology are highly synergistic, as exemplified by the urgent need to identify reliable endpoints, biomarkers, natural history, and cross-species similarities. The development of a successful therapeutic for a single gene disorder (the best-case scenario) would galvanize the field to further understand neurobiology and enhance therapeutic development since it demonstrates that such a quest can yield tangible results and likely provide important lessons and caveats. A successful therapeutic could also serve as a tool for neurobiological inquiry, enabling interrogation of critical period windows and helping to exclude neurobiological processes that are not targeted by the therapy. Characterizing normal development in animal models and humans (e.g., via transcriptomics and neuroimaging) is vital to interpreting how rare variants impact development. We are now poised at a critical juncture, as a multitude of therapies for neurodevelopmental and neuropsychiatric disorders are currently under development. To realize these goals, we urgently need systematic and standardized data, analyzed in rigorous ways. This requires careful experimental design, well-powered analyses, researchers focused on rigor, and an emphasis on replication. We propose an optimal experimental design that matches gene prioritization to assay throughout to generate a data set that can be used to identify convergent patterns of neurobiology, assess the validity of model systems at different levels of analysis, and accelerate therapeutic development.

Acknowledgments

Funding sources for associated research: MH122678, DA053628, MH116488 (NS), U54-NS092090, P50-HD105351 (MS); MH108528, MH109885 (LMI); MH129395 (SAK), U01MH119736, R21MH116473, R01MH085953 (CEB), U01MH122681, R01MH129751, R01MH125516 (SJS). Special thanks to Ioana Ciuperca for valuable assistance with references and formatting.

6

Promises and Challenges of Precision Medicine in Rare Neurodevelopmental Disorders

Mustafa Sahin

Abstract

Rare deleterious variants with large effect sizes offer a unique opportunity to understand the pathophysiology of neurodevelopmental and psychiatric disorders and provide insights into mechanism-based therapies. Single gene disorders may, in particular, be addressable with gene-based technologies even in cases where we may not understand the pathophysiology completely, as has been the case for spinal muscular atrophy. This chapter reviews the therapeutics development process in several modalities, including small molecules, antisense oligonucleotides, and viral vector-mediated gene replacement using examples of rare genetic disorders such as tuberous sclerosis complex, Fragile X syndrome, Rett syndrome, and Angelman syndrome. Finally, a strengths, weaknesses, opportunities, and threats (SWOT) analysis is included to guide the use of rare genetic variants to develop treatments. Identification of rare genetic variants has changed the landscape of research in this field; however, to translate these discoveries into rational, mechanism-based, safe, and effective treatments for neurodevelopmental and psychiatric disorders will require building and sustained support of networks/consortia that work closely with patient communities and industry partners.

Introduction

It is now well established that many psychiatric neurodevelopmental disorders (NDD), such as autism spectrum disorder (ASD, schizophrenia, and bipolar disorder, have high heritability (Hebebrand et al. 2010). Advances in genetics and genomics, in particular the wider application of exome and genome sequencing to ever larger cohorts of individuals with ASD, have revealed that both common and rare variants contribute to autism risk. Most of the genetic risk for ASD is accounted for by the presence of multiple common variants (Gaugler et al. 2014) that individually have small effect sizes. In contrast, rare deleterious variants with large effect sizes can be the primary determinant in specific individuals; these variants are often associated with intellectual disability. According to a Swedish epidemiological database (the Population-Based Autism Genetics and Environment Study or PAGES), up to ~27% of individuals with ASD have pathogenic or likely pathogenic rare variants (Mahjani et al. 2021). Recent meta-analyses have recommended the use of exome or genome sequencing as first line testing for neurodevelopmental disorders such as ASD (Manickam et al. 2021; Srivastava et al. 2019). In this chapter, I will evaluate current understanding of the NDD genetic landscape from the perspective of therapeutic development and provide a strengths, weaknesses, opportunities, and threats (SWOT) analysis to guide the use of rare genetic variants to develop treatments.

Genetic Landscape of Autism Spectrum Disorder

Individuals who suffer from ASD can harbor rare disruptive variants in genes that are intolerant of loss of function and/or variation in the broader population. This finding has enabled statistical analysis of genetic variants in large ASD cohorts compared to the general population. Analysis of ever larger research cohorts has increased the number of genes for which we have high confidence from 65 in 2015 (Sanders et al. 2015) to 102 with FDR <0.01 in 2020 (Satterstrom et al. 2020) to 183 genes with FDR <0.05 in 2022 (Fu et al. 2022). According to these statistical analyses, the odds ratio of carrying one of these variants can be 10- to 20-fold higher in the ASD cohort compared to the general population. These estimates are based, however, on small numbers of individuals in the ASD cohort and even smaller or none in the control cohort. Therefore, clinical confirmation of such findings is extremely important. There is a strong ascertainment bias in these types of studies; therefore, learning the full phenotype and penetrance of the genetic variants will almost always require the collection of a larger number of individuals with that variant identified through clinical testing and potentially population-level analyses using birth cohorts or health system registries (Sanders et al. 2019).

Much research in neuropsychiatric disorders has focused on copy number variants (CNVs). For many CNVs, it has been difficult to identify a single critical gene within the chromosomal region that is driving the effect. In fact, for many recurrent CNVs, multiple genes with smaller individual effect sizes seem to contribute to the overall risk. For example, the typical 22q11.2 deletion, a CNV associated with variable and complex behavioral and medical syndromes including autistic features, encompasses around 50 genes, 10 of them intolerant to haploinsufficiency. Taken together, single gene disorders are likely to be easier to address with gene-based therapies than multigenic CNVs.

The assertion that a gene is implicated in syndromic versus nonsyndromic intellectual disability or ASD is often based on methods of ascertainment and extent of detailed phenotyping. A syndrome is a group of traits that tend to occur together and characterize a recognizable disease. Some syndromes (such as FXS, Rett syndrome, and tuberous sclerosis) have been recognized for decades. Several genes, initially implicated in syndromic conditions, were later reported in subjects with nonsyndromic forms of intellectual disability (e.g., *ARX, CASK, JARID1C, FGD1*, and *ATRX*). There has also been some debate about whether there is sufficient evidence for "autism-specific" genes (Buxbaum et al. 2020; Myers et al. 2020a, b; Satterstrom et al. 2020). Regardless, it is unequivocally clear that there is a significant overlap between "ASD-predominant" and "ASD with NDD" genes from both a statistical and a clinical genetics perspective. For the purposes of therapeutics, this debate is not particularly productive.

Before considering the advantages and disadvantages of targeting rare genetic variants for therapeutics development, one needs to briefly review the process of drug development in neuroscience. The translational pipeline necessary to bring a therapy to the clinic requires several steps: correct target, correct molecule, correct dose, correct duration of drug treatment, correct subset of patients, correct stage of disease, correct sample size, correct endpoints, and acceptable side effect profile. There is potential for failure at each of these steps (Figure 6.1). Even if every step is successful, the traditional drug discovery process (from target discovery to approval) can take 10–17 years (Ashburn and Thor 2004). Recently, alternative drug development approaches have come to the forefront. One of them, drug repurposing, can reduce the time to approval. Another is gene-based therapies for genetic disorders. The application of each of these approaches to rare genetic variants will be discussed below with representative examples.

Therapeutic Modalities

Small Molecules

The drug industry has traditionally focused on small molecules, although the drug discovery toolbox has grown from protein-based therapeutics (proteins, peptide, and antibodies) to, more recently, gene-based therapies: antisense oligonucleotides (ASOs), small interfering RNAs (siRNAs), gene replacement, and gene editing. Small molecules remain the most well-established platform and have many advantages, including low cost and scale of synthesis, multiple routes of administration, bioavailability, controlled dosing, and stability. Small molecules could theoretically target all tissues, although exposure depends on the chemical structure, especially for penetrating the blood–brain barrier. Certain targets, such as G protein-coupled receptors or kinases, have proven tractability with small molecules, but recently other mechanisms, such as correction of misfolding/trafficking (e.g., CFTR protein in cystic fibrosis)

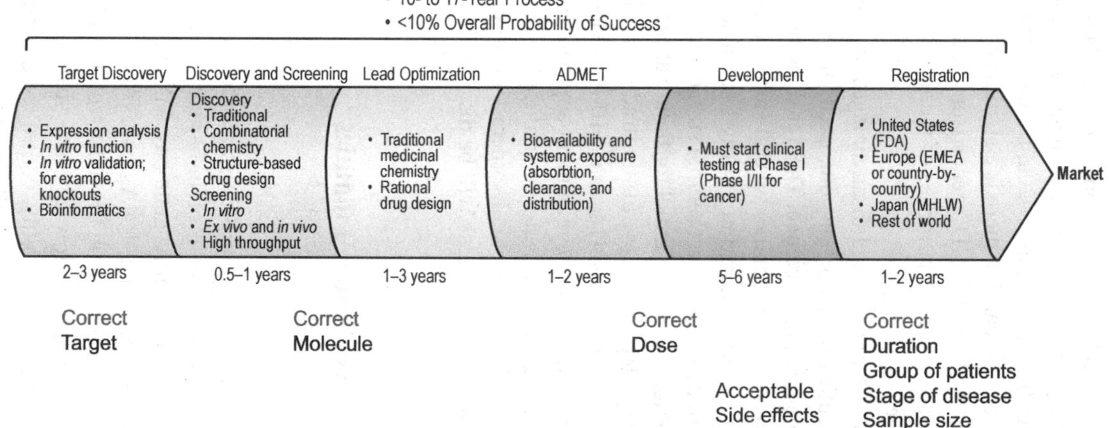

Figure 6.1 Stages in the traditional drug discovery process and potential pitfalls. The probability of success is ~10%. Absorption, distribution, metabolism, excretion, and toxicity (ADMET), European Medicines Agency (EMEA), Food and Drug Administration (FDA), intellectual property (IP), Ministry of Health, Labor, and Welfare (MHLW).

or modulation of splicing (e.g., *SMN2* gene in spinal muscular atrophy), have proven successful. One of the unique advantages of rare genetic diseases for small-molecule drug development is the ability to perform phenotypic screens, including the possibility of drug repurposing. A case in point is amyotrophic lateral sclerosis (ALS): a phenotypic screen performed in iPSC-derived ALS motor neurons demonstrated that retigabine, an FDA-approved drug for epilepsy, decreased hyperexcitability and increased survival of human motor neurons. This drug is now in Phase II trial for ALS patients (Wainger et al. 2014).

Both whole animal and cell-based disease models can play crucial and complementary roles in the development of therapeutics (Figure 6.2). Although animal models are necessary to study behavior, their relevance in brain disorders has been an area of rigorous debate (Howe et al. 2018; Pankevich et al. 2014). One point of agreement, though, is that for findings to be translationally impactful, better pharmacokinetic/pharmacodynamic studies need to be encouraged in animal models (Kleiman and Ehlers 2016). Using iPSCs can circumvent species-related issues, but the promise of using iPSCs for drug discovery also comes with some caveats; most importantly, variability and reproducibility. Several recent papers have analyzed these important issues and provided recommendations for accelerating translation (Anderson et al. 2021; Engle et al. 2018; Germain and Testa 2017; Volpato et al. 2018). The consensus is that both animal and human neuronal models can represent part

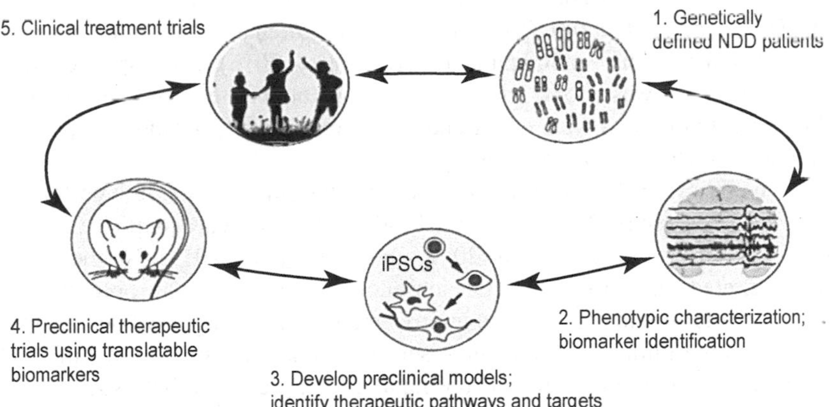

Figure 6.2 The translational cycle for precision therapies in neurodevelopmental disorders (NDDs): (1) identification of patients, (2) phenotypic characterization, (3) cellular models, (4) animal models, and (5) clinical trials. Successful development of safe and effective treatments is likely to take several cycles. Modified from Sahin and Sur (2015).

of the evidence for target validation, but neither alone is sufficient to predict success before starting proof-of-concept clinical trials, as long as the experimental compounds are safe.

mTOR Inhibitors and Tuberous Sclerosis Complex

Rapamycin is a natural compound that was first identified in soil samples from Easter Island in 1964 as a potential fungicidal compound. Rapamycin turned out to have immunosuppressant and antiproliferative properties and in 1999 received FDA approval as an immunosuppressant for organ transplants. Everolimus (Afinitor®, Novartis), an analog of rapamycin, was approved for the treatment of patients with advanced renal cell carcinoma. Around 2002, several groups around the world discovered that loss of function of *TSC1* or *TSC2* genes, which are the causal genes in tuberous sclerosis complex (TSC), leads to hyperactivation of mTOR (mechanistic Target of Rapamycin, a protein kinase that controls cell growth, proliferation, and survival). The first open-label clinical trial, performed by David Franz and colleagues, treated six patients who had a rare type of brain tumor (SEGA) seen in TSC patients with rapamycin. All the tumors stopped growing or shrank (Franz et al. 2006). This was followed by a Phase II trial with everolimus, another drug targeting mTOR, in 28 patients; similar results were shown, leading to approval of everolimus for SEGA (Krueger et al. 2010).

Epilepsy, another major symptom in TSC, was the next indication, and detailed preclinical pharmacokinetic/pharmacodynamic studies as well as treatment trials on several different mouse models of TSC supported the notion that mTOR inhibitors could rescue the seizure phenotype in mice (Meikle et al. 2008; Zeng et al. 2008). Clinical evidence required a double-blind placebo-controlled trial with over 300 patients (French et al. 2016). The response rate in the placebo arm was ~15%, while the response rate in the low-dose and high-dose everolimus arms were ~30% and ~40%, respectively, leading to approval of everolimus for refractory epilepsy.

Two clinical trials (one in the U.S.A., the other in Europe) were performed to test whether mTOR inhibitors could also improve neurocognitive deficits in TSC patients (Krueger et al. 2017; Overwater et al. 2019). Neither study demonstrated superiority of mTOR inhibitors over placebo. One potential reason for the failure to demonstrate improvement in neurocognitive deficits may have been the timing of treatment onset. In fact, in an animal model of TSC, early mTOR inhibitor treatment (postnatal day 7) prevented both social interaction deficits and repetitive behaviors (Tsai et al. 2012). In contrast, treatment later in life (6 weeks of life) rescued the social deficits but not the repetitive behaviors. Treatment beyond 10 weeks rescued neither outcome (Tsai et al. 2018). Based on such preclinical as well as clinical data, there are now two trials testing the hypothesis that early pharmacological intervention can improve neurocognitive outcomes in TSC (NCT05104983, NCT02849457). Another outstanding question is whether cellular pathways such as mTOR signaling or translational regulation (see below) may be a point of convergence among different genetic causes of ASD (Figure 6.3). True testing of this concept will only be possible by applying interventions successful in one disorder to others and seeing if they succeed.

The Metabotropic Glutamate Receptor Theory of Fragile X Syndrome

Fragile X syndrome (FXS) is one of most common monogenic disorders associated with intellectual disability and ASD. In almost all cases, FXS arises from a CGG trinucleotide repeat expansion in the 5′ untranslated region of the *FMR1* (Fragile X messenger ribonucleoprotein 1) gene, which silences the production of its protein product, Fragile X messenger ribonucleoprotein (FMRP). There are at least two major functions of FMRP in neurons: (a) regulation of protein synthesis and (b) interaction with ion channels. Most of the focus has been on alteration in protein synthesis, which has led to the "metabotropic glutamate receptor (mGluR) theory of fragile X." This theory is based on the observations that mGluR activation leads to the rapid protein synthesis in the postsynaptic dendrites and that protein synthesis is exaggerated in the absence of FMRP. Large numbers of studies in multiple animal models of FXS have demonstrated that diverse phenotypes thought to model aspects of disease can be corrected by inhibiting a subtype of mGluR, mGluR5 (Bhakar et al. 2012). Despite preclinical successes, early clinical trials in adolescents and adults with FXS have not shown efficacy (Berry-Kravis et al. 2016). These

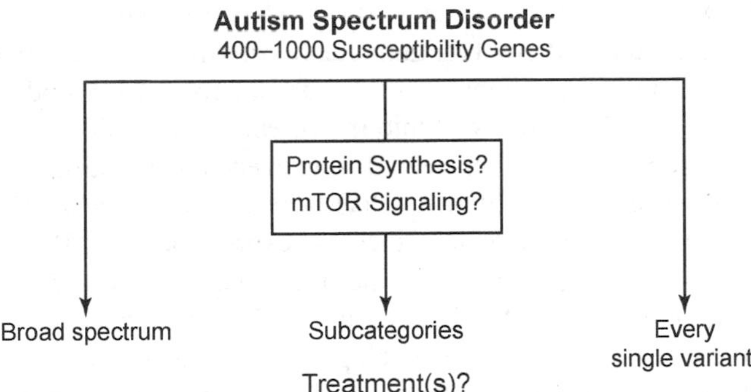

Figure 6.3 The scenario of "convergence" among the etiologies underlying ASD. In terms of the development of treatments, one can think of several scenarios. One possibility is that a single treatment will work for all etiologies (unlikely, especially for conditions where either under- or overexpression of a gene results in symptoms). Another scenario is that we will have to develop a unique treatment for each gene or even each variant (highly labor and resource intensive). A potential opportunity may arise if certain conditions have a shared pathophysiology such that a treatment developed for one condition may be effective in several similar etiologies. Such convergence may occur at the level of cellular or circuit functions.

trials have raised critical questions in the field about optimal clinical trial design, whether younger individuals should be treated, whether the trials should be performed with longer treatment duration and longer placebo run-ins, and whether biomarkers could help assess behavioral and cognitive benefits earlier and in more objective and reproducible ways. To address some of these issues, another mGluR5 inhibitor trial is currently being funded by the NIH in younger children in combination with a language-based intervention and an EEG-based biomarker (NCT02920892).

For both TSC and FXS, the studies reviewed above are based on the repurposing of small molecules, initially developed for other indications. The advantage of this approach is that these drugs have well-known safety and dosing profiles, reducing risks and development times (Ashburn and Thor 2004). NIH has an initiative, entitled "Discovering new therapeutic uses for existing drugs" that aims to accelerate this approach.

Oligonucleotide Therapies

In recent years, there has been considerable interest in oligonucleotide-based therapeutics that alter gene function at the level of the RNA molecule. The most extensively investigated of these are ASOs and siRNAs, which can bind to complementary RNA and lead to its degradation. ASOs can also be used for other manipulations, including exon skipping, cryptic splice restoration, and alternative splicing. One major advantage of oligonucleotides is that their specificity is based on gene sequence such that theoretically any gene could be targeted. Sequence specificity, however, can also be a disadvantage, such as when different patients with the same disease have different gene sequences and therefore require different oligonucleotides. Another drawback for the treatment of NDD is that oligonucleotides do not cross the blood–brain barrier, so they need to be introduced into the cerebrospinal fluid (CSF), e.g., by lumbar puncture, and require repeated dosing every few months.

The most successful use of ASOs has been for spinal muscular atrophy. An ASO, nusinersen, was shown to increase expression of SMN protein and improve neurological symptoms in spinal muscular atrophy, a disease that is often fatal in early childhood (Finkel et al. 2017). The success of nusinersen has opened the possibility of rapid development of "n-of-1" treatments for rare variants (Kim et al. 2019). Acceleration of ASO applications in the clinical trial setting has also uncovered adverse events that were unanticipated under certain cases (Stoker et al. 2021). Previous studies have, for example, documented sequence-specific pro-inflammatory effects of phosphorothioate modified ASOs (Bennett et al. 2017; Krieg 2006).

Angelman syndrome provides a unique opportunity for the use of ASOs. It occurs due to defects in the maternally derived *UBE3A* gene, which is imprinted exclusively in the brain. The paternally derived copy of *UBE3A* is normally silenced by an antisense transcript (*UBE3A-ATS*) but could be reactivated by targeting the antisense Ube3a-ATS transcript using ASOs. In a UBE3A-deficient mouse model, treatment with ASOs that were designed to absorb the *UBE3A-ATS* transcript resulted in increased UBE3A production in neurons throughout the brain (Meng et al. 2015). There are now several initiatives to test this strategy in a clinical trial. The first, being developed by GeneTx, had shown promising results in a few patients, but the Phase 1/2 open label had to be paused due to a severe side effect, acute inflammatory polyradiculopathy (Davidson et al. 2022).

Viral Vector-Mediated Gene Replacement

In theory, for monogenic diseases with loss-of-function variants, the delivery of a wild-type copy of the mutated gene to cells which lack functional protein represents the most curative approach. There are two major types of gene delivery: *ex vivo* and *in vivo*. A common *ex vivo* gene delivery approach is to use lentiviruses to genetically modify extracted patient cells (e.g., hematopoietic stem cells) prior to re-infusion. Inherited metabolic disorders affecting lysosomal and peroxisomal metabolic activity are amenable to *ex vivo* therapies. Altered progeny of hematopoietic stem cells, including microglia, overexpressing the gene of interest that has been introduced by a lentivirus can achieve stable levels of the missing enzyme in the mouse brain (Matzner et al. 2005). There are now ongoing trials for X-linked adrenoleukodystrophy (X-ALD), metachromatic leukodystrophy (MLD), mucopolysaccharidosis (MPS) type I and type III, and Fabry disease (Eichler et al. 2017; Ellison et al. 2019; Fumagalli et al. 2022; Gentner et al. 2021). It is not yet clear whether *ex vivo* gene therapy can be used more broadly for NDDs that are not metabolic in origin.

For most forms of gene delivery in NDDs, the target is likely to be neurons, which will require *in vivo* gene delivery. For that application, a different method will be required to deliver genetic payloads. Recombinant adeno-associated virus vectors (rAAVs) are the most widely used in the neuroscience community. In mouse models, AAV-mediated gene therapy appears remarkably successful. AAV-mediated UBE3A expression rescued the cognitive deficits in a mouse model of Angelman syndrome (Daily et al. 2011). Several papers have reported improvement in the phenotype of mouse models of Rett syndrome by re-expression of *Mecp2,* the gene missing in Rett syndrome (Gadalla et al. 2013; Sinnett and Gray 2017; Tillotson et al. 2017). However, both Angelman and Rett syndromes are representative of conditions where the level of gene expression seems to have a narrow physiological range and either down-regulation or up-regulation of gene expression can result in a neurodevelopmental disorder, posing a considerable dosing challenge.

Rett syndrome (RTT) is one of the most common monogenic causes of intellectual disability and is an X-linked disorder predominantly affecting girls. The main cause is a deleterious mutation of the *MECP2* gene on one of the X chromosomes. Classic RTT is characterized by a brief period of stagnation after normal or near-normal development up to 6–18 months, followed by rapid loss of skills before stabilization or slowing of regression. The phenotype can be affected by skewed X-inactivation, leading to more or less X chromosomes with the intact *MECP2* gene to be active in patients. *MECP2* duplication syndrome predominantly affects males, but females who carry the duplication on one X chromosome (heterozygotes) may exhibit some signs of the disorder. This syndrome is characterized by global developmental delay, recurrent respiratory infections, epilepsy, and progressive spasticity. *MeCP2* has been implicated in a wide range of molecular functions, including transcriptional repression and activation, chromatin architecture, alternative splicing, miRNA processing and translational regulation, thus similar to *TSC1/2* genes and FMRP, it also modulates the expression of a large number of proteins.

Although the exact pathways are unknown, deficient brain-derived neurotrophic factor (BDNF) expression has been proposed to be involved in RTT pathogenesis, leading to the hypothesis that restoration of BDNF function might treat the disorder. BDNF, however, does not cross the blood–brain barrier. A related growth factor, insulin-like growth factor 1 (IGF-1), can cross the blood–brain barrier and like BDNF can promote the development and maintenance of neural circuits. IGF-1 administration reversed some RTT-related phenotypes in a mouse model of RTT but failed to improve neurological symptoms in girls with RTT. A large number of therapeutic trials have been pursued in preclinical and clinical studies in RTT (Leonard et al. 2017). Recently, trofinetide, a synthetic analog of a naturally occurring neurotrophic peptide, which is the terminal tripeptide of IGF-1, was approved by the FDA for RTT. Some of these have targeted the neurotransmitter systems disrupted in RTT; others have involved growth factors, cell metabolism, and homeostasis. However, given the very large number of proteins whose expression is regulated by MECP2 and the many cellular processes that are aberrant in MECP2-deficient cells, it is difficult to imagine that targeting one particular neurotransmitter system or growth factor will be sufficient to change the natural history of this disorder. Therefore, more recently, attention has turned to gene-based therapies.

The fact that healthy brain development appears to require just the right amount of MECP2 expression creates a daunting challenge to development of a treatment for this X-linked disorder. Brains of girls affected with RTT contain a mosaic of wildtype and reduced MECP2 expression based on X-inactivation in each cell. Therefore, re-expression of MECP2 may rescue some cells from too little MECP2 expression to the normal range while being toxic for other cells which were expressing MECP2 in the normal range prior to treatment. Therefore, controlling deleterious overexpression of MECP2 is a crucial goal in gene therapy development for RTT. Several approaches have been developed in preclinical models to overcome this obstacle. One approach is to add a miRNA target cassette to the transgene to regulate the expression of the exogenous MECP2, which could regulate gene expression levels on a cell-by-cell basis (Sinnett et al. 2021). When MECP2 is overexpressed, it would increase the levels of certain miRNA that would in turn bind to the 3′UTR of the transgene and reduce its expression.

While RTT is a particularly difficult disorder to treat with AAV-mediated gene delivery due to X-inactivation and a narrow physiological window of expression, the rate-limiting step in the development of successful AAV gene therapy is biodistribution. Although certain AAV9-derived variants (e.g., PHP.B or PHP.eB) can cross the blood–brain barrier and transduce neurons in mice, the receptor that mediates their transport across the blood–brain barrier is not expressed in primates. Therefore, AAV9 delivery into the CSF is often used. Recent quantitative studies compared biodistribution of AAV9 associated expression of green fluorescent protein (GFP) in juvenile cynomolgus macaques either infused intrathecally via lumbar puncture or the intra cisterna magna. In both cases, GFP expression was observed primarily in perivascular astrocytes in the brain, but relatively little in neurons (Meseck et al. 2022). Therefore, developing novel AAVs or other delivery systems that have improved central nervous system (CNS) cell tropism after direct or peripheral delivery is a major ongoing effort (Chen et al. 2022; Davidsson et al. 2019; Deverman et al. 2016; Lin et al. 2020; Lukashchuk et al. 2016; Nonnenmacher et al. 2021; Wang et al. 2019).

Aside from the issues of toxicity due to overexpression, there are also other risks with AAV-mediated gene delivery. A major issue is the low efficiency of gene delivery to the CNS by viral vectors that requires large vector doses and consequently brings the risk of immune reaction. The presence of preexisting neutralizing antibodies can also be a problem (Foust et al. 2009; Gray et al. 2011). Moreover, while AAV vectors typically remain outside of the host genome in a stable, episomal form, the AAV genome can sometimes integrate into the host at low frequency. If it is inserted into the DNA in the wrong location, it could possibly cause harmful mutations to the DNA (Donsante et al. 2007), although this seems to be rare in human genome (see discussion in Wang et al. 2019). A more common problem with AAV administration into the CSF has been dorsal root ganglia (DRG) toxicity, which may affect spinal cord function. DRG toxicity has been reported in both preclinical and clinical studies (Hinderer et al. 2018; Hordeaux et al. 2018; Mueller et al. 2020).

A number of additional gene therapy platforms are being tested in preclinical studies, though none have yet reached clinical testing for CNS disorders. These approaches include (a) gene editing that alters nucleotide sequence in the genome directly, such as CRISPR, base editing, prime editing (Chen et al. 2021; Koblan et al. 2021; Wolter et al. 2020), and (b) gene activation or deactivation by using small molecular drugs or CRISPR and other technologies (Matharu et al. 2019; Monteys et al. 2021). In conclusion, the therapeutic armamentarium for rare genetic diseases affecting the CNS is likely to expand even further in the near future.

SWOT Analysis of Rare Variants

Strengths

The advances in mechanism-based therapies for rare genetic disorders discussed above highlight several of the advantages of using these variants to develop therapies (Figure 6.4). The scientific knowledge base regarding underlying genetic mechanism, mutational spectrum, and tolerance to haploinsufficiency or overexpression provides a significant advantage over less well characterized "idiopathic" and heterogeneous conditions such as ASD. In theory, for loss-of-function recessive disorders, re-expressing the correct sequence in the right cells at the right time at the right doses should provide a marked improvement in the phenotypes. Spinal muscular atrophy is an example of such success, even though we still do not fully understand the cellular function of SMN protein.

Such knowledge about the genetics also enables the creation of cell-based and animal models, another opportunity often missing in "idiopathic" conditions. These models allow for experiments aimed at clarifying the neurobiology underlying these disorders as well as the testing of therapeutic approaches *in vitro* and/or *in vivo* before clinical testing, providing some confidence about the safety and potential efficacy of the approach. Unbiased phenotypic screens can also be used in such models, enabling genome-wide investigations or very large, small-molecule compound library screens.

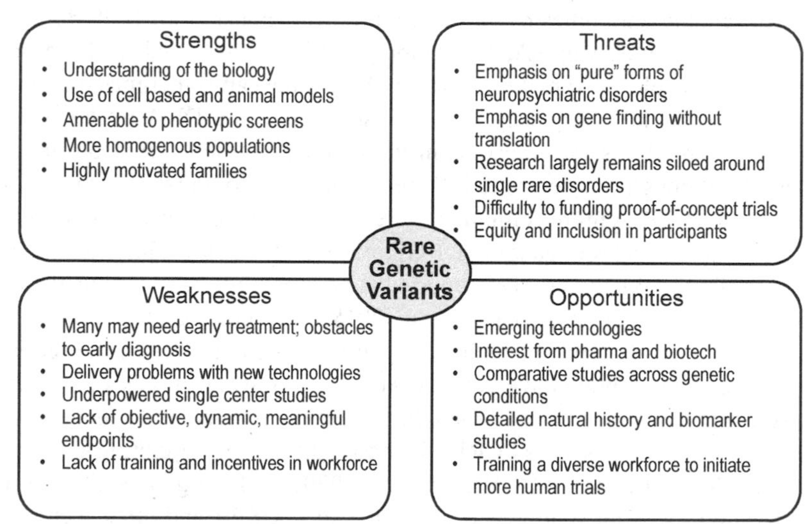

Figure 6.4 SWOT analysis for using rare genetic variants in development of precision therapies.

In terms of translation to clinical trials, rare genetic variants also provide a more homogenous cohort of participants to enroll, potentially reducing the variability in response to the intervention and correspondingly increasing statistical power.

Weaknesses

Despite the promise noted above, research in rare genetic variants in neurodevelopmental and psychiatric disorders has not yet produced as many successes as anticipated. One potential reason is that these variants are by definition rare and can be difficult to identify. This challenge is especially acute since treatments for many of these variants would need to be delivered in the early postnatal period. There are many systemic obstacles to access to genetic testing for such conditions, creating lengthy "diagnostic odysseys." Partially, but not exclusively, because of these challenges, many of the proof-of-concept trials have been performed in very small cohorts and at single centers. While such open-label trials often yield promising results, subsequent larger, controlled clinical studies frequently fail.

Some of the new technologies available for delivery of therapeutics are hampered by limited bioavailability. Even for small molecules, evidence that they engage brain targets may be limited. Another significant obstacle in clinical trials is the lack of sensitive, quantitative, and meaningful outcome measures to gauge the success of the intervention. Finally, the diverse workforce needed to perform such trials has not been developed in clinical settings, and the incentives to develop such a workforce are not well aligned with academic careers.

Opportunities

The combination of emerging technologies with disease-modifying potential, a better understanding of the underlying mechanisms to limit the risk of therapeutics development, and the incentives provided for the industry by the Orphan Drug Act provide an opportunity for major progress in rare genetic disorders. What could accelerate such progress are detailed natural history cohorts developed by multi-center networks that are well coordinated and use standardized acquisition/analysis. Remote assessment may be a way to be more inclusive in the populations studied, reducing obstacles to access. Translational biomarkers can also be tested and validated in multiple disorders and at multiple centers, providing tools for stratification of participants and/or assessing target engagement (Sahin et al. 2018). To realize the full promise of using rare genetic variants to develop treatments for neurodevelopmental and psychiatric disorders will require integration and sustained support of networks/consortia that work closely with patient communities and industry partners.

Threats

There is a list of external factors that have limited the impact of therapeutics based on rare genetic variants. First of all, certain groups and funding agencies have excluded syndrome forms of disorders (i.e., those that arise from specific rare variants) when seeking to understand and investigate the more common forms of neurodevelopmental disorders. Others have focused predominantly on gene-finding studies with little or no support for clinical translation. Such approaches have made it extremely difficult for investigators to initiate proof-of-concept trials and test hypotheses in rare disease populations. Furthermore, there is insufficient convergence of approach and of knowledge across different specific rare genetic conditions. Partly, this is because much of the research is supported by patient advocacy groups focused on a specific condition. Finally, research cohorts typically lack representation from medically underserved communities, limiting the impact of the research and posing a challenge to the equitable application of medical advances. Taken together, this analysis clearly highlights the fact that rare genetic diseases provide a unique opportunity for both understanding the pathophysiology of neurodevelopmental disorders and developing mechanism-based therapies in the near future. By addressing the weaknesses and threats outlined above, the investigators, patient advocacy groups and funding agencies will further enhance this opportunity and help improve the lives of individuals and families affected with these disorders.

Disclosures

M. Sahin reports grant support from Novartis, Roche, Biogen, Astellas, Aeovian, Bridgebio, Aucta and Quadrant Biosciences. He has served on Scientific Advisory Boards for Novartis, Roche, Celgene, Regenxbio, Alkermes, and Takeda.

7

Experimental Model Systems for Rare and Common Variants

Kristen J. Brennand and Steven A. Kushner

Abstract

Resolving the target genes, pathways, cellular phenotypes, and circuit functions impacted by the hundreds of genomic loci significantly associated with psychiatric disorders is a major challenge. Applications of genomic engineering in human-induced pluripotent stem cells (hiPSCs) and mice are widely used to study the impact of psychiatric risk variants within defined cell types of the brain. As the scale and scope of functional genomic studies expands, so must our ability to resolve the complex interplay of the many risk variants linked to psychiatric disorders. Here we discuss the current state of the field, with particular emphasis on hiPSC and mouse models, which have facilitated efforts to understand the pathophysiology of psychiatric disorders and translate genetic findings into disease-relevant biology in the service of advancing diagnostics and therapeutic development.

Introduction

Mental illness is a major contributor to global disease burden (GBD 2016 Disease and Injury Incidence and Prevalence Collaborators 2017). Successful efforts toward improved diagnosis, prognosis, treatment, and prevention require integrated efforts in a multitude of disciplines ranging from governmental legislation and public health strategies to biomedical innovation and pathophysiological insights. Here we discuss experimental approaches widely utilized in uncovering the molecular mechanisms underlying neurodevelopment and pathophysiological dysfunction of the human brain, with an emphasis on leveraging human genetic variation to elucidate the biology of mental illness through experimental model systems. We consider two widely used model systems for investigating the biology of genetic risk factors for human psychiatric disorders: genetically modified mice and human-induced pluripotent stem cells (hiPSCs).

Most pharmacotherapies currently used in psychiatry were introduced to the clinic in the second half of the twentieth century. In 1949, lithium was discovered as a psychotropic medication with mood stabilizing effects, and in the following decade, the major classes of other pharmacotherapies (antipsychotics, benzodiazepines, and antidepressants) were introduced (Hyman 2012). Like many medications used in medicine, these medications were not rationally designed based on a known mechanistic pathophysiology to specifically target disorder mechanisms for modifying causal biological processes. Rather, most therapeutic discovery in psychiatry has emerged from serendipitous observations. Many of the seminal mechanistic "insights" into psychiatric disorder pathophysiology derived from uncovering the molecular targets of these serendipitously discovered therapeutic compounds. For instance, the findings that monoamine oxidase inhibitors are efficacious antidepressants and that D2-receptor antagonists are effective antipsychotics offered entry points for studying the neurobiology of depression (Hirschfeld 2000) and schizophrenia (Kendler and Schaffner 2011), respectively. However, emerging psychiatric genetic findings have paved a novel road forward with regard to cell type-specific disease etiology (Skene et al. 2018).

Heritability of Psychiatric Disorders

A critically important insight into the etiology of psychiatric disorders became known a century ago when the tendency for mental illness to aggregate in families was observed. This observation was statistically confirmed in the second half of the twentieth century in a large number of family, twin, and adoption studies aimed at quantitatively distinguishing environmental from nonenvironmental (i.e., genetic) disorder risk (Polderman et al. 2015). These studies revealed a relatively high, but varying degree of heritability for the major psychiatric illnesses (Visscher et al. 2008). For example, major depressive disorder has an estimated twin heritability of 0.37, autism spectrum disorder (ASD) 0.75, bipolar disorder 0.72, and schizophrenia (SCZ) 0.81 (Sullivan and Geschwind 2019). Overall, psychiatric disorders reflect the additive impact of hundreds of risk variants, each of which confer only a tiny increase of risk and are common in the population at large, coupled with that of highly penetrant rare mutations that underlie a fraction of cases.

Common Variation in Psychiatric Disorders

Genome-wide association studies (GWASs) were a promising design to overcome some of the obstacles encountered in linkage and candidate gene designs. After their introduction, single nucleotide polymorphism (SNP) microarrays quickly became inexpensive, which enabled researchers to investigate relatively large cohorts of cases and controls. Furthermore, with SNP markers being distributed widely across the genome, loci could be investigated in an unbiased fashion. Despite these advantages, the first years of GWASs in psychiatry were characterized by failures to identify reproducible loci that reached the threshold for genome-wide statistical significance. For example, nine GWASs on major depressive disorder (published between 2010 and 2013 with sample sizes ranging between 1,000–9,500 cases) did not reveal any genome-wide significant loci (Flint and Kendler 2014).

Successes using the GWAS approach began to emerge as sample sizes increased (Hyde et al. 2016; Major Depressive Disorder Working Group of the Psychiatric GWAS Consortium 2013; Wray et al. 2018a), and phenotypes were more narrowly defined (Converge Consortium 2015). This development was facilitated by the formation of global research consortia, such as the Psychiatric Genomics Consortium, which allowed for the analysis of very large cohorts with consistent genotype quality control. To date, GWAS has yielded:

- 287 loci for SCZ (Pardinas et al. 2018; Trubetskoy et al. 2022).
- Over 100 for major depressive disorder (Howard et al. 2019; Levey et al. 2021; Wray et al. 2018b).
- 12 for ASD (Grove et al. 2019).

Biologically, risk variants linked to SCZ (Fromer et al. 2014; Marshall et al. 2017; Pardinas et al. 2018; Purcell et al. 2014), ASD (De Rubeis et al. 2014; Sanders et al. 2015; Satterstrom et al. 2020), and more broadly across the neuropsychiatric disorder spectrum (Cross-Disorder Group of the Psychiatric Genomics Consortium 2019; Lee et al. 2019d; Schork et al. 2019; Sey et al. 2020; Watanabe et al. 2019a) are enriched for genes involved in synaptic biology and transcriptional regulation (De Rubeis et al. 2014; Neale et al. 2012; O'Roak et al. 2012a, 2014; Sanders et al. 2012; Talkowski et al. 2012).

The GWAS design is suited to discover SNPs associated with diseases that are common in a population, where the minor allele frequency is >1%. Individually, each SNP typically confers only a small risk to disease status, with odds ratios ranging between 1.05–1.15, but in aggregate, common variants explain approximately 24% of the variance in SCZ liability (Trubetskoy et al. 2022). In recent years, an increasing number of publications have investigated multiple SNPs that are differentially present in cases versus controls, leading to the generation of polygenic risk scores for psychiatric disorders (International Schizophrenia Consortium et al. 2009) as predictors of diagnosis, clinical severity, and/or drug responsiveness (Hess et al. 2021; Ruderfer et al. 2016; Zhang et al. 2019). For SCZ, for example, when sorted on effect size (odds ratios), inheriting the top 10% versus the bottom 10% of SNP-risk variants increases one's chance for developing SCZ nearly fortyfold. Although informative with respect to the role of SNPs on the biology of SCZ, as well as the shared polygenic risk architecture across psychiatric disorders (Cross-Disorder Group of the Psychiatric Genomics Consortium 2019; Lee et al. 2019d; Schork et al. 2019), the sensitivity and specificity of these polygenic risk scores are currently too low to contribute meaningfully to individual-level psychiatric diagnoses (Zheutlin et al. 2019).

Rare Variation in Psychiatric Disorders

The discovery of the architecture of rare genetic variation in psychiatric disorders has progressed in parallel with the elucidation of common SNP associations. The first wave of findings implicating rare genetic variation in psychiatric disorder risk were large copy number variants (CNVs) that disrupted the function of one or multiple genes and were found in patients with ASD and SCZ (Iossifov et al. 2012; Karayiorgou et al. 1995; Marshall et al. 2017; Sebat et al. 2007). Following these early discoveries, whole-exome and whole-genome sequencing continued to reveal novel, rare, and highly penetrant variants implicated in psychiatric disorder risk. Rare variant discovery has been most successful for ASD, for which over 100 high-confidence genes have been described to date (Satterstrom et al. 2020); these are typically *de novo* protein-truncating variants (PTVs) that are individually rare, but jointly account for around 15% of individuals with ASD. For SCZ, ten genes have been identified thus far with the same degree of statistical confidence (Singh et al. 2016, 2022; Steinberg et al. 2017; Takata et al. 2014). Among rare variants, evidence of their association with SCZ risk has been strongest for PTVs. However, missense variants have also been implicated in ASD, although effect sizes are typically smaller than for PTVs (Ruzzo et al. 2019; Sanders et al. 2015). For major depressive disorder and bipolar disorder, very little is known about the contribution of rare variants to risk (Palmer et al. 2022).

Rare variants are frequently pleiotropic and show robust overlap across psychiatric disorders (Rees et al. 2021), although different mutation types are implicated in some shared genes (Ben-Shalom et al. 2017). In addition, it is increasingly recognized that common and rare genetic risk factors converge at least partially on the same underlying pathogenic biological processes (Chang et al. 2018; Jia et al. 2018; Nehme et al. 2021; Singh et al. 2022).

Functional Genomic Studies of Psychiatric Disorder Pathophysiology

Understanding the heritability and genetic architecture of psychiatric disorders is only the first step in understanding the underlying pathophysiology and successfully translating this knowledge into clinically effective treatments. Although the contribution of common variation to the heritability of most psychiatric disorders appear collectively to exceed that of rare variation, mechanistic biological insights into rare variants has thus far been technically more feasible to investigate using gene targeting approaches in experimental model systems. However, increasingly sophisticated methods are yielding exciting new advances and insights into the biology of common variants and polygenic risk.

Mouse Models of Psychiatric Genetic Risk

Much has been learned from mouse models with modifications in genes associated with psychiatric disorders. For ASD, gene knockouts include the mouse homologues of *CHD8* (Katayama et al. 2016), *TSC1* (Goorden et al. 2007), *SCN2A* (Spratt et al. 2019), *SHANK3* (Peca et al. 2011), *NRXN1* (Etherton et al. 2009), *CNTNAP2* (Penagarikano et al. 2011) as well as *16p11.2* microdeletion (Brunner et al. 2015), all of which are causal to syndromic or non-syndromic ASD in humans (Satterstrom et al. 2020). These rodent models have partially overlapping behavioral phenotypes reminiscent of human ASD-related behavior, including impaired social interactions and vocal communication, repetitive grooming, and seizures. Commonalities in these models across the molecular, cellular, and circuit levels include neuronal morphology deficits as well as altered cellular signaling (PI3K, mTOR) and excitation/inhibition imbalance (de la Torre-Ubieta et al. 2016). Rodent models for ASD have been particularly useful because of their relatively high degree of genetic homology to humans, their practical advantages as experimental animals, the availability of phenotypic batteries for core behavioral phenotypes, and the possibility for experimental inquiry at multiple levels of organization, from molecule to circuit to behavior.

For SCZ, the number of valid and therefore useful genetic rodent models has been fewer than for ASD because of the time required to identify *high-confidence* risk genes or CNVs for SCZ. Moreover, given that historical candidate genes for SCZ have largely failed to validate in more recent genomic studies (Farrell et al. 2015; Sullivan 2013), many long-standing animal models of SCZ (notably *DISC1* KO) have questionable credibility today. The two genetic risk factors that confer the highest risk for SCZ—the *22q11.2* microdeletion (Sigurdsson et al. 2010) and *SETD1A* (Mukai et al. 2019; Nagahama et al. 2020)—have therefore yielded genetic rodent models with a higher *a priori* chance for robust face and construct validity. Moreover, a mouse model of the well-replicated *16p11.2* microduplication SCZ genetic risk variant has also yielded novel biological insights (Bristow et al. 2020; Horev et al. 2011). Overall, behavioral phenotypes for SCZ models include deficits in working memory and prepulse inhibition, hypothesized to be reminiscent of cognitive and negative SCZ symptoms.

The ability to spatiotemporally manipulate genetically defined cell types and neuronal circuits *in vivo* has been a critical advance for understanding the complexity of network connectivity, perception, and behavior. Genetically engineered mouse lines and viral vectors utilizing common strategies for cell type-specific expression of transgenes has enabled a diverse set of tools to monitor, label, and manipulate genetically defined brain cell types. The

Cre/loxP system, in which Cre recombinase efficiently catalyzes recombination at genomically integrated *loxP* sites, is the most widely employed strategy for cell type-specific transgene expression and endogenous genome manipulation, enabling cell type-, temporal-, and region-specific control through cell type-specific gene promoters combined with an ever-expanding suite of fluorescent proteins, optogenetic tools, and genetically encoded calcium indicators. Increasing numbers of well-characterized Cre driver lines with CNS expression have been generated through large-scale initiatives such as GENSAT (Gong et al. 2007), NIH Neuroscience Blueprint Cre Driver Network (Taniguchi et al. 2011), and the Allen Institute (Madisen et al. 2012), as well as by independent investigators. Limited effort has been given, however, to implement next-generation genome-wide screens for novel cell type-specific enhancers (Shima et al. 2016). Thus, the full potential and utility of the various driver lines and enhancer elements currently available for providing genetic access to defined cell populations across the entire brain have not yet been fully realized. Continued efforts to discover cell type-specific gene promoter driver lines will provide increasing precision to the classification of cell types, dissection of neural circuit function, and pathophysiological understanding of psychiatric disorder risk variants.

Modeling psychiatric disorders in rodents also comes with caveats and limitations, the foremost being the complex phenotype of mental disorders. Despite high hopes and expectations, other than rare pathogenic mutations for SCZ and ASD (which only account for ~2% and ~10% of cases, respectively, based on current best estimates), psychiatry still lacks objectively measurable biomarkers with sufficiently high positive and negative predictive values to contribute meaningfully to clinical diagnosis for the majority of common psychiatric disorders. Therefore, we remain dependent on cognitive and behavioral phenotypes as outcome measures. Psychiatric disorders typically affect higher-order brain processes, including cognition, emotion, and perception for which the current diagnostic criteria are heavily reliant on self-report of subjective experiences. Accordingly, a substantial proportion of mouse models of genetic risk for neurodevelopmental and psychiatric disorders generated to date have struggled to yield robust behavioral phenotypes that have been reliably replicated across multiple independent laboratories. Although many aspects of brain development appear to be conserved across mammalian species (Defelipe 2011), mice and humans are separated by an estimated 85 million years of evolution. Moreover, species-specific differences in neurobiology appear to be especially apparent in the cerebral cortex. For example, the human neocortex has approximately a thousandfold increase in both neuronal numbers and surface area compared to mice (Herculano-Houzel et al. 2006). At the tissue-organizational level, superficial layer neurons appear to be expanded in numbers in humans (Hill and Walsh 2005), as is the case for outer radial glial cells that are scarcely present in mice (Hansen et al. 2010; Shitamukai et al. 2011; Wang et al. 2011). Single nucleus RNA sequencing has recently corroborated some of these histological observations and has revealed other notable transcriptomic differences across putatively homologous cell types (Hodge et al. 2019). Furthermore, although coding sequence and linear gene sequence are reasonably well conserved between mice and humans, noncoding sequence is highly divergent, which has proven highly problematic for mouse modeling of common variant polygenic risk. Moreover, the recent emergence of molecular genetic therapeutics, such as antisense oligonucleotides, might also be difficult to model in mice for modalities that have very stringent genomic target sequence requirements (e.g., Angelman syndrome mouse models; Milazzo et al. 2021; see also Bearden et al., this volume).

hiPSC-Based Modeling of Psychiatric Disorder Risk

Human embryonic stem cell lines, first grown in 1998, were immediately recognized as a nearly limitless source of material for studies of human disease (Thomson et al. 1998). Studies to uncover the molecular networks regulating pluripotency (i.e., their capability to differentiate into every cell type in the human body) found four genes that, when overexpressed, are sufficient to reprogram adult somatic cells into hiPSCs (Takahashi et al. 2007), making it possible to generate donor-specific cells. This opened novel avenues of human disease modeling, in particular for neuropsychiatric disorders, that otherwise have limited opportunity for physiological studies with patient-derived CNS cell types and tissue. Early studies of psychiatric disorders largely focused on idiopathic cohorts of ASD (Mariani et al. 2015) and SCZ (Brennand et al. 2011). To reduce heterogeneity between cases, hiPSC-based studies frequently contrast hiPSC-derived neurons generated from cases that share a highly penetrant rare mutation with, for example, *MECP2* (Marchetto et al. 2010), *FMR1* (Zhang et al. 2018), *CACNA1C* (Paşca et al. 2011), *SHANK3* (Shcheglovitov et al. 2013), *NRXN1* (Flaherty et al. 2019), *NLGN4* (Marro et al. 2019), and *22q11.2* microdeletion (Khan et al. 2020). These studies report cellular phenotypes such as altered neuronal development and/or synaptic function. Likewise, engineered deletions of risk genes—such as *FMR1* (Zhang et al. 2018), *SHANK3* (Yi et al. 2016), and *NRXN1* (Pak et al. 2015)—yield similar cellular phenotypes compared to those derived from patients carrying equivalent mutations. Despite the relatively subtle effects predicted for SCZ-associated GWAS SNPs, several have been validated using case-control cohort designs; for example, *C4* (Sellgren et al. 2019) and *CACNA1C* (Yoshimizu et al. 2015).

Neural differentiation from hiPSCs can yield all major cell types of the brain:

- glutamatergic neurons (Yu et al. 2014),
- GABAergic neurons (Shao et al. 2019),
- dopaminergic neurons (Hook et al. 2014),
- neural progenitor cells (Brennand et al. 2015),

- astrocytes (Windrem et al. 2017),
- oligodendrocytes (McPhie et al. 2018), and
- microglia (Sellgren et al. 2019).

These hiPSC-derived brain cells recapitulate many aspects of gene expression (Brennand et al. 2015; Hoffman et al. 2017; Mariani et al. 2012; Nicholas et al. 2013; Paşca et al. 2015; Qian et al. 2016), cellular diversity (Velasco et al. 2019), and micro-architectural features of the developing human brain (Kadoshima et al. 2013; Paşca 2019), but have thus far shown resistance to *in vitro* differentiation into later neurodevelopmental stages. Notably, the rare and common risk genes associated with psychiatric disorders are enriched for those expressed during fetal cortical development (Gulsuner et al. 2013; Loohuis et al. 2015; Schork et al. 2019; Talkowski et al. 2012). Both ASD and SCZ involve pathophysiological mechanisms with antecedents substantially earlier than the onset of clinical symptoms. In conclusion, hiPSC-derived models are particularly well-positioned to investigate the neurodevelopmental impact of psychiatric risk variants, particularly those predicted to influence fetal cortical development.

CRISPR Methods for hiPSC-Based Psychiatric Risk Modeling

CRISPR-associated proteins (Cas) use short, easily synthesized, clustered regularly interspaced short palindromic repeats (CRISPR) sequences to guide RNAs to recognize specific complementary strands of DNA. Together, they form the basis of a technology known as CRISPR/Cas genome engineering with which it is possible to edit DNA sequences efficiently (Anzalone et al. 2019; Hsu et al. 2014), activate or repress endogenous gene expression (Ho et al. 2017), cleave RNA (Konermann et al. 2018), methylate DNA (Liu et al. 2018b), modify histones (Hilton et al. 2015; Thakore et al. 2015), or alter chromatin interactions (Liu et al. 2018a) on a near genome-wide scale (Sanson et al. 2018). Altogether, this makes it possible to comprehensively introduce or correct the risk architecture associated with psychiatric disorders, alone or in combination, across the major cell types of the brain.

Moreover, because CRISPR engineering yields comparisons across a shared genetic ("isogenic") background, the mechanism of action of SCZ SNPs can be resolved in a cell type-specific and even context-dependent manner, through enhancer-promoter looping (*CACNA1C*; Roussos et al. 2014), 3D-genome folding (*PCDH*; Rajarajan et al. 2018), miRNA abundance (*miR-137*; Forrest et al. 2017), and mRNA levels (*FURIN*; Schrode et al. 2019).

High-throughput methods facilitate the comprehensive survey of the loci associated with psychiatric disease (Townsley et al. 2020). Massively parallel reporter assays evaluate the regulatory activity of the thousands of loci associated with psychiatric disorder risk (Mulvey and Dougherty 2021; Myint et al. 2020; Uebbing et al. 2021) and/or human cortical development (Geller et al. 2019; Inoue et al. 2019), albeit not at endogenous loci. For examining regulatory elements within their original genomic context, CRISPR expression quantitative trait loci (eQTL) mapping can identify SNPs that differentially regulate proximal (Gasperini et al. 2019) and distal (Fulco et al. 2019) target gene expression. Likewise, population-scale village-in-a-dish experiments—whereby single-cell RNA sequencing is applied to pooled populations of hiPSC-derived neurons or glia from dozens of genotyped donors (Cuomo et al. 2020; Jerber et al. 2021; Mitchell et al. 2020; Neavin et al. 2021a)—are well-powered to uncover transcriptomic and/or phenotypic impacts of common and rare variants.

Traditional functional genomic approaches assess one variant or gene at a time in a hypothesis-driven manner. Large-scale screens systematically manipulate many variants or genes in an arrayed format, characterizing those that result in specific changes, but requiring substantial investments of time and resources. In contrast, pooled designs can identify variants or genes that impact phenotypes such as proliferation, survival, or fluorescence; this allows for isolation of "hits" from the cellular population using fluorescent-activated cell sorting. Moreover, coupling CRISPR-based pooled perturbations to single-cell RNA sequencing (Dixit et al. 2016; Mimitou et al. 2019) expands the questions that can be queried. Altogether, this makes possible the comprehensive interrogation of candidate disease genes (Cederquist et al. 2020) or gene lists (Liu et al. 2018c; Lu et al. 2019; Tian et al. 2019).

Fundamental Questions Lacking Answers

A major challenge in the field is connecting disease-associated risk genes to their respective pathways and functions (Sullivan and Geschwind 2019). Risk variants are predicted to converge at the pathway level (Ballouz and Gillis 2017). Might this represent a novel point of therapeutic intervention? Perturbation of a dozen SCZ risk genes in human neurons revealed convergent changes in gene expression among a subset of genes and subnetworks involved in synaptic function (Townsley et al. 2022). Evaluation of an overlapping set of ASD genes *in vivo* (35 genes) in fetal mouse brains (Jin et al. 2020) and *Xenopus tropicalis* (10 genes) (Willsey et al. 2021), and *in vitro* in human neural progenitor cells (27 genes) (Cederquist et al. 2020) and human brain organoids (3 genes) (Paulsen et al. 2022) revealed convergent impacts on gene expression (Jin et al. 2020; Paulsen et al. 2022), WNT signaling (Cederquist et al. 2020), and neurogenesis (Cederquist et al. 2020; Jin et al. 2020; Paulsen et al. 2022; Willsey et al. 2021). Taken together, multifaceted evidence suggests that asynchronous development of inhibitory GABAergic neurons and deep-layer glutamatergic projection neurons contribute meaningfully to the etiology of severe psychiatric illness through distinct molecular pathways (Paulsen et al. 2022).

Because psychiatric disorders arise through iterative pathological changes in circuit function (Südhof 2017a), an important challenge is to assemble more physiologically relevant *in vitro* models. How do risk variants impact cellular function within circuits? To answer this, we must incorporate critical aspects of neuronal circuitry (Birey et al. 2017; Xiang et al. 2019), glial support (Abud et al. 2017; Dezonne et al. 2017; Marton et al. 2019), vasculature (Cakir et al. 2019; Mansour et al. 2018), and blood–brain barrier functions (Vatine et al. 2019) but retain the capacity to resolve cell type-specific effects. For example, mutations in *CACNA1C* associated with Timothy syndrome cause deficits in calcium signaling in both glutamatergic (Birey et al. 2017; Paşca et al. 2011) and GABAergic (Birey et al. 2017) neurons, which specifically lead to perturbations of interneuron migration into cortical assembloids (Birey et al. 2022).

Risk variants linked to psychiatric disorders show cumulative effects (Tansey et al. 2016; Weiner et al. 2017). Will understanding how risk variants combine to yield a greater impact in aggregate improve genetic diagnosis and/or indicate new drug targets? Despite evidence to the contrary at the population level (Visscher et al. 2008; Wray et al. 2018b), within individual patients, genetic risk factors may combine in patterns dependent on whether their target genes are co-expressed in the same cell types or act within the same biological functions. For example, when SCZ risk genes are manipulated together in neurons, an unexpected combinatorial effect occurs that cannot be predicted from single gene perturbations alone, and this effect is concentrated within synaptic function and psychiatric disorder risk genes (Schrode et al. 2019). Likewise, interactions of multiple target genes at a single SCZ GWAS risk locus result in synergistic contributions to molecular and synaptic phenotypes observed in neurons (Zhang et al. 2021).

Disease-associated variants may regulate their target genes in context-dependent manners. How do risk variants interact with the environment across the diverse cell types that comprise the human brain? Gene–environment interactions in GWAS may be especially critical in studies of those psychiatric disorders that require specific exposures (e.g., substance use disorders) or stressors (e.g., posttraumatic stress disorder). For example, glucocorticoid signaling is highly associated with trauma response (Daskalakis et al. 2014), for which *in vitro* studies reveal that brain organoids exposed to excessive glucocorticoid show impaired neuronal maturation (Cruceanu et al. 2021), and hiPSC neurons derived from cases with posttraumatic stress disorder can be distinguished from controls by glucocorticoid hypersensitivity (Breen et al. 2021).

Finally, the extent to which clinical drug responsiveness is heritable and/or stable throughout the lifetime requires further investigation, but promising examples, such as lithium-responsive bipolar disorder (Hou et al. 2016), have been identified (Stern et al. 2018). Is clinical treatment response predictable? In hippocampal neurons derived from lithium-responsive (but not nonresponsive) patients with bipolar disorder, hyperexcitability is ameliorated following lithium treatment (Mertens et al. 2015). A similar phenotypic analysis was able to predict with 92% accuracy whether hippocampal granule cell neurons were derived from a patient with or without clinical responsiveness to lithium. An improved drug-screening strategy would better recapitulate disease pathophysiology and integrate advances in psychiatric genetics. Moving toward this, proof-of-concept application of transcriptomic drug screening, using hiPSC-based models, have demonstrated that drug-induced differences in SCZ patient-derived neural progenitor cells could reverse postmortem SCZ transcriptional signatures and were enriched for genes related to SCZ biology (Readhead et al. 2018). Altogether, these studies reveal major advantages of incorporating cell type- and patient-specific platforms in drug discovery.

Summary

Each patient represents a unique aggregation of risk factors with distinct expression patterns, biological convergence, and cumulative effects. A functional genomics approach that integrates stem cell and animal models with genome engineering might resolve some of the major questions regarding the impact of patient-specific variants across cell types, genetic backgrounds, and environmental conditions. Striving to translate risk "variants to genes," "genes to pathways," and "pathways to circuits" has the potential to reveal unexpected causal relationships between risk factors within and between the cell types of the brain. These insights could identify therapeutics tailored to an individual's specific risk profile and fuel the development of novel, personalized approaches to mental health care.

Understanding Common Variation

8

Common Alleles

Next Steps in the Study of Common Variants

Hyejung Won, Naomi R. Wray, Elisabeth B. Binder, Kristen J. Brennand, Barbara Franke, Michael J. Gandal, Beth Stevens, Thomas Südhof, and Michael J. Ziller

Abstract

Common allele associations provide the starting point for delineating biological pathways that could progress understanding of psychiatric disorders. Multiple genomic approaches have been synergistically used to identify key contributing biological pathways that show evidence of convergence. Crucial next steps entail identification of causal risk variants, identification of causal risk genes, and identification of causal biological pathways. While a small number of genes could be prioritized and studied using the experimental paradigms applied to rare allele (large-effect) associations, this approach is neither feasible nor relevant for common variant associations where each person at high risk of disease carries a unique portfolio of risk variants, and where risk variants are carried by all of us. New experimental paradigms are needed that exploit the natural genetic variation present in populations and seek to understand why these unique portfolios of risk variants converge to disturb biological homeostasis, which lead to a common disease diagnosis. Recommendations for pathways forward are made, including new experimental paradigms that are specifically focused on combinations of risk-associated variants supported by new brain-specific data resources.

Introduction

The challenge of taking common risk allele associations into biological hypotheses and actionable outcomes applies to genome-wide association study (GWAS) results for all common diseases and disorders. Despite the complexity of the challenge, it is estimated that results from human genetic studies have contributed to 66% of drugs achieving FDA approval in 2021 (Ochoa et al. 2022). While the route from maps to mechanisms to medicines is never likely to be linear (International Common Disease Alliance 2020), this is particularly true for psychiatric disorders. Studies of brain disorders involve an organ that is much more difficult to access than for nonbrain-related disorders. Accordingly, in this chapter we focus on roadmaps and resources needed to clarify the role of common variation in psychiatry.

Translation of common allele associations requires a different approach from characterization of rare large-effect alleles for the following reasons:

1. Common single nucleotide polymorphisms (SNPs) have correlation structures that make it difficult to pinpoint causal variants based purely on association statistics.
2. Over 90% of common risk alleles significantly associated with psychiatric disorders are in the noncoding space (Watanabe et al. 2019a).
3. Combinations of variants together contribute to the risk of disorders.

In this chapter, we discuss existing knowledge gaps in the translation of GWAS discoveries and recommend experimental approaches, cellular models, and (genomic) resources which could help fill those gaps (see Figures 8.1 and 8.2). Specific recommendations are listed in the final section.

Pathway: Common Risk Allele to Causal Variant

The most significantly associated common risk allele in a genomic region identified in GWAS is not necessarily the functionally relevant variant. When many SNPs are in perfect linkage disequilibrium ($r^2 = 1$), it is not possible from statistical analysis to distinguish between them. Knowing, however, which SNP (or other classes of DNA variants) is functionally relevant is often the first step in understanding the mechanism of risk. The problem of fine mapping a GWAS locus to causal variants is a consideration for any GWAS and is not restricted to psychiatric disorders. Below, we discuss strategies to identify causal variants from the GWAS locus.

Increase GWAS Sample Size

In 2017, it was estimated that at least 80% of GWAS associations were within 33.5 kb of causal variants and that the mapping precision would increase both with larger GWAS sample sizes and larger imputation reference panels (Wu et al. 2017). As sample size increases, haplotypes with recombination events between tightly correlated alleles are increasingly likely to be present in the data set, which allows improved statistical fine mapping. While increased sample sizes will happen organically (see Ronald et al., this volume), current sample sizes are insufficient to infer causal variants purely from association statistics.

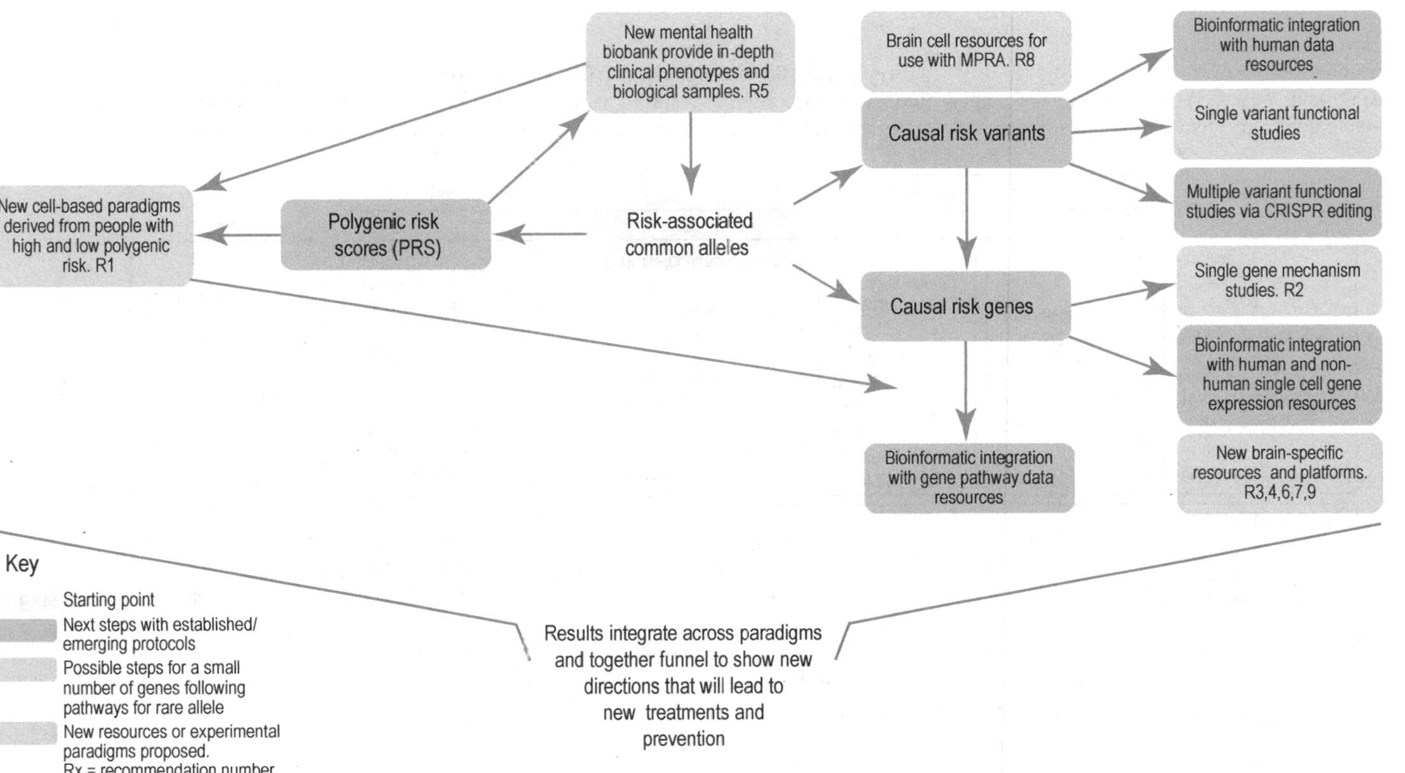

Figure 8.1 Overview of pathways forward from common risk alleles to potential clinical impact in the future. R1–R9 refers to specific recommendations listed below (see section, Recommendations).

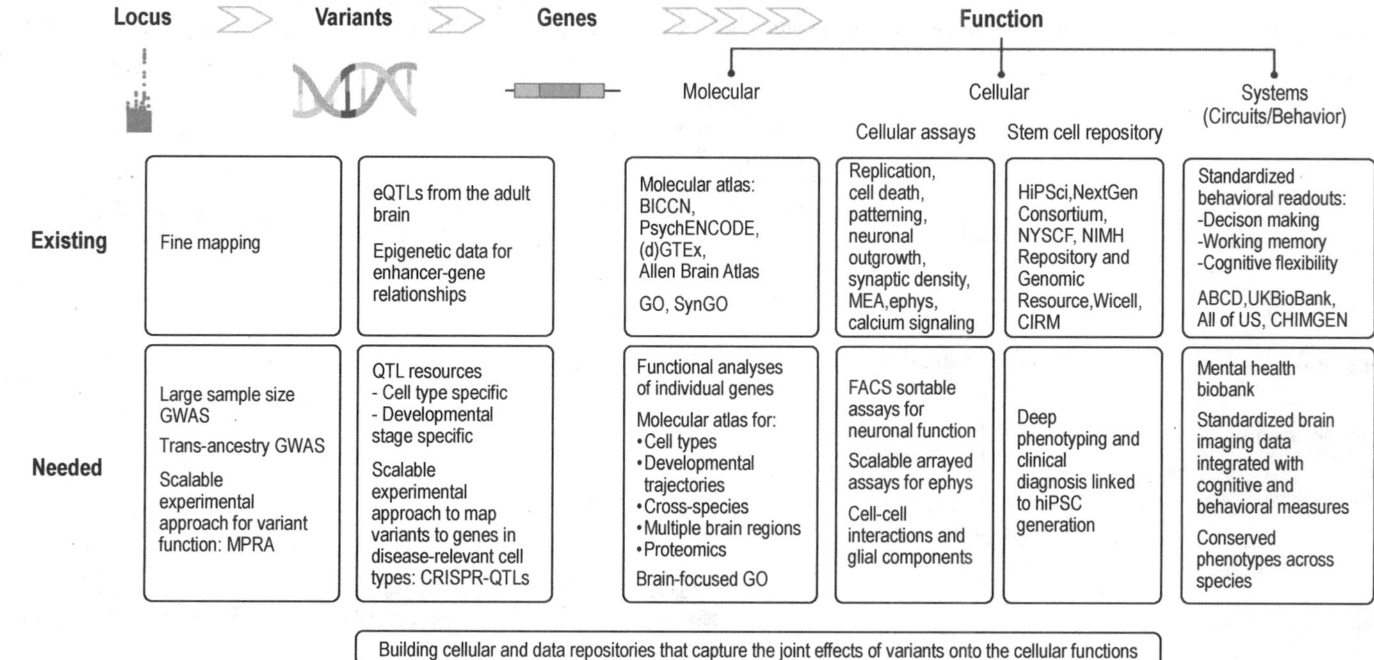

Figure 8.2 Existing and needed resources to distill biological hypotheses from common risk alleles. Electrophysiology (ephys), expression quantitative trait loci (eQTL), fluorescence-activated cell sorting (FACS), gene ontology (GO), genome-wide association studies (GWAS), massively parallel reporter assay (MPRA), multielectrode array (MEA), synaptic gene ontology (SynGO).

Experimental approaches to identify functional variants out of schizophrenia GWAS loci suggest that SNPs with the strongest association signals are functional only in ~10% of loci (McAfee et al. 2022b).

Meta-Analyze GWAS across Ancestries

Common causal variants are likely shared across ancestries, but because ancestries have different population histories, linkage disequilibrium blocks and allele frequencies differ between them. Notably, linkage disequilibrium blocks are much smaller in individuals of African ancestry. Hence, the most associated SNP from cross-ancestry meta-analysis is more likely to be the causal risk variant. The need to increase GWAS sample sizes across ancestries has already been recognized (Martin et al. 2019b; Ronald et al. and Appelbaum, this volume).

Statistical Fine Mapping

A number of statistical fine-mapping tools have been developed which attempt to prioritize the underlying candidate causal variant(s) at a given GWAS locus with some posterior inclusion probability (Schaid et al. 2018). These are statistical predictions, however, and empirical evaluation of results from different fine-mapping algorithms give different sets of credible SNPs (Mah and Won 2020). Challenges can arise, in particular, when fine mapping is performed on aggregated summary statistics across multiple cohorts, when true causal variants are not directly measured and when algorithms assume only one causal variant is present at a given locus. Furthermore, the functionality of these predictions is largely untested. The recent schizophrenia GWAS systematically addressed some of these issues and provided fine-mapping results along with GWAS summary statistics (Trubetskoy et al. 2022). Still, the field needs improved means for prioritizing the most likely candidate causal variant at a given locus, before more costly follow-up experimentation steps are taken. While this issue may ultimately be resolved through trans-population meta-analyses, different fine-mapping approaches are needed in the near term and should be benchmarked against a standard set guided by experimentally validated SNPs.

Experimental Validation of Variant Function

Common SNPs associated with psychiatric disorders are enriched within active regulatory elements and are thought to play a role in gene regulation. Massively parallel reporter assays (MPRA) offer a scalable approach to experimentally test the gene regulatory activity of thousands of elements in a single assay (see Hu and Won as well as Brennand and Kushner, this volume). Such high-throughput screens for regulatory element activity have only recently been applied to measure allelic regulatory activity of variants (Deng et al. 2023; Matoba et al. 2020; McAfee et al. 2022b; Myint et al. 2020; Tewhey et al. 2016) and are increasingly being applied to evaluate putative causal expression quantitative trait loci (eQTL) that overlap with GWAS loci for complex disorders (Abell et al. 2022). It should be noted, however, that the majority of such experiments have been performed in cancer cell lines rather than brain cells, which makes it difficult to apply the findings to interpret GWAS of psychiatric disorders.

Given the enormous tissue- and cell-type specificity of active regulatory elements in which common SNPs reside, adapting MPRA for use in brain cells is critical if we are to understanding cell type-specific models of regulatory logic in psychiatric disorder risk variants (see section on Recommendations). The successful use of MPRA in human embryonic stem cell-derived neural precursor cells and neurons (Deng et al. 2023; Geller et al. 2019; McAfee et al. 2022b; Uebbing et al. 2021) is a promising step toward their wider application in identifying causal variants from psychiatric GWAS. Particularly exciting is the potential for development of massively parallel sequencing protocols in models based on patient-derived human-induced pluripotent stem cells (hiPSCs) that would enable cell type-specific identification of regulatory elements in polygenic background. Similarly, since hiPSC-derived neurons are already used to model human cortical development, applying these techniques in temporal analyses of hiPSC-derived cells may elucidate early developmental factors involved in the etiology of psychiatric disorders.

While MPRA offers a scalable approach to screen regulatory activity of noncoding variants at an unparalleled scale across diverse cell types of the brain, it does not provide information on the impact of the endogenous loci or identify the genes of action. This limitation can be mitigated by combining the MPRA strategies with other complementary approaches, such as CRISPR-mediated genome editing. The Impact of Genomic Variation on Function (IGVF) Consortium aims to validate experimentally the functional impact of SNPs via the combination of MPRA and CRISPR engineering in more physiologically relevant cell types (see section on Recommendations).

Given the lack of evolutionary conservation of noncoding elements (Han et al. 2018), hiPSCs provide a unique system to study the impact of noncoding variation on cellular features. CRISPR editing in hiPSC-derived cell types can resolve the molecular and cellular impacts of perturbing individual SNPs. Of the 108 schizophrenia GWAS loci identified initially by the Schizophrenia Working Group of the Psychiatric Genomics Consortium (2014), 19 harbored colocalized GWAS and eQTL signals in postmortem brain RNA sequencing (Fromer et al. 2016). Of the five loci predicted to involve a single protein-coding gene, only one locus (*FURIN*) was the most significant GWAS SNP (rs4702) and also the most significant eQTL-SNP. Fine-mapping analysis strongly suggests this to be a single putative causal *cis*-eQTL (posterior probability = 0.94) (Schrode et al. 2019). CRISPR-based allelic conversion resulted in decreased *FURIN* expression in hiPSC-derived glutamatergic neurons accompanied with reduced neurite length and altered population-wide neuronal activity patterns (Schrode et al. 2019). This example illustrates the power of hiPSC-derived cell types in studying molecular and cellular impacts of individual noncoding variants, although the mechanistic link to disease remains unclear.

Pathway: Causal Risk Variant to Gene

Mapping a causal risk variant in the noncoding space of the genome to the gene it modulates remains a major challenge in the field. This difficulty is rooted in the large number of parameters that determine a variant's effect and the distinct mechanisms of action an individual variant can have. Noncoding genetic variants can disrupt the function of noncoding gene regulatory elements that modulate distinct genes to different extents (Fulco et al. 2019). Roughly 80% of noncoding variants also regulate "non-nearest" genes (Sey et al. 2020), suggesting that variant-gene relationships cannot be simply captured in the context of the linear genome. Moreover, the effects of noncoding variants on genes have been shown to be mediated through multiple distinct mechanisms of action, such as modulating gene expression levels, splicing patterns, chromatin accessibility, transcription factor and microRNA binding as well as alternative polyadenylation (GTEx Consortium 2020; Huan et al. 2015; Li et al. 2021b; Wang et al. 2018). Adding another layer of complexity, noncoding variants frequently operate in a highly cell-type-, developmental stage, and condition-specific manner. Thus, tailored high-throughput assays and context-specific cellular model systems are required to systematically associate individual variants with their downstream targets. The resulting data sets require advanced computational approaches to facilitate discovery and integration of respective results. Below, we summarize existing and urgently needed resources, methods, and assays to start tackling these questions, relevant to both common and rare associated alleles (see also Bearden et al., this volume).

Bioinformatic Integration with QTL Resources

Systematic integration of GWAS with experimentally defined quantitative trait loci (QTL), for molecular features profiled within the human brain, provides an important way to prioritize the candidate causal gene at a given GWAS locus. This can be achieved without identifying the causal risk variant. Large-scale efforts have been undertaken to identify gene expression and splicing QTLs in the adult human brain. As sample size and tissue are the most critical factors for QTL discovery, this has largely been done in bulk adult cortex samples through mega- and meta-analysis (de Klein et al. 2023; Wang et al. 2018; Zeng et al. 2022). Despite these concerted efforts, brain eQTLs alone cannot link all GWAS loci to targetable genes (Zeng et al. 2022). Hu and Won (this volume) and Robinson et al. (this volume) describe currently available QTL resources in both adult and developing human brains as well as critical next steps, such as developing cell type-specific QTL resources and expanding splicing QTL and isoform-level resources. We recommend that more brain-specific gene expression resources be generated (see section on Recommendations).

Bioinformatic Integration with Other Genomic Resources

Compared to current eQTL resources, which lack cellular and developmental resolution, epigenomic profiling provides an alternative resource to address the cell type and nature of variant-gene relationships specific to development. Multi-omic data sets are particularly useful to link variants to genes. Existing multi-omic resources and approaches to link enhancers (and variants) to genes are described in detail by Hu and Won (this volume). One key benefit of using epigenomic assays to infer target genes of variants is that enhancer-gene relationships are robust to linkage disequilibrium (Whalen and Pollard 2019). Furthermore, a growing number of epigenetic data sets are being generated at cellular resolution through the advancement of single-cell genomics, which allows cell type-specific target gene identification. To facilitate growth in this area, brain-specific omics resources and ear-marked funding for data integration would be beneficial (see section on Recommendations).

Experimental Validation of Variant-Gene Relationship

Inferences regarding variant-gene relationships from transcriptomic or multiomic approaches need to be functionally validated. One approach to confirm the effects of variants in regulatory elements involves CRISPR screening. Coupling CRISPR editing with single-cell RNA sequencing readouts can validate the regulatory impact of GWAS SNPs on predicted target genes at cellular resolution, yielding rich and high-dimensional phenotypes (Gasperini et al. 2019). To date, however, many CRISPR screens have been conducted in cancerous cell lines. Similar assays will need to be conducted in brain cell types. In particular, CRISPR screens that target noncoding variants in brain cell types across multiple differentiation time points will allow us to systematically interrogate the variant-gene connection in a cell type and developmental context-specific manner. Current CRISPR screens are designed to measure gene expression changes upon perturbing a regulatory element rather than a single nucleotide change. Therefore, CRISPR screens alone may not provide the directionality of effects of the variants. As discussed earlier, CRISPR screens can be complemented by other experimental validation assays: MPRA provides causal variants and directionality of effects, whereas CRISPR provides target genes of variants.

Beyond Gene Expression Readouts

The functional impact of noncoding variants could involve multiple mechanisms (e.g., splicing regulation, UTR function, RNA localization), yet most experimental assays focus on enhancer function. There has been a considerable progress in the development of high-throughput functional genomic strategies to measure the impact of individual genetic variants on splicing (Cheung et al. 2019; Rosenberg et al. 2015), mRNA degradation (Rabani et al. 2017), UTR function (Griesemer et al. 2021), and subcellular RNA localization (Mikl et al. 2022). Adapting such high-throughput assays for distinct molecular layers will enable comprehensive understanding of the functional impact of variants that exert their effects through different molecular mechanisms. In contrast, advances in the identification of *trans*-mediated effects of individual genetic variants have been much more limited.

In addition, the dependence of the molecular consequence of a single genetic variant on the genetic background of a specific individual remains unclear. To study the variant effects in the context of a polygenic background, new experimental and computational strategies are required to better identify *trans*-effects of individual genetic variants beyond simply acquiring larger cohorts of individuals profiled for gene expression. Moreover, systematic efforts are needed to evaluate the impact of genetic background on single variant-gene association by performing the assays discussed earlier in cellular contexts from distinct genetic backgrounds and ideally across species (see section on Recommendations).

How to Prioritize Genes for Validation

Once we identify target genes implicated by the common risk variants, we must understand their functional role in the brain. This step can follow the same experimental paradigms used to investigate the functional role of genes identified from rare-variant, large-effect associations (see Bearden et al., this volume). Gandal (this volume) provides an example of how the common allele association at the major histocompatibility complex locus led to a detailed analysis of the function of the *C4A* gene. Despite this success, the majority of psychiatric GWAS loci have not yielded testable biological hypotheses. Unlike rare variation that disrupts protein function, the exact mechanisms through which common SNPs act on the genes remain unknown. Moreover, GWAS results implicate hundreds of genes that may act together in a combinatorial fashion within the polygenic background. Therefore, not all genes implicated by GWAS may reveal clear mechanistic insights into disease when investigated individually (see section on Recommendations).

Pathway: Gene to Function and Phenotype

Once variants are mapped to genes, the next steps are to identify disease-relevant biochemical pathways with which to generate and test mechanistic biological hypotheses. This is where the strategies to study rare-variant associations and common variant associations clearly diverge. For most common risk alleles, it is simply not feasible to generate biological hypotheses from individual variants, since the role of risk variants likely depends on the genetic context in which they are present. New strategies are needed to identify the biological convergence associated with the heterogeneous set for risk variants (unique to each individual) which are associated with high risk of disease. To achieve this, we need new experimental paradigms and new omics reference data sets that can be integrated with GWAS results, supplemented with a platform that facilitates multimodal data integration (see section on Recommendations). This, in turn, requires a better understanding of the cell types and circuits as well as the relevant developmental periods. Some of this information may emerge from ongoing (single-cell) transcriptomic studies of human and animal model brain tissue. However, diverse cellular and animal-based systems are needed to study gene function and candidate disease mechanisms (Figures 8.1 and 8.2).

Molecular Function and Biological Pathways

The functional impact of genes targeted by common SNPs can be interrogated within biological contexts by bioinformatic integration of disease-associated gene lists with annotated gene sets (e.g., gene ontology, GO). Most available gene sets, however, are not curated with respect to brain function, which makes it challenging to decipher brain-relevant disease biology from psychiatric variants. Whereas some data sets already exist through initiatives such as the BRAIN Initiative Cell Census Network (BICCN) (2021), the GTEx Consortium (2020), the Allen Brain Atlas, and the PsychEncode Consortium et al. (2015), integrating multimodal data sets acquired from different initiatives can be challenging. Concerted efforts aimed at systematic annotation of genes and pathways can be powerful, as illustrated by SynGO, an approach to integrating data in synapse biology (Koopmans et al. 2019). Its success argues strongly for the establishment of a more comprehensive brain ontology consortium which would extend the SynGO approach to a central "brain-centric GO" repository (see section on Recommendations). This would host not only manually curated brain-relevant biological pathways but also the growing list of gene sets derived from perturbation experiments (e.g., CRISPR screens, drug treatment response).

Cellular Function

Given the lack of evolutionary conservation of noncoding elements (Han et al. 2018), animal models may not provide the necessary context to explore the variant-gene-function continuum. However, hiPSCs provide a unique system to study the impact of noncoding variation on cellular features. As described above, CRISPR editing can be used to investigate the function of individual risk variants. To understand the impact of unique portfolios of thousands of risk variants, multiple biologically functional variants need to be simultaneously introduced, and it is not straightforward to scale via CRISPR editing. One potential alternative mode to measure the joint effects of variants on cellular phenotypes would be to create a large collection of hiPSCs representing a range of genetic backgrounds and disease conditions. There are several ongoing initiatives relevant to fast-track this approach. The Human Induced Pluripotent Stem Cells Initiative (HipSci) includes more than 700 hiPSC lines from ~300 individuals, the vast majority of which are from control donors of British ancestry (Kilpinen et al. 2017). The NextGen Consortium (a US-based team) generated a large collection of hiPSCs in parallel; although not focused on neuronal cell types, their focus on polygenic metabolic disorders may provide insights relevant to neuropsychiatric disease (Warren et al. 2017). The New York Stem Cell Foundation (NYSCF) has likewise assembled a large trans-ancestry collection of hiPSCs with a focus on Parkinson disease. Individual researchers are contributing their hiPSC collections to a variety of repositories, such as the NIMH Repository and Genomics Resource, and WiCell, yielding a bank of patient-specific hiPSCs generated across a variety of laboratories via an assortment of methodologies. The California Institute of Regenerative Medicine (CIRM) hiPSC collection is one of the largest US-based single-derived collections of genotyped hiPSCs (1,618 donors), generated by a standardized, non-integrating episomal reprogramming approach in a single production facility. Scalable approaches to culture and differentiate hiPSC lines from different donors are emerging for systematic investigation of variant-cellular function relationship. Village-in-a-dish approaches mix hiPSCs from dozens of donors together for transcriptomic (single-cell RNA sequencing) and/or phenotypic (FACS-based) assays in pools (Jerber et al. 2021; Mitchell et al. 2020; Neavin et al. 2021b), making it possible to test the genotype-dependent effects at scale.

Since the pioneering study by Dobrindt et al. (2021; see also Brennand and Kushner, this volume), which utilized a high versus low polygenic risk score (PRS) design, another study has extended the paradigm to compare 13 high PRS neuronal cell lines derived from people diagnosed with schizophrenia against 15 neurotypical individuals with low PRS (Page et al. 2022). The latter study identified altered Na+ channel function, action potential interspike interval, and GABAergic neurotransmission as being associated with high PRS. While these early results need further validation, the ability to identify basic neuronal physiological properties that can be related to core clinical characteristics of illness may be a critical step in understanding mechanism of polygenic disease and generating leads for novel therapeutics. Widespread adoption of a common set of hiPSC lines with extreme schizophrenia PRS will not only help evaluate the reproducibility of functional genomic studies, it will also facilitate the integration of data sets generated by different laboratories, revealing any convergent impacts of independent schizophrenia-associated variants. This leads to our recommendations for a high/low PRS cell-line study conducted at scale and for the establishment of a mental health biobank to generate the cell-line resource linked to in-depth clinical, longitudinal phenotypes (see section on Recommendations).

Systems Level: Circuits and Behavior

Brain Circuits

Having the ability to link molecular and cellular phenotypes to brain structure, function, and connectivity as well as cognitive and behavioral phenotypes would enable the translation of polygenic effects and enhance our understanding of psychiatric disease. Early studies of circuit-relevant phenotypes were plagued by small sample size, but now the field of genetic imaging has seen immense progress through the formation of large-scale consortia, such as ENIGMA (Thompson et al. 2022) and CHARGE (Psaty et al. 2009), with an emphasis on the development of open-source protocols and resources to improve standardization of data analysis workflows in the field of magnetic resonance imaging (MRI) and electroencephalogram (EEG). Similarly, efforts such as the UK Biobank and the ABCD Study have provided large data sources with standardized neuroimaging data. The brain measures used in these studies are moderately to highly heritable, and while obtained largely from individuals without disease, they show associations with psychiatric disease phenotypes, although the genetic overlap between them is small (Grasby et al. 2020). The need for large sample sizes has so far limited the range of phenotypes assessed to relatively crude measures of global and regional morphology, brain activity, and structural and functional connectivity. While the costs of generating omics data are expected to decline, the cost of generating imaging data is likely to remain high. Thus, due to cost considerations, we are unable to recommend the purpose-driven generation of MRI data sets of the scale required (Marek et al. 2022) for gene discovery. If generated in the context of other large-scale efforts, however, they may be useful for integrative analyses of common variant associations.

Cognitive and Behavioral Phenotyping

Large-scale data collections of cognitive and behavioral phenotypes are becoming available through population-wide initiatives (e.g., the UK Biobank, the ABCD Study, All of US Research Program), but the depth of psychiatry-relevant phenotypes is, to date, insufficient. It is well-recognized that large-scale population, volunteer-based initiatives underrepresent people with psychiatric disorders. Notably, most cohorts provide limited longitudinal measures even though the importance of longitudinal trajectories of these measures is increasingly recognized (Shah et al. 2020). The human connectome project for early psychosis is a good example of a cohort (N = 200 with early psychosis and

N = 100 controls) with in-depth multimodal phenotyping and potential for a hiPSC resource (Demro et al. 2021).

Clearly, the field needs initiatives directed at defining the most disease-relevant imaging and behavioral traits. While progress is being made (e.g., the Psychiatric Genomics Consortium conducts analyses of secondary phenotypes including cognitive measures), sample sizes are much smaller than for case/control analyses. New data collection is urgently needed, including in-depth, longitudinal phenotyping across multiple dimensions and biobanking of samples, not only for DNA and other omics analyses, but processed to allow future generation of hiPSCs. We recommend that a mental health biobank be initiated to provide longitudinal information on individuals with psychiatric disorders (see also section on Recommendations).

Phenotypes that Transcend Experimental Paradigms

Since cognitive, behavioral, and imaging phenotypes (unlike psychiatric disorders) can be measured in animal models, efforts to increase translatability of phenotypes across species are important. At the brain imaging level, development of whole brain function ultrasound in awake-behaving animals may permit generation of phenotypes that parallel human fMRI (Brunner et al. 2020; Brunner et al. 2021), including brain network activity changes at rest or under specific tasks that emerge as highly relevant for psychiatric disorders. Such translatability across species could also be achieved with EEG-based measures, with increased availability of wireless EEG in rodents, including sleep EEG (Karamihalev et al. 2019), where headband-based ambulatory EEG methods are now increasingly available for humans. At the level of behavioral and physiological assessments, current technical developments in human and animal phenotyping (e.g., touch screen, actimetry, startle responses) allow better cross-species alignment.

With increased research focus on cell-based models, phenotypes that can be measured *in vivo* an *in vitro* are of particular interest. For instance, measures captured at the electrophysiological level in hiPSC-derived neuronal models (Page et al. 2022) can be related to the *in vivo* context in animals using next-generation electrodes (e.g., Neuropixels probes) that are increasingly translatable to EEG or even MEG in humans (e.g., Schulte et al. 2021). Similarly, circadian rhythm phenotypes measured in cell lines have been associated with circadian rhythms of bipolar disorder patients from whom the cell lines were derived (Sanghani et al. 2021). Likewise, synaptic density, a feature associated with psychiatric disorders in postmortem brains and *in vitro*, can now be measured *in vivo* through positron emission tomography imaging of synaptic density using synaptic vesicle glycoprotein 2A (SV2A) in animal models and humans (Cai et al. 2019; Toyonaga et al. 2022). We recommend specific focus on phenotypes that can be meaningfully measured across multiple experimental paradigms (see section on Recommendations).

Pathway: Context

Genes and genetic variants may have different functions under different biological and environmental contexts. For example, variant and gene function may vary in different cell and tissue types, across development, aging, and in response to stressors. Having a map of context-dependent annotations will be invaluable in guiding our understanding of variant to function connections. Context changes could unmask previously unrecognized variant to gene, gene to function, or polygene to function connections that are not apparent in a baseline state. Context needs to be a key consideration in all experimental approaches, and challenges represent any stimuli acting as stressors that would deviate cells/organisms from maintaining homeostasis. For instance, MPRA screens (discussed above) used for functional validation of risk variants should be conducted in different cell types as well as after exposing cell lines to stimuli. Supporting this claim, MPRA in the context of activating the glucocorticoid receptor (a key mediator of the stress response) unveiled a novel function of genetic variants associated with psychiatric disorders specific to stress hormone exposure (Penner-Goeke et al. 2022). In designing perturbation experiments, "stressors" can be summarized into major categories of metabolic stress, oxidative stress, action of hormones (e.g., glucocorticoids), and inflammatory stress. Other stimuli particularly relevant to neuronal function could be neuronal activation as well as the action of certain neurotransmitters. Incorporation of gene–environment interactions may be especially critical in studies of neuropsychiatric disorders, which may require or include specific stressors (e.g., posttraumatic stress disorder) or exposures (e.g., substance use disorder) among diagnostic criteria, or may count exposure to illicit substances or extreme stress as among the most critical risk factors for disease development (e.g., schizophrenia). Toward deciphering complex gene–environment interactions, there is an urgent need to explore the additive impact of environmental stressors on the effects of risk variants and genes within individuals, and extending PRS approaches to include the gene–environment interactions at the population level. Importantly, sex-specific effects and sex-environment/perturbation interactions are likely to be needed. While increasing the complexity of the proposed experiments, they are essential for ensuring generalizability of results (see section on Recommendations).

A systematic interrogation of gene–environment interactions could be achieved by initiatives such as Connectivity Map (CMAP). This platform provides a comprehensive catalog of molecular and cellular signatures elicited across multiple cell lines by systematic perturbation of cell lines by pharmacological perturbations. CMAP serves as a database resource to investigate the modes of action in a wide range of drug perturbations. Researchers can purchase the cell lines used in CMAP to conduct perturbation experiments and can benchmark gene expression perturbations induced by new compounds against the CMAP perturbation experiments. CMAP, however, is not well curated to address gene–environment interactions in the context of psychiatric disorders. It only includes a small portfolio of drugs relevant to psychiatric disorders and does not cover brain cell lines.

Recommendations

The biological robustness implied by the polygenic architecture of psychiatric disorders provides a major challenge in translating genetic association results into meaningful outcomes for those whose lives are, or will be in the future, affected by psychiatric disorders. Common risk allele associations provide multiple new directions for research. In describing the pathways forward (Figure 8.1) we have uncovered the need for data resources and experimental paradigms, many of which must be undertaken at scale as well as collaboratively across groups and even nations (Table 8.1). Guiding principles for building such resources include transparency, accessibility (e.g., open source), strong emphasis on quality control, and community building. In this section, we provide nine recommendations (R1–R9) for future research priorities. Given our focus on pathways forward for common alleles, we have ordered the recommendations around this goal. We believe the results from these proposed studies, regardless of actual outcomes, will propel the field forward and expose

Table 8.1 List of existing and needed resources.

	Existing Resources	Resources Required
Molecular atlas	• Brain Initiative Cell Census Network (BICCN) • PsychENCODE consortium • Genotype-Tissue Expression (GTEx) • Developmental GTEx • Allen Brain Atlas	• Cross-species • Multiple brain regions beyond cortex • Inclusion of data beyond expression and proteomics
Gene ontology	• GO • SynGO	• Brain ontology consortium
Stem cell resources	• HipSci • NextGen consortium • NYSCF • NIMH Repository and Genomics Resource • WiCell • CIRM	• Deep phenotyping • Clinical diagnosis linked to the cell lines
Longitudinal behavioral phenotyping	• ABCD Study • UK Biobank • All of US Research Program	• Mental health biobank

new avenues of research that will ultimately drive progress to the key goals of improved prevention, diagnosis, and treatments.

R1: A New Experimental Paradigm That Can Capture Polygenicity

We need an experimental paradigm that goes beyond the analysis of individual genetic variants and assesses instead the aggregated impact of naturally occurring combinations of common risk variants that jointly act, integrating over *cis*- and *trans*-effects, and results in high (or low) risk of disease (Figure 8.3). hiPSC-based model systems provide the unique opportunity to identify consistently dysregulated genes and pathways associated with diagnostic groups. To maximize power for a given budget, we propose a high/low polygenic risk experimental design that has already been piloted on a small scale (Dobrindt et al. 2021; Page et al. 2022). Although the scale of study we propose stretches current technical limits, scalability in hiPSC-based model systems is a fast-moving field and will be driven further by need. The power of the design increases with the strength of selection on polygenic risk. Currently, there is a 39-fold difference (95% confidence 29–53) in risk of schizophrenia between the top and bottom centile of polygenic risk, but only a 16-fold difference (95% confidence 15–17) between the top and bottom decile (Trubetskoy et al. 2022). To achieve an extreme PRS design with sufficiently large N, a very large cohort of participants needs to be collected with genotype data to measure PRS. Unfortunately, recontact with participants, necessary to establish hiPSC models, is likely to be more difficult in psychiatry compared to other branches of medicine; hence, biobanking of blood processed to enable generation of cell lines must be done early in study participation. This links to the need for a mental health biobank, discussed below (see R5). The experimental approach we propose will pave the way for precision medicine in psychiatry, similar to approaches already pioneered in cancer, heart, or kidney disease: optimal treatments personalized to an individual will be determined through responses to perturbations applied to person-specific cell lines or organoids. The model is described in Figure 8.3. Table 8.2 provides a justification for the underlying experimental design, and Table 8.3 presents a SWOT analysis. Although the design is set up for schizophrenia (SCZ) because the genetic discovery to date is highest (PRS explain 10% of variation in liability), the design could be implemented for any disease.

- *Vision*: To establish a novel and well-powered experimental paradigm that uses cellular measures to identify biological signatures that correlate with diagnosis. A cellular platform is a simplification of real biological processes because different sets of risk loci likely to have biological impacts in multiple cell types and at multi-developmental time points in response to biological environments. We believe this platform will provide a tractable model in which different sets of risk

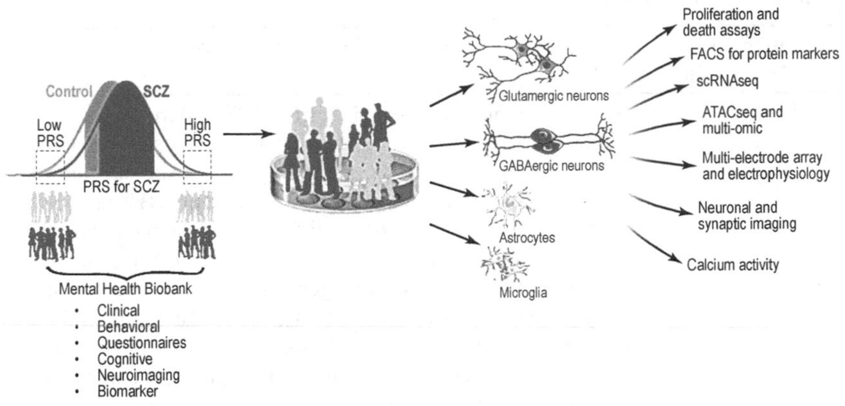

Figure 8.3 Experimental model system to identify biological correlates of genetic risk and diagnosis.

variants generate convergent biological readouts. This paradigm would allow us not just to better understand relationships between risk variants, function, and phenotype, and to causally query these hypotheses across disease relevant contexts.

- *Major goals:* To translate polygenicity into biological and cellular pathophysiology; to establish protocols for repeatable cellular phenotypes that can inform disease mechanisms; to provide protocols for repeatable perturbation studies applied to at scale that expose convergent biological responses; and to provide a framework for precision medicine in psychiatry.
- *Design:* Generate hiPSC lines using a 2×2 design of high and low PRS with/without SCZ diagnosis, justified in Table 8.2. The extreme PRS design is cost-effective and the 2×2 design generates combinations of comparisons that together are more informative than simpler designs.
- *Which cell type*: Variant function can diverge in different cell types, so identification of the disease-relevant cell type will be essential for the success of the proposed experimental system. Analyses of GWAS and emerging single-cell transcriptomic data nominate excitatory neurons for prioritization (Sey et al. 2020; Skene et al. 2018). Hence, initial focus could be on excitatory neurons and later expanded to other cell types, as well as more complex organoid models.
- *Which model*: The hiPSC village-in-a-dish model can increase scalability, minimize variability, and might be more affordably implemented across laboratories. This model is well suited to sequencing measures as individual cells can be identified through genomic data. For other

Table 8.2 Justification of the 2 × 2 design: high vs. low polygenic risk score (PRS), with or without a schizophrenia (SCZ) diagnosis.

PRS with SCZ	PRS no SCZ	Justification of comparison
High	Low	Since all people carry risk alleles for SCZ, differences at the biological level between cases and controls are expected to be subtle. This design utilizes PRS data to accentuate the biological differences between case and control groups. Based on current PRS, there is a 39-fold difference in risk based on top vs. bottom centiles. In this comparison we expect to observe or construct perturbations that generate strong differences in cellular measures between the two groups. The observed differences may reflect general case/control status or something more specific to polygenicity. Results from the pairwise comparisons will help differentiate these scenarios.
High	High	Here, all individuals have high PRS for SCZ, so differences in cellular measures will provide information about functional pathways associated with SCZ over and above those associated with the identified polygenic risk. A parsimonious hypothesis is that nonidentified genetic risk variants (i.e., those with high PRS and SCZ compared to those with high PRS but without SCZ) will impact the same biological pathways in the same way as currently identified risk variants. Empirical evidence is needed to support or reject this hypothesis.
Low	Low	This comparison is underpinned by parsimonious hypotheses: Those with low PRS and SCZ must be enriched for genetic risk variants not yet identified (see exclusions). Nonidentified genetic risk variants will impact the same biological pathways as currently identified risk variants. Cellular measures that differ between low PRS with/without SCZ should be the same as cellular measures that differ between high PRS with/without SCZ. Empirical evidence is needed to support or reject these hypotheses.
Low	High	This comparison is underpinned by parsimonious hypotheses: Those with low PRS and SCZ must be enriched for genetic risk variants not yet identified, which have a stronger biological signal than those with high PRS but no disease diagnosis. Cellular measures that differ between low PRS with SCZ and high PRS without SCZ should be the same as cellular measures that differ in at least one of the other pairwise combinations. Empirical evidence is needed to support or reject these hypotheses.
Exclusions		In all comparisons, those carrying large-effect rare-variant alleles will be excluded. Such alleles are often associated with syndromic phenotypes and/or are nonspecific to SCZ. We propose that they should be studied in add-on cell-line comparisons and excluded from the baseline 2 × 2 design.

Table 8.3 SWOT (strengths/weaknesses/opportunities/threats) for the 2 × 2 cell-based experimental paradigm designed to understand the molecular mechanisms associated with common allele polygenic risk.

Strengths	Weaknesses
• Captures polygenic background in the absence of confounds • The 2 × 2 design provides multiple comparisons which together will generate more robust conclusions • Regardless of results, new biological insights will be obtained • Village-in-a-dish model improves scalability of the approach • Systematic platform to test interplays between genes and environmental challenges	• Scaling to sample sizes desired will be challenging • Relevant readouts are not yet available • Readouts can be noisy and difficult to interpret • Lack of tools for analyzing and integrating different phenotypic modalities • Will be challenging to set up to be representative of all ancestries; other ancestry-specific studies will be needed to inform this
Opportunities	**Threats**
• Multimodal integration • Provides possibility for development of diagnostic biomarkers in psychiatry • Provides possibility of linking cellular phenotypes to clinical phenotypes (e.g., electrophysiology translating to EEG) • Motivates collection of a mental health biobank future-proofed to benefit from outcomes • New methods will be developed which will be valuable in many research domains • Globally shared platform • Fosters collaboration	• Sample sizes may be too small given actual effects sizes and multiple comparisons • Identification of individuals with extreme PRS with/without disease requires large cohorts genotyped and with biological samples for hiPSC • Ethical concerns associated with hiPSC research

technologies, the participant identity is integral if cell lines are held individually.

- *What to measure*: Phenotypic assays need to be carefully selected so that they are orthogonal and allow high-throughput characterizations:
    1. Genomics: single-cell RNA sequencing and single-cell sequencing assay for transposase-accessible chromatin
    2. Morphology: High-content imaging for neurite outgrowth and synapse density
    3. Electrophysiological property: multielectrode array, optical electrophysiology

Measures need to be repeatable (which could be achieved through testing of protocols across multiple labs) and heritable (i.e., phenotypic variation is associated with genetic variation), which could be verified in parent/offspring or sibling designs.

- *What perturbations to apply*: In the first instance, we propose a small number of perturbations which could be informed by CMAP type experiments (see below, R4).
- *Sample size:* Pilot studies demonstrate that significant differences can be identified from sample sizes of less than 20 in each group (Dobrindt et al. 2021; Page et al. 2022). The power of the study also depends on the strength of selection that can be applied to the PRS. Our expectation is that the platform will be used to test multiple hypotheses. Moreover, our knowledge of common disease establishes a baseline expectation of complexity. Hence, suggestions for the number of samples required for each comparison are unknown. Since we expect the strongest differences in cellular measures from the high PRS with SCZ/low PRS without SCZ, this comparison could be tested in a pilot phase that develops protocols to determine which cell types to generate, and which cellular measures and which perturbations generate reproduceable and repeatable results. Ultimately, we anticipate that a design with N = 500 per group balanced by sex, is the minimum sample size required.

R2: New Scalable Platforms for Functional Analyses

Complementing R1, this recommendation is based on the need to understand the functional implications of common genetic variants associated with neuropsychiatric disorders in a well-controlled and reproducible approach. We acknowledge that the functions of most protein-coding genes as well as of most noncoding genomic loci are incompletely understood. Even for genes with apparently clear-cut functions and involvement in psychiatric disorders (Dai et al. 2019; Singh et al. 2022), such as those encoding subunits and regulators of NMDA-type glutamate receptors (NMDARs), the field does not yet understand the synaptic and extra-synaptic functions of these genes. We do not know, for example, what the various types of NMDAR subunits do, how they are regulated, and how the interplay of different types of glutamate receptors (AMPA, NMDA, and kainite receptors) informs neural circuits. Functional analyses with a range of relevant readouts are needed for studying the functional effects of individual common genetic variants and combinations of common variants in multiple genetic backgrounds. This can be achieved by having shared cell lines each of known genetic background, to allow comparisons across laboratories.

To meet this challenge, new scalable platforms for functional analyses are necessary that are currently not available. The challenge is made difficult because several key processes in brain, such as various synaptic functions (receptor composition, release probability, short- and long-term plasticity), neuronal excitability, myelination, and microglial immune responses, are not (yet) amenable to high-throughput assays. For example, current scalable approaches, such as multielectrode arrays or calcium imaging, provide an excellent readout of neuronal activity but do not provide insight into either any synaptic function or neuronal excitability. In view of these needs and limitations, it is recommended to invest in tools that achieve scalable analyses either by developing completely new high-throughput assays or enabling a medium-scale analysis of various brain processes. Such tools, for example, could (for synaptic functions) consist of automated measurements of miniature synaptic responses using robotic patching or optical measurements of specifically pre- and postsynaptic calcium transients using dual color calcium sensors. The proposal complements the Brain Initiative's focus on scalable cellular/molecular approaches (BRAIN Initiative Cell Census Network 2021).

R3: Facilitate Data Integration Research

Many brain-omics data sets have been, and will be, generated through a wide range of research projects funded internationally. Progress in understanding biological mechanisms associated with polygenic disease can be made through intelligent bioinformatic integration of data sets. The underlying omics data sets can be expensive to generate, so the integrative analyses will be integral to maximize the utility of the data at relatively low (but not zero) additional cost. To facilitate research integrating data sets, a platform should be established that brings together multimodal data sets. This will allow researchers to query and contribute to data sets. An example platform for hosting multimodal data sets is the Alzheimer Disease Forum (AlzForum). An example platform for comparing machine learning algorithms or statistical models to standardized data sets is Kipoi. Similar platforms need to be established to underpin research in psychiatric disorders.

R4: Establish a Brain CMAP

The CMAP study has proven to be a useful resource for investigating mode of action of drugs, with 4,435 Google cites to the primary paper (Lamb et al. 2006). We recommend that this study be extended to generate gene expression changes that result from a catalog of psychiatry-relevant cell types, cellular assays, and pharmacological agents, as we believe this could reveal new layers of convergence which, in turn, could inform biology of psychiatric disease. The resulting data base and resource would be relevant to many research studies of the brain. Brain CMAP perturbation could inform which types of stimuli would most likely unmask relevant functional differences in brain cells with different polygenic risk background.

R5: Establish a Mental Health Biobank

Our high/low PRS design is dependent on relatively large samples with and without recorded diagnosis (e.g., SCZ) together with genotype data to generate

PRS and biological samples to allow generation of cell lines. The impact of the design is maximized if cellular phenotypes can be correlated with in-person phenotypes, because it prepares for a future cell-based precision medicine platform. To support this design, we recommend that a mental health biobank be established to provide longitudinal clinical phenotypes and matched biological samples of people diagnosed with psychiatric disorders. Such a biobank would have considerable impact across the breadth of research in psychiatry. Common disease research has benefited massively from the UK Biobank project, where 500,000 people have been measured for hundreds of phenotypes as well as genome-wide genotypes. Such volunteer biobanks, however, underrepresent people with psychiatric disorders. Thus, the biobank needs to be established in collaboration with participants and other relevant stakeholders to ensure engagement with such an initiative. Avoiding pitfalls of stigmatization, the mental health community deserves the same opportunities to benefit from technological advances applied in other branches of medicine.

R6: Establish a Cross-Species Brain Gene Expression Resource

Having a comprehensive gene expression atlas will benefit the field if it captures multiple brain regions (e.g., prefrontal cortex, hippocampus, basal ganglia, cerebellum) at cellular resolution (e.g., neurons, oligodendrocytes, microglia, astrocytes), across developmental time points (e.g., embryonic, postnatal, adolescence, adult), and matched across multiple species (e.g., human, marmoset, mouse) (Figure 8.4). Some research questions cannot be addressed in human cellular models, and different species provide different experimental paradigms for the investigation of mechanisms. The resource could be designed to include gene expression changes resulting from specific perturbations that can be imposed in more than one species, in conjunction with phenotypes that transcend species. A matched resource for gene expression across species would support integration of results across paradigms and ensure early establishment of the direct relevance of results from animal models for human disease.

R7: Establish a Human Brain-QTL Resource

Extending the GTEx resource to include brain cell types brings another general benefit to the field. The SNP-gene eQTL associations from GTEx are a key resource for integration with GWAS SNP-trait associations. GTEx includes data from 11 brain regions, although the associations are at the level of bulk tissue rather than individual cell type. GTEx has demonstrated that highly significant associations can be identified from relatively small sample sizes (N ~100). Although postmortem brains are a scarce resource, the power of a brain-QTL study could be enhanced by sourcing different brain regions from different individuals so that gene expression measures from different brain regions are not correlated; this would increase the specificity with which cell type-specific

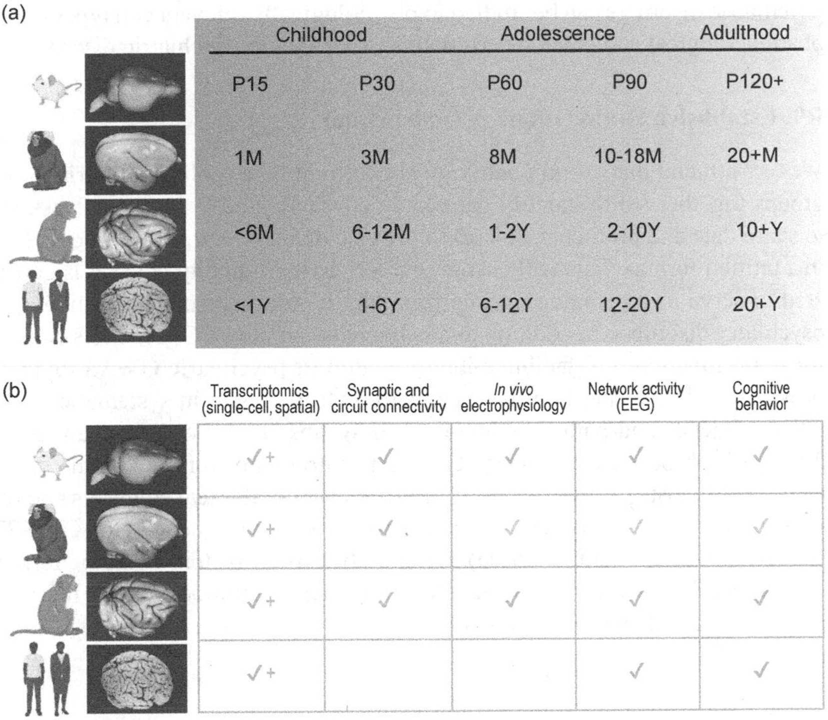

(a)

Childhood		Adolescence		Adulthood
P15	P30	P60	P90	P120+
1M	3M	8M	10-18M	20+M
<6M	6-12M	1-2Y	2-10Y	10+Y
<1Y	1-6Y	6-12Y	12-20Y	20+Y

(b)

Transcriptomics (single-cell, spatial)	Synaptic and circuit connectivity	*In vivo* electrophysiology	Network activity (EEG)	Cognitive behavior
✓+	✓	✓	✓	✓
✓+	✓	✓	✓	✓
✓+	✓	✓	✓	✓
✓+			✓	✓

Figure 8.4 Neurodevelopmental timing in mouse, marmoset, macaque, and human. Approximate cross-species alignment of postnatal developmental ages is based on brain transcriptomics (Kang et al. 2011; Zhu et al. 2018), structural neuroimaging (Sawiak et al. 2018), and cellular neuroanatomy (Charvet 2020; Charvet and Finlay 2018; Charvet et al. 2022). Species icons from Biorender.com; brain images from brainmuseum.org. Figure prepared by Matthew Johnson.

QTL could be identified. The same resource could be used for expression and chromatin accessibility QTL. For a discussion of the existing gaps in brain-QTL resources, see Hu and Won (this volume).

R8: Establish a Brain-IGVF

We recommend that the scope of the Impact of Genomic Variation on Function (IGVF) Consortium be broadened to include a focus on brain cell types. IGVF was launched (a) to interrogate the functional impact of variants via; perturbation experiments such as MPRA and CRISPR engineering, (b) to establish cell type-specific regulatory networks, and (c) to develop a computational model to predict the variant function on phenotypes. The initiative, however, is not focused on generating brain-centric data sets. Thus, resulting data may not be readily applicable to risk variants of psychiatric disorders. We propose a Brain-IGVF consortium in which the functional impact of variants associated with psychiatric disorders can be studied in physiologically relevant cell types under pharmacological and genetic perturbations relevant to psychiatric disorders.

R9: Establish a Brain Ontology Consortium

We recommend that a brain ontology consortium be established to bring core groups together (a) to identify gaps and coordinate and synergize efforts, (b) to share data and protocols, and (c) to provide quality control and process data in a unified format. This will ensure that a rich, high-quality data set is generated to serve as a resource for interrogating the mechanisms which underpin psychiatry disorders. In addition to the manually curated GO, gene sets curated for brain function will facilitate interpretation of psychiatric GWAS. SynGO provides a clear example of how concerted efforts result in systematic annotation of genes and pathways involved in synapse biology (Koopmans et al. 2019). We propose extending SynGO, as a central repository of "brain-centric GO," which hosts manually curated brain-relevant biological pathways and the growing list of gene sets derived from perturbation experiments (e.g., CRISPR screens, drug treatment response). Ultimately, this repository could be further expanded to serve as a central data platform where multimodal data is held and accessible for integrative analyses.

9

Hypotheses of How Common Variants Create Risk for Psychiatric Disorders

Naomi R. Wray

Abstract

Over the last 15 years, genome-wide association studies have demonstrated that psychiatric disorders, like other common diseases, are highly polygenic. The traditional toolbox of approaches used to characterize functional effects of causal genetic variants has been constructed for monogenic disease, where a single variant is associated with a high probability of disease risk at some point in the lifetime. This toolbox has limited utility for studying risk variants of small effect. To develop new experimental paradigms requires a deep understanding of polygenic architectures. First, many risk variants have small effect, which means most people with each variant do not have the disease associated with the risk. Disease is associated with carrying a high burden of risk variants, implying that the function of each risk variant is dependent on its genetic context. Second, each person diagnosed with a common disease is expected to carry a unique, or almost unique, portfolio of risk variants. Yet despite this heterogeneous genetic architecture, diagnostic classes do have some biological validity. Third, as observed for other common diseases, we expect there to be multiple pathways that contribute to increased risk of disease across many cell types and impacting over the lifespan. The key question then is how to penetrate this polygenic complexity.

Introduction

Genome-wide association studies (GWASs) have identified hundreds of loci associated with psychiatric disorders. A key question for the field is how to translate these findings into clinical utility. Traditional laboratory approaches are tailored for studying rare variants of very large effect associated with rare diseases. Even then, when large effect mutations have been identified, the journey from discovery to actionable outcomes for prevention or treatment can be long. For example, causal variants in *HTT*, *SOD1*, *BRCA1*, and

APOE associated with Huntington disease, amyotrophic lateral sclerosis, breast cancer and Alzheimer disease, respectively, were all discovered around two decades ago. While these discoveries have furthered mechanistic understanding of their diseases, translation to new treatments has been limited. New approaches are starting to be developed that aim to penetrate the complexity of how a polygenic architecture creates risk for psychiatric disorders. Here, I explore the fundamental concepts of a polygenic architecture, contrast psychiatric disorders with other polygenic diseases and traits, and consider experimental designs that embrace this polygenicity.

The Different Facets of Polygenicity

The face value description of a polygenic disease, that thousands of DNA variants contribute to risk of disease, seems straightforward. But what does this population description mean for individual people within the population? How do we reconcile the key observations of thousands of risk loci, increased risk in relatives (reflecting the heritability of the disease), and the fact that even common diseases only affect a minority of people? Key to understanding the nature of polygenic disease are some fundamental concepts of quantitative genetics, summarized in this section; for a more in-depth discussion, see Baselmans et al (2021). The term "polygenic" covers many different genetic architectures defined as the number of risk variants, the population frequency of those risk variants, and their effect sizes. How does the polygenicity of psychiatric disorders contrast to that of other diseases and disorders, and can we learn anything from this?

Each Person Has a Unique Portfolio of Risk Variants

A key feature of polygenic disease is that each person with the same disease diagnosis is expected to have a unique portfolio of risk variants, some of which may include variants of relatively large effect. In fact, it is now recognized that even classical monogenic diseases are more accurately classified as polygenic diseases that include a very large effect variant. For example, consider Huntington disease, which is the textbook example of monogenic autosomal dominant disease. All those affected have an expanded copy number of a trinucleotide repeat near the gene *HTT*, with a higher expansion number associated with age of onset. Nonetheless, the Genetic Modifiers of Huntington Disease Consortium has identified 21 independent single nucleotide polymorphisms (SNPs) associated with age of onset from a sample size of 15,000 cases (Lee et al. 2019b), thus illustrating how genetic context of the *HTT* mutation is important. Moreover, genetic architecture signals from these data are consistent with an expectation that more associated SNPs will be identified with larger sample size. In studies of large effect variants associated with common disease (e.g., familial hypercholesterolemia variants associated with heart disease, *BRCA1* or *BRCA2* variants associated with breast or ovarian cancer, and colorectal cancer Lynch syndrome), high estimated risk constructed from the polygenic burden is associated with earlier age of onset or greater severity of disease compared to monogenic variant carriers with low estimated polygenic risk (Fahed et al. 2020). Examples more relevant to psychiatry are the copy number variants such as deletions in 1q21.1, 15q13.3, or 16p11.2 seen in the context of epilepsy, autism, mental retardation, or schizophrenia diagnoses. The association with multiple diagnoses likely reflects the genetic background in which the deletion events have occurred. An important consideration for polygenic disease is that all people carry a burden of risk variants for each disease, but only those that carry a high burden of risk variants (and other risk factors) will develop symptoms that lead to disease diagnosis. A polygenic model is consistent with biological robustness since the vast majority of risk variant portfolios carried by individuals does not increase risk of disease.

Additive on Liability Scale but Nonadditive on the Disease Status Scale

Modeling polygenicity suggests that complex biological interactions govern the relationship between polygenic variation and disease. The liability threshold model (LTM) is a working model for common polygenic disease. The model was developed over 70 years ago (Falconer 1965) and is based on the infinitesimal model (all DNA variants contribute a small effect to each trait). The last decades have not provided empirical data to reject the LTM as a useful working model even though estimates from genetic architecture modeling suggest only 1–5% of common SNPs are likely to contribute to each disease (Zeng et al. 2021), but estimates are higher for psychiatric disorders than other diseases discussed below. Indeed, the estimated number of contributing variants is still exceptionally high (tens of thousands) and so the conceptual utility of the model is retained (and in fact the utility of the LTM holds even if there are as few at ten risk variants). The LTM is just one of a suite of models that all imply the same shape of relationship between polygenic burden and risk of disease (Slatkin 2008), but it is usually the model of choice because of its mathematical tractability. The shape of this relationship is very nonlinear, which is the only way to reconcile the two key parameters defining disease: heritability and relatively low lifetime risk of disease. The nonlinear relationship between polygenic burden and disease risk is more nonlinear for diseases that are less common and/or that have heritability. Hence, interaction effects are expected for the biological function of risk variants acting together. However, since all people carry a different portfolio of risk loci, the traditional tools for studying interaction which investigate interactions between only a few loci (usually only two) is unlikely to be useful. The interaction is on a scale of so many variants and many different combinations of variants that disease modeling focuses on additivity to liability disease. Hence a key concept is that polygenic disease implies additivity of effects on the liability to disease scale and massive nonadditivity on the risk of disease scale. In a recent review (Baselmans et al. 2021), I tried to explain these concepts in depth in the context of psychiatric disorders.

Are Psychiatric Disorders More Polygenic than Other Common Diseases and Disorders?

In the post-GWAS era, many methods have been developed to evaluate genetic architecture from the distribution of SNP effects reported in GWAS summary statistics. For example, for any trait, the SbayesS (summary-based Bayes method estimating the S-parameter) provides estimates of the contribution of common SNP variation to the trait (SNP-based heritability), the proportion of all SNPs that contribute to the trait (polygenicity), and the correlation between minor allele frequency and effect size ("S," an indicator of selection pressure) (Zeng et al. 2021). These values can be meaningfully compared across traits when the same common SNP set is used. In an SbayesS analysis applied to 18 common diseases (Figure 9.1), GWAS summary statistics for both schizophrenia and bipolar disorder provided strong evidence for negative selection S (~ -0.7). Notably, this was similar to, but not greater than, the estimates for other diseases. It also showed exceptionally high polygenicity (consistent with estimates from other methods, e.g., Ripke et al. 2013). The average polygenicity across the 44 traits studied was ~1%, compared to 5% for schizophrenia and 3% of bipolar disorder, which were significantly higher than for other diseases (Zeng et al. 2021).

It could be argued that high levels of polygenicity for disorders of the brain are to be expected; the brain is such an important organ that many backup pathways exist, consistent with biological robustness. However, it is worth considering whether any artifact could contribute to the observation of the exceptionally high levels of polygenicity. Psychiatric disorders are always described as being very heterogeneous. Thus, we must consider the possibility that empirical estimates of polygenicity are a reflection of the same disease labels being attached to biologically distinct disorders. To illustrate this, Wray and Maier (2014) considered the following toy example: Imagine that a disease labeled A with population lifetime risk of ~1% is actually comprised of two biologically distinct diseases, B and C, each with a population lifetime risk of 0.5% that are impossible to differentiate based on clinical presentation. Assume diseases B and C have a heritability of 80% but being biologically distinct have independent risk variants. The heritability of composite disease A would be estimated to be substantial (~65%), using the standard approach of increased risk observed in first degree relatives (the estimate would be lower if increased risks from more distant relatives are used). In a GWAS, however, the composite disease A has much reduced power compared to the biologically distinct diseases of B and C. If the true SNP-based heritabilities of diseases B

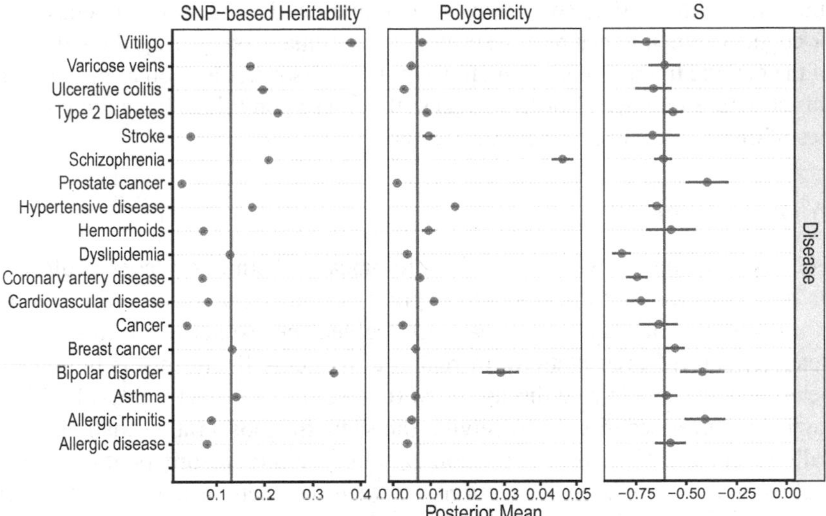

Figure 9.1 Genetic architecture parameters for 18 common diseases, showing the posterior means (dots) and standard errors (horizontal bars) of the parameters for each trait. Data from Zeng et al. (2021; see Figure 2) estimated from GWAS summary statistics using SBayesS. SNP-based heritability is the proportion of variance in liability attributable to common SNPs. The polygenicity parameter is an estimate of the proportion of common SNPs associated with the disease. S is a selection parameter and represents the relationship between allele frequency and effect size (negative values imply selection against the disease).

and C were the same, then the SNP-based heritability of disease A would be estimated as 50% of the value, and it would make sense to infer that estimates of polygenicity would be higher for A than if estimated separately for B and C.

As we consider the genetic architecture of psychiatric disorders, it is worth keeping in mind the potential heterogeneity of biological disease that underpins a diagnosis applied to symptoms. We should not forget to challenge basic assumptions made in our foundational analyses. That said, the toy example described is extreme and, in fact, implies nonadditivity on the liability scale of disease A, which would likely give unusual properties of the joint distribution of GWAS effects which have not been observed. Data sets which include deep phenotyping are needed to provide an evidence base to conclude if the higher polygenicity estimated for psychiatric disorders than for other diseases is inherent or a reflection of biological heterogeneity not reflected in current nosology.

The Relationship between Polygenicity and Disorder

The complexity and polygenicity revealed by genetic studies of psychiatric disorders raise the question whether they are true disorders as opposed to difficult-to-differentiate collections of multiple conditions, or even behavioral or cognitive phenotypes best described as continua. Considering the structure of the genetic findings pertaining to psychiatric disorders as well as comparing this structure to other disorders suggest that these conditions have the properties of disorders, however heterogeneous.

What Is a Disorder?

The toy example above, where two biologically distinct diseases could not be distinguished in clinical settings, points to an important question: What is a disorder label, and is it meaningful given the extensive discussions of heterogeneity of presentation? In real life, it seems likely that if biological heterogeneity underpins a disease, then this would happen at the level of biologically correlated diseases receiving the same diagnosis rather than biologically independent diseases. In the context of psychiatric disorders, it is notable that estimates of genetic correlations between data sets of the same disorder are consistently higher than estimates of genetic correlations between different psychiatric disorders (Cross-Disorder Group of the Psychiatric Genomics Consortium et al. 2013), implying that the standard nosology does have biological support. Moreover, estimates of genetic correlations between data sets of the same disorder, which are expected to be 1, are notably less than 1 for major depression and attention deficit hyperactivity disorders (Cross-Disorder Group of the Psychiatric Genomics et al. 2013), likely a reflection on the recognized heterogeneity in diagnosis within and between data sets.

Genetic analyses of rare and common variants in developmental delay and autism spectrum disorder clearly demonstrate that genetic architecture and diagnostic labels are not perfectly aligned. For example, girls with a diagnosis of autism are more likely to harbor a large effect copy number variant than boys, despite a higher rate of diagnosis in boys. This is explained by the female protective effect, such that boys who carry the same large effect copy number variant are more likely to be diagnosed with of developmental delay (Robinson et al. 2014). Within those diagnosed with developmental delay, autistic behavior is found to be significantly associated with the polygenic score of autism ($p=2.5 \times 10^{-4}$), and severity of intellectual disability is significantly associated ($p=4.0 \times 10^{-3}$) with the polygene score educational attainment (Niemi et al. 2018).

Learning from Other Common Complex Diseases

Practicing psychiatrists always emphasize the heterogeneity in clinical presentation associated with each diagnostic category and that few individuals fit the classic textbook definitions of disorder diagnoses. Since diagnosis within psychiatry is based on interview criteria rather than any gold standard biological biomarker, there may be a perception that this heterogeneity is not present in other disorders. In fact, heterogeneity in presentation seems to be the norm in all common diseases. Let us take type II diabetes as an example. Arguably, more is understood about the functional impairment of insulin secretion from the pancreas than is known about functional causes or consequences of psychiatric disorders within the brain. Yet multiple pathways are known to contribute to type II diabetes (Udler et al. 2019), including pathways of insulin secretion, insulin resistance, and dyslipidemia (Figure 9.2). One appealing hypothesis has been to use these pathways to allocate people to diabetes subtypes; however, recent research rejects this as being naïve (McCarthy 2017). To understand a polygenic disorder with many contributing pathways, McCarthy (2017) introduced the concept of the palette model as a visual analogy. An artist's paint palette comprises a set of primary colors (representing biological mechanisms), and each person has a personal mix of these colors, allowing many combinations to reach the diagnosis (McCarthy 2017). It is unlikely for a person's color to be dominated by a single color, so by analogy few people can be allocated to specific subtypes defined by these pathways. This conceptualization is consistent with the long-held view of polygenicity and can be equally relevant and helpful when representing psychiatric disorders. Learning from the type II diabetes research community, it would be unwise to invest heavily in research on a pathway-specific model for psychiatric disorders. If pathway-specific considerations are relevant in the identification of personalized treatments, then these

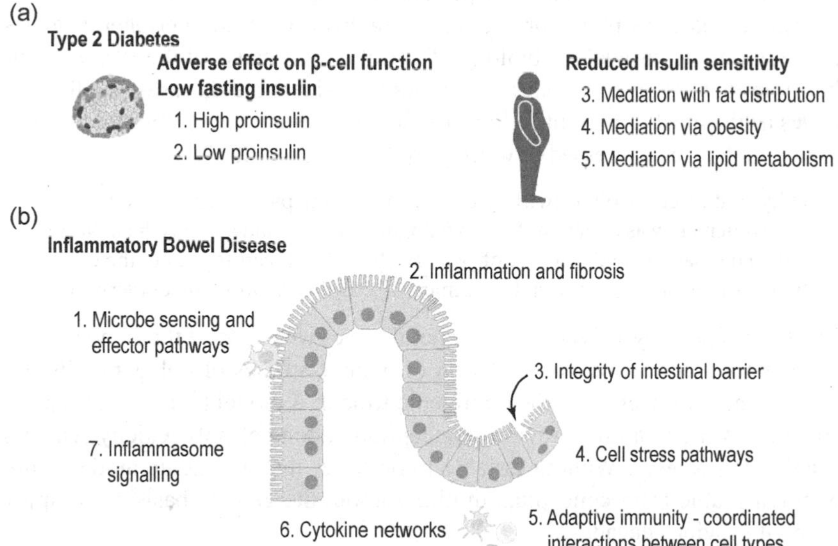

Figure 9.2 Pathway paradigms highlighted by genetics: (a) type II diabetes (Udler et al. 2019) and (b) inflammatory bowel diseases (Graham and Xavier 2020). Created with BioRender.com.

will likely emerge through research that does not specifically set out with this goal in mind.

Another useful benchmark for psychiatric disorders is to consider inflammatory bowel diseases, for which much more is known about the functional mechanisms underlying genetic associations. Graham and Xavier (2020) show seven pathways that contribute to risk of these diseases (summarized in Figure 9.2). We anticipate a similar complexity for psychiatric disorders, implying that the heterogeneous diagnostic construct is likely unavoidable. Research clarifying the contributing mechanistic pathways is emerging and will be important in understanding mechanistic pathways, but it is unlikely that these will contribute to disease subtyping.

Common Diseases Are More Complex than Implied by the Omnigenic Model

For over 100 years the infinitesimal model has been used to conceptualize polygenic traits and diseases, and its utility has not been rejected despite extensive empirical testing. In 2017, the omnigenic model was introduced as a conceptual framework to offer a mechanistic explanation for why so many variants spread across the genome can be responsible for the genetic variation between people observed for complex traits and common disease (Boyle et al. 2017). In brief, the underlying logic is that variants with *cis* effects on genes considered "peripheral" to disease pathways perturb the regulation of a smaller class of core genes via *trans*-regulatory networks. In this way, these "peripheral" genes are important to unravel the biology of a trait only because of their *trans*-regulatory influences on core genes. The model considers the disease-specific core genes as the most important for disease-specific research. A common response to the model was expressed in writing by Nancy Cox (2017):

> [M]y first reaction to the swirling discussions of the paper was to wonder what the excitement was all about. How would anyone who understands the nature of polygenic liability and is aware of what we have been learning about the contribution of regulatory variation to common disease heritability think otherwise?

The terms core, key, driver, and peripheral genes were part of the standard vernacular for mechanistic interpretation of genetic studies of polygenic disease prior to the introduction of the omnigenic model. A model that is a conceptual advance over and above previous conceptualizations of polygenicity requires testable hypotheses. Without testable hypotheses the omnigenic model is not distinguishable from conceptual thinking about the genetic basis of complex traits of previous decades.

Sinnott-Armstrong et al. (2021) set out to test one major component of the model, namely the identities and roles of core genes. Recognizing that this cannot be achieved with data from common disease, they took a step back in complexity and looked at molecular traits, where a strong relationship between trait variation and DNA variation can be expected and for which the omnigenic model is more plausible. They chose three blood traits from the UK Biobank: urate, IGF-1, and testosterone. As has been shown by others for blood-derived measures (e.g., Ruth et al. 2020), many of the lead association signals are very highly significant and interpretable in terms of the known physiology of the traits. Hence, the genes identified can rightly be considered core genes that reflect core pathways. Despite this level of interpretability, these traits are also highly polygenic, with the association signal attributed to core pathways explaining < 10% of the SNP-based heritability. Moreover, Sinnott-Armstrong et al. (2021) conclude that testing the second part of the omnigenic model (that most of the genetic association passes through *trans*-regulatory networks) is intractable given the sample sizes needed, even for these molecular traits. From their work, it seems clear that the omnigenic model is too simplistic to explain common disease, which likely comprises the overlaying of hundreds of these simple molecular traits. There is no need to abandon the existing models of polygenic disease, which better describes the complexity of common disease (Wray et al. 2018b). One reason to speak out against the omnigenic model is that it has been used as a call-to-arms for the identification of core genes for common disease and for reinvigoration of experimental paradigms used for monogenic disease. New experimental designs that embrace the polygenic architecture of disease are needed to further understand common diseases, including psychiatric disorders.

Experimental Designs that Embrace Polygenicity

Drawing on some of the key observations of polygenic disease discussed above, let us consider how these can inform new designs for understanding functional mechanisms of complex diseases:

1. Common diseases are highly epistatic on the scale of disease risk, which means that the function of the variant is dependent on its genetic context. In most genetic backgrounds, the risk variant does not lead to a disease status.
2. Each person diagnosed with a common disease is expected to carry a unique or almost unique portfolio of risk variants. Despite this, individuals share a diagnosis that has some biological validity (i.e., higher genetic correlations between cohorts of the same disorder than between cohorts with different disorders).
3. As observed for other common diseases (e.g., type II diabetes and inflammatory bowel diseases), we expect there to be multiple pathways that contribute to an increased risk of disease across many cell types and impacting over the lifespan.

The question is: How can we penetrate this polygenic complexity?

It is likely that different subsets of risk variants act in different cell types at different time points throughout development and aging. The consequence of any one such subset could be very subtle. For example, some risk variants could set up a vulnerable cellular infrastructure simply through the speed of cell differentiation, the composition of cell types, or cell morphology and function. A vulnerable basic infrastructure could then compound the impact of other genetic risk variants associated with synaptic pruning during adolescence and these effects could be enhanced through environmental stress exposures. While studying one gene at a time (as is traditionally done for monogenic disease) will add value to our knowledge base, I believe that to impact the lives of those affected by psychiatric disorders more quickly (both now and in the future), experimental designs that embrace the polygenicity better must be developed. Below we consider two relevant paradigms.

Extreme of Polygenic Score Design

An experimental design which acknowledges that all people carry risk variants, that those affected carry a higher burden, and that each person carries a unique portfolio requires us to study the cellular/organoid phenotypes of those at the extremes of the polygenic score (PGS) distribution. Based on current GWASs, there is a fortyfold difference in risk between those in the top centile versus bottom centile of the PGS distribution (Trubetskoy et al. 2022). Of course, this approach requires collection of genetic data on very large cohorts of individuals to identify those at the extremes, and the recontacting of participants is likely needed to generate cell lines. The extreme PGS approach has been pioneered in the Brennand lab (Dobrindt et al. 2021) selecting six high and six low PGS lines from existing population-based cell lines (from healthy individuals). Going forward it makes sense to contrast high/low PRS lines using those who do and do not have disease. Given that each individual has a different portfolio of risk variants, cellular phenotypes need to be associated with all (or a high proportion) of those in the group "high PRS and disease" compared to those with low PRS. Induced pluripotent stem cell phenotypes are starting to be associated with clinical phenotype (e.g., circadian rhythm phenotypes in the context of bipolar disorder) (Sanghani et al. 2021).

Integration of GWAS Results with Single-Cell RNA Sequencing

The GWAS era has generated a host of post-GWAS analyses in which many different types of independently collected reference data can be integrated with the GWAS associations linked via SNPs or SNPs annotated to genes (Pasaniuc and Price 2017). At the level of the gene unit, integration allows reference data sets to be generated in animal models. For many other common diseases much is known about the most relevant cell types within specific tissues most affected by the disease (e.g., see Figure 9.2). However, for psychiatric disorders where the prefrontal cortex is recognized as the brain region of relevance, knowledge of the role of specific cell types is less clear. A number of methods have been proposed that integrate GWAS gene associations with genes enriched with expression in specific cell types (Timshel et al. 2020; Zhu et al. 2020). Disassociation of single cells from human brain tissue is more difficult than for other tissues, so RNA sequencing data sets for brain tend to be from single nuclei if using human brain and only from the whole cell if using mouse brain (which, of course, may not have the complete suite of cell types or cell subtypes present in humans). Application of these methods to diseases where specific, relevant cell types have been identified by histology and other research methods provides verification of these approaches. For example, GWAS for inflammatory bowel disease point to cells in the colon and ileum, whereas for diverticular disease (sac-like protrusions of the colon sigmoid) they point to cells in the colon sigmoid, consistent with known pathology (Wu et al., submitted). When these methods are applied to schizophrenia, pyramidal neurons are identified from both human and mouse tissue, with the evidence strengthening with larger GWASs (Trubetskoy et al. 2022). A limitation of these studies is that they are dependent on the cell types present in the data sets. More reference data sets are needed to build a more complete picture of the cell types in which the genetic risk factors likely operate.

Conclusion

Psychiatric disorders, like other common diseases, have a polygenic genetic architecture. This implies that all individuals likely carry thousands of risk variants for each disease, but those most vulnerable carry a higher burden, each with a unique portfolio. Under this architecture, the consequences of each associated variant or gene seems irrelevant since disease only results when the variants are present in the context of other genetic or nongenetic risk factors. New experimental paradigms are needed to study sets of genetic variants jointly.

Acknowledgment

I acknowledge funding from the Australian National Health & Medical Research Council 1113400, 1173790.

10

From Common Variant to Function

State-of-the-Art Approaches

Ellen Hu and Hyejung Won

Abstract

Genome-wide association studies (GWASs) have been integral to our understanding of the polygenic architecture of psychiatric disorders, yet distilling disease biology from GWAS remains a challenge because GWAS-identified genomic regions often contain dozens of variants with highly correlated structure. The majority of variants within these loci are located within the noncoding genome, so their functional consequences are not immediately apparent. Moreover, to characterize thousands of such variants requires a highly scalable experimental approach. Such systematic interrogation of the functional consequences of variants is enabled by population-scale molecular assays (e.g., quantitative trait loci) or scalable genomic perturbation assays (e.g., massively parallel reporter assays or CRISPR screens). This review describes available genomic resources and cutting-edge experimental approaches that have been adopted to infer functional consequences of risk variants. Additionally, it outlines gaps in defining causal variants, linking variants to target genes, interrogating combinatorial effects of variants within the polygenic background, and considering the context-specific nature of variants. Extended efforts to fill these gaps will enable more comprehensive interpretation of GWAS and ultimately reveal the fundamental biological context behind polygenic psychiatric disorders.

Introduction

Despite the success of genome-wide association studies (GWASs) in identifying common variants associated with psychiatric disorders, specific properties of common risk variants pose a unique challenge for interpreting their functions. The traditional strategy to link (*de novo*) rare variants to function is to identify their impact on protein function. Since rare variants are often located in protein-coding sequences, this strategy is often straightforward. Nonetheless, two unique features of common variants distinguish them from rare variants, making the scientific approach to linking them to function extremely challenging. First, common variants exhibit a correlation structure with nearby variants due to linkage disequilibrium. Thus, a typical GWAS locus contains dozens to hundreds of variants with strong association signals, making it difficult to identify which variants are playing a causal role in disease etiology. Second, over 90% of common variants are in the noncoding genome (Watanabe et al. 2019b). Unlike variants located in protein-coding genes, we often do not know the function of noncoding variants, as they are likely involved in complex, cell-type, and context-dependent gene regulatory activities. Strategies that have been used to decipher the impact of rare variants on psychiatric disorders are thus not directly applicable to common variants where we do not expect direct impact on single protein function by coding sequence changes but effects on the regulatory fine-tuning of gene expression.

What Is the Definition of Causal Variants?

A challenge in the field is a lack of consensus on the definition of causal common variants. Computational fine mapping was initially used to identify putative causal or "credible" variants, which refer to the smallest set of variants that can explain the association statistics of a given GWAS locus including many correlated variants. We have previously shown that different fine-mapping algorithms can predict different sets of credible variants (Mah and Won 2020). This lack of reproducibility raises questions on how accurately any given fine-mapping algorithm can predict the most likely causal variants.

To address this issue, experimental approaches that measure the functional consequences of noncoding variants are now being increasingly used. For example, effects on gene regulatory activity can be assessed using massively parallel reporter assays (MPRA) and CRISPR editing. These assays measure the functional impact on gene regulation of a large number of risk variants simultaneously, based on the hypothesis that causal variants likely act through altered gene expression. MPRA adopts the design of a traditional luciferase assay, which has been used to study the regulatory activity of noncoding elements. A luciferase assay examines the ability of small sections of DNA that contain the variants of interest to modulate the expression of the reporter gene, luciferase, which can be read out via luminescence. Whereas luminescence of luciferase is measured as readouts for regulatory activity in luciferase assays, random barcode expression is measured as readouts for regulatory activity in MPRA via RNA sequencing, greatly increasing its throughput (Figure 10.1a). MPRA permits rapid testing of regulatory effects of many variants in a single experiment and identifies variants with differential allelic regulatory effects (McAfee et al. 2022a).

CRISPR screens utilize nuclease-dead Cas9 (dCas9) fused with a repressor domain (KRAB; Yeo et al. 2018). After introducing guide-RNAs (gRNA) that target dCas9-KRAB to loci containing the variants of interest, gene expression profiles of nearby genes are measured by RNA sequencing (Figure 10.1b). If a certain gene is up- or downregulated after introducing a gRNA, we can conclude that the targeted locus can contain a regulatory variant that affects expression of that gene. Therefore, regulatory regions carrying the variants of interest and many potential target genes can be interrogated in a single assay. While CRISPR screens also allow the testing of allele-specific differences, the scale of such experiments is far below those which just target putative regulatory regions that contain the variant.

Joint use of MPRA and CRISPR screens can comprehensively illuminate the variant function, at least with regard to gene regulatory functions. When used together, MPRA can identify variants with allelic regulatory activity at a scale beyond the capacity of CRISPR, whereas CRISPR screens can supplement the endogenous regulatory context and target genes of the variants.

Note again that the MPRA and CRISPR screens are powerful experimental strategies that depend on a prevailing hypothesis in the field; namely, that "functional regulatory variants" are "causal variants." It remains unknown, however, whether all functional regulatory variants with significant association signals are causal variants or whether causal variants are always engaged in gene regulatory function. Other options include indirect effects on gene regulation via noncoding RNAs or regulation of alternative splicing.

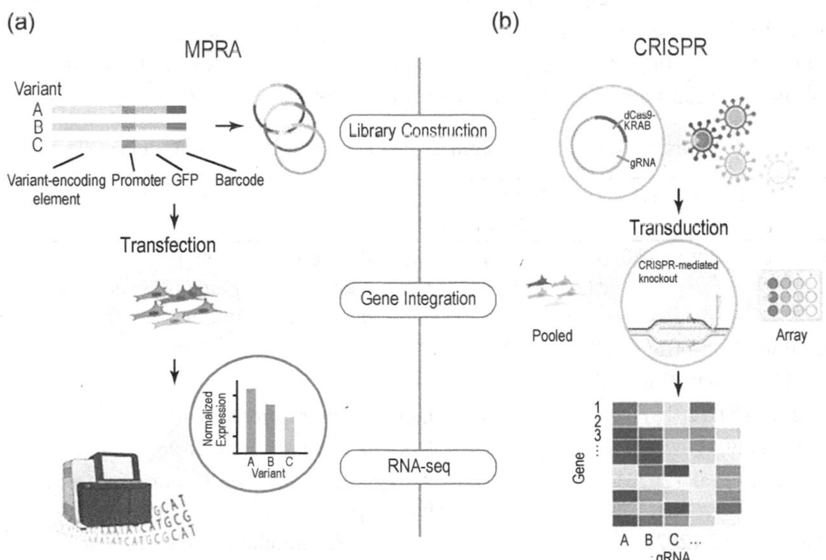

Figure 10.1 Schematic workflow of experimental assays (MPRA and CRISPR) for large-scale functional validation of genetic variants.

Development of additional experimental and computational strategies, as well as a standardized benchmark to define causal variants against, will be pivotal to unravel the role of variants in disease etiology. Alternative approaches are also discussed below.

Next we discuss how multi-omic data sets generated and made available through consortia-level efforts have enabled functional annotation of noncoding variants.

Population-Scale Molecular Assays to Link Variants to Genes

Population-scale RNA sequencing data combined with genotype provides a resource for expression quantitative trait loci (eQTL) that can correlate variants with gene expression levels. Because eQTLs can translate variant information to quantified gene expression, they have played a pivotal role in addressing the functional consequence of variants associated with human traits and diseases. Accordingly, compiling large eQTL resources has been the focus of many groups and consortia (Table 10.1). The NIH-funded GTEx Consortium was a pioneering effort that gathered RNA sequencing data from 838 individuals across 49 tissues that include multiple brain regions, such as the cortex, cerebellum, hippocampus, striatum, amygdala, and substantia nigra (GTEx Consortium 2020). The PsychENCODE Consortium generated a more comprehensive catalog of brain eQTLs by amassing dorsolateral prefrontal cortex (DLPFC) RNA sequencing data acquired from 1,387 individuals (Wang et al. 2018). Meta-analysis of multi-ancestry eQTLs further expanded this resource by profiling RNA sequencing data from 2,119 individuals, with focus on diverse ancestries for more non-European representation (Zeng et al. 2022).

Table 10.1 Existing resources of brain expression quantitative trait loci (eQTL).

Resources	Number of Individuals	Brain Regions or Cell Types
GTEx Consortium (2020)	≤209	Amygdala, cortex, cerebellum, hippocampus, hypothalamus, nucleus accumbens, putamen, substantia nigra
BrainSeq Consortium (2015)	738	Dorsolateral prefrontal cortex, hippocampus
PsychENCODE Consortium		
Wang et al. (2018)	1,387	Dorsolateral prefrontal cortex
Zeng et al. (2022)	2,119	Dorsolateral prefrontal cortex
de Klein et al. (2023)	6,518	Amygdala, basal ganglia, cortex, cerebellum, hippocampus, hypothalamus
Bryois et al. (2022)	196	Astrocytes, endothelial cells, excitatory/inhibitory neurons, microglia, oligodendrocytes, oligodendrocyte precursor cells, pericytes

More efforts are being undertaken to create a more comprehensive eQTL catalog that covers seven brain regions (de Klein et al. 2023) or different cell types (Bryois et al. 2022). Indeed, eQTL catalogs are now transitioning from sequencing bulk tissue to obtaining data with cell-type resolution using single-cell sequencing approaches.

While eQTL resources have been central to functionally interpreting GWAS-identified variants, currently available eQTL resources cannot explain all GWAS loci. According to current data, many genetic variants associated with psychiatric disorders do not exhibit detectable effects on gene expression in eQTL studies. For example, colocalization analysis between multi-ancestry brain eQTLs and joint GWAS of schizophrenia and bipolar disorder assigned only 20 out of 144 loci to genes (Zeng et al. 2022). One way to address this gap is to increase the scale of eQTL studies. However, increasing sample size to detect additional eQTLs in steady-state adult brain samples using bulk sequencing is approaching saturation (Wang et al. 2018; de Klein et al. 2023), so other strategies that target unexplored aspects of regulatory mechanisms may be a more effective target of focus. Below, we discuss some of the missing QTL resources that may be pivotal to closing the gap in the QTL approach to GWAS functional interpretation.

Quantitative Trait Loci for Different Molecular Assays

Changes in transcriptional regulation are only one kind of potential functional consequence of common or noncoding genetic variation. RNA species besides polyadenylated RNA, such as long noncoding RNA (lncRNA) and microRNA, have also been shown to play a critical role in gene regulation. However, single nucleotide polymorphism (SNP) associations with lncRNA and microRNA have not yet been evaluated comprehensively at the genome-wide level. QTLs that target these RNA species may identify unexplored mechanisms underlying psychiatric disorders. Promisingly, transcriptomic profiling of postmortem brain samples with psychiatric disorders has shown that many lncRNAs are dysregulated in psychiatric conditions (Gandal et al. 2018b). In addition, other noncoding RNAs, such as circular RNAs, should also be explored.

Another important transcriptional control occurs at the level of alternative splicing. Postmortem brain samples with schizophrenia show widespread dysregulation of splice isoforms (Gandal et al. 2018b), and processes involved with RNA splicing are associated with various psychiatric disorders (Sey et al. 2020), indicating that RNA splicing can provide imperative insights into disease biology. Variants associated with RNA splicing or isoform usage in the human brain have been identified by the detection of splice-QTLs and splicing-isoform QTLs (Li et al. 2016; Wang et al. 2018).

Chromatin QTLs (cQTLs) propose another functional explanation for the association between risk loci and disease mechanism. Specifically, analyzing variant effects on profiles of open-chromatin (from ATAC sequencing) gives chromatin accessibility QTLs (caQTLs), while that for specific chromatin marks (from ChIP-seq) gives histone QTLs (haQTLs). PsychENCODE pioneered the large-scale identification of brain caQTLs (Bryois et al. 2018) and haQTLs (Wang et al. 2018). Overlapping cQTLs with eQTLs can provide mechanistic insight into (a) how chromatin changes facilitate downstream effects on gene expression and (b) on the level of impact of the genetic variant.

Cell Type-Specific Quantitative Trait Loci

Another key limitation in the current eQTL resources is attributed to bulk RNA sequencing, where expression quantification is heavily affected by cellular heterogeneity. Since gene expression varies with cell type, QTL resources obtained from the bulk brain homogenate may lack cell type-specific regulatory variants that could have a strong impact on psychiatric disorders. Hence, identifying cell type-specific QTLs can help prioritize cell types with the largest impact on disease development.

A significant advancement in the identification of cell type-specific QTLs could be achieved by single-cell (sc)RNA sequencing, which solves the cellular heterogeneity issue with bulk sequencing by measuring gene expression at cellular resolution (Bryois et al. 2022). QTLs can be combined with scRNA sequencing to catch otherwise undetectable functional effects of variants that are specific to particular cell types. Large-scale scRNA sequencing data, however, is very expensive and suffers a low signal-to-noise ratio due to the sparsity of the data set; hence conducting such studies on large samples with robust expression profiles represents a practical challenge. When such a large-scale scRNA sequencing resource is not available, computational deconvolution methods by which cell type composition is inferred from bulk data can provide a potential alternative to the existing RNA sequencing data sets generated from the bulk brain samples. While current deconvolution methods are only modestly accurate (Kim-Hellmuth et al. 2020), once improved, they may provide a resourceful way to extract cell type-specific signatures from abundant existing bulk sequencing data.

In addition to cell type-specific QTLs, SNPs may affect the disease biology by regulating cellular proportions within tissue; in the case of brain tissue, this could have a large impact. The PsychENCODE Consortium has identified cell fraction QTLs, which indicate SNPs associated with variance in cell-type proportions, by deconvolving bulk RNA sequencing data with scRNA sequencing signatures as a reference (Wang et al. 2018). Fraction QTLs were found to explain a large portion of gene expression variability in the brain samples, implying that changes in cell composition can shape bulk expression profiles. This result suggests the possibility that variant impact on cell-type composition could provide additional insights beyond variant function within a cell type. Such fraction QTLs may emerge from genetic variants related to cell-type differentiation during development and may also moderate cell-type proportion changes over age. Taken together, cell type-specific QTLs and fraction QTLs can elucidate unexplored facets of variant function in psychiatric disorders.

Quantitative Trait Loci that Span Developmental Stages

Many psychiatric disorders are thought to have neurodevelopmental origins. Both gene expression and the regulatory landscape are highly variable across developmental stages (Kang et al. 2011; Li et al. 2018), supporting the idea that psychiatric disorders need to be characterized across critical stages of brain development. Enhancers in the developing human brain were found to be enriched in variants associated with psychiatric disorders, illustrating the importance of the regulatory landscape during neurogenesis to the etiology of psychiatric disorders (de la Torre-Ubieta et al. 2018; Spiess and Won 2020; Won et al. 2016).

To expand QTL resources across developmental stages, eQTLs have been compiled from fetal brains (Walker et al. 2019; Werling et al. 2020). Though many of these eQTLs are not entirely distinct to the fetal brain, their enrichment in psychiatric risk variants implies that mechanisms contributing to neuropsychiatric disease start as early as the fetal stage (Werling et al. 2020). The existence of fetal-specific eQTLs and identification of temporal-dominant eQTLs (prenatal- or postnatal-dominant; Werling et al. 2020) suggests that eQTLs exert varied effects on expression across developmental stages. Therefore, large-scale expression data across multiple developmental stages will be necessary to understand a crucial window for the development of psychiatric disorders.

Context-Specific Quantitative Trait Loci

Regulatory variants may require an external stimulus, such as a drug or environmental factor, to become activated. Response eQTLs and caQTLs have been identified in macrophages upon immune activation, demonstrating that some variants affect gene regulation only upon stimulation (Alasoo et al. 2018). Context-specific profiling of the human brain is sparse due to a lack of large data sets with environmental exposures and gene expression. Further exploration of context-specific QTLs may help explain why some GWAS loci have been linked to target genes but were not associated with changes in expression (Javierre et al. 2016); the loci may not have been studied under conditions necessary to activate variants, so experimenting with various stimuli may reveal the true variant function on gene expression.

Are Quantitative Trait Loci Gold Standards to Link GWAS to Function?

While refined QTL studies, such as those noted above, are needed to elucidate the full picture of variant effects on gene regulation, the importance of eQTL studies for linking GWAS hits to biological function has not been definitively established. For example, recent studies have suggested that eQTL studies and GWAS may identify different sets of variants driven by selective pressure (Mostafavi et al. 2022). Supporting this finding, over 60% of schizophrenia risk variants whose regulatory functions are validated by MPRA do not exhibit eQTL signals (McAfee et al. 2022b). Furthermore, MPRA-validated variants do not overlap with eQTLs mapped to genes with higher mutational constraints and richer functional annotations, compared to those that do overlap with eQTLs. The observed discrepancy can be partially explained by selective pressure: the episomal design of MPRA may not be subject to the selective pressure that depletes eQTLs around mutation-intolerant genes. Since eQTLs remain a dominant strategy to link GWAS to function, there is a need to develop and adopt additional genomic approaches for linking variants to genes that are immune to linkage disequilibrium structure and selective pressure. In the next section, we review how other types of functional genomic data sets offer such alternatives to investigate variant function and disease mechanism.

Functional Genomic Approaches to Annotate Variants

Studying chromatin architecture (e.g., chromatin accessibility, histone modifications, chromatin interaction profiles) provides a complementary opportunity to link GWAS variants to genes. For example, chromatin architecture may be well-suited for linking variants to genes that are under selective pressure. Mutation-intolerant genes associated with various human diseases (including schizophrenia; see Pardiñas et al. 2018) were shown to be depleted of eQTLs because deleterious regulatory variants for these genes may occur at low frequency in the population (Mostafavi et al. 2022). In contrast, mutation-intolerant genes were shown to have more complex regulatory architecture (e.g., enhancer-gene interactions) to buffer them from deleterious regulatory variants (Wang and Goldstein 2020). For those genes, chromatin architecture may allow for more comprehensive annotation of disease-associated variants.

Here, we will first use chromatin interaction profiles as an example to show how chromatin architecture has facilitated functional annotation of GWAS. Thereafter, we show how integration of multi-omics data sets can further improve variant-gene relationships.

Chromatin Interaction Profiles

Chromatin interaction maps, defined by chromosome conformation capture techniques (e.g., Hi-C), can supply insight on functional consequences of noncoding variants by linking them to the target genes. For example, if a variant A forms a loop with a gene B, it is postulated that the variant A may regulate gene B given their physical proximity (Figure 10.2).

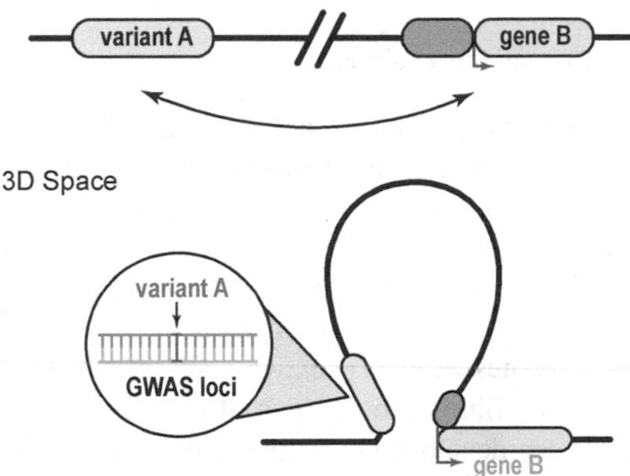

Figure 10.2 Three-dimensional proximity of variant A to gene B in a loop configuration suggests that variant A holds a regulatory role in the expression of gene B (e.g., via an enhancer-promoter interaction).

Chromatin interaction profiles have shown that over 80% of noncoding variants physically interact with distal genes (Sey et al. 2020). This underscores the importance of distal regulatory relationships in mapping variants to genes. Notably, chromatin interaction maps have been built across brain development and in different cell types (Pratt and Won 2022). These maps potentially facilitate the identification of genes associated with psychiatric disorders in a developmental stage and cell type-specific manner (Table 10.2).

The genome-wide nature of Hi-C allows unbiased characterization of interacting targets of all variants. This, together with the genome-wide gene mapping tool MAGMA, led to the development of H-MAGMA, which converts the search space from variants of unknown function to genes of well-characterized function leveraging chromatin interaction maps (de Leeuw et al. 2020; Sey et al. 2020). H-MAGMA aggregates variant-level association statistics to

Table 10.2 Existing resources of brain chromatin interaction profiles.

Reference	Brain region	Cell types	Developmental Stage
Won et al. (2016)	Cortex	Germinal zone, cortical plate	Fetal
Song et al. (2020)	Cortex	Radial glia, intermediate progenitors, excitatory and inhibitory neurons	Fetal
Nott et al. (2019)	Cortex	Neuron, microglia, oligodendrocyte	Pediatric
Wang et al. (2018)	Cortex	Brain homogenate	Adult
Hu et al. (2021)	Cortex	Neuron, glia	Adult
Sey et al. (2022)	Midbrain	Dopaminergic neuron	Adult

gene-level summary in a genome-wide fashion, allowing characterization of subthreshold loci or relatively low-powered GWAS.

Integrative Multi-omic Approaches

Advances in multi-omic experimental approaches and computational integrative analytic tools allow us to refine regulatory relationships between variants and genes. For example, chromatin interaction profiles can be combined with other epigenomic profiling to capture a specific type of chromatin interaction. HiChIP, a hybrid of Hi-C and ChIP-seq, not only identifies likely target genes of genetic variants on the basis of enhancer-promoter interactions, it also functionally annotates variants (i.e., whether variants reside in enhancers) (Mumbach et al. 2017). Similar to the idea of HiChIP, the activity-by-contact (ABC) model has been developed to combine enhancer activity and chromatin contact frequency to infer variant function (Fulco et al. 2019). This model proposes that the magnitude of variant effect and its target gene can be better predicted by taking both enhancer activity and chromatin contact frequency into account. The resulting ABC score was shown to outperform alternative models for predicting enhancer-promoter relationships. In addition, single-cell multi-omic profiling that integrates scRNA sequencing with scATAC sequencing allows us to infer relationships between chromatin accessibility and gene expression, which can be further extended to refine variant-gene expression relationships (Ma et al. 2020). Together, simultaneous dissection of multilayered molecular phenotypes can synergistically bridge the gap between variants and genes.

Beyond Cataloging

Assigning variants to genes they regulate is the first step to understand mechanisms by which common variants contribute risk for psychiatric disorders. The next step is to study the function of risk genes, which is in itself a challenge, especially considering the large number of genes identified from GWAS (e.g., H-MAGMA identified >5,000 genes associated with schizophrenia; Sey et al. 2020). Furthermore, different genomic approaches can give different sets of risk genes, resulting in a growing list of risk genes reported from different studies. So far, the field lacks a gold standard set of risk genes that can be benchmarked against risk genes identified from different genomic approaches. Transcriptomic data sets can be used to create such benchmarks by checking whether GWAS risk genes are dysregulated in psychiatric conditions. However, the majority of transcriptomic data sets are obtained from postmortem brain tissue, which does not accurately represent the onset of disease. Indeed, differential expression signatures from postmortem brain samples of schizophrenia showed weak to moderate association with schizophrenia heritability. This suggests that the accumulation of environmental exposures over the life course can dilute the effects of genetic risk factors on transcriptomic signatures (Yu et al. 2021). Human-induced pluripotent stem cells (hiPSCs) derived from individuals with psychiatric disorders could fill this gap by providing transcriptomic signatures in the early phase of the disease directly impacted by genetic risk factors. While hiPSC-based disease models have limitations, such as reduced cell maturity and inter-lab variance due to nonstandardized differentiation protocols, they still offer an accessible way to explore molecular landscapes of polygenic disorders that cannot be recapitulated by animal models. To implement transcriptomic signatures from hiPSC-derived models as a benchmark for GWAS risk genes, a standardized differentiation protocol as well as a large collection of hiPSCs with psychiatric disorders will be integral.

Once GWAS risk genes are prioritized, their function can be interrogated using traditional toolkits developed for studying monogenic disorders (e.g., knocking out a gene and measuring cellular and behavioral phenotypes). However, given the polygenic architecture of psychiatric disorders, their functional characterization demands a systems genetics approach. One such approach, Perturb-seq, provides a scalable method to test the functional impact of dozens of genes in a single assay by combining CRISPR gene perturbation with scRNA sequencing (Jin et al. 2020) (Figure 10.3). Single-cell expression profiling after CRISPR-mediated gene editing enables us to identify cell type-specific alterations in the transcriptomic architecture upon perturbation of psychiatric risk genes. Furthermore, *in vivo* application in animal models of Perturb-seq across developmental epochs or in response to specific external stimuli would allow temporal frame- and context-specific dissection of gene function.

Conclusion

A large compendium of common variants has been identified via GWAS to be associated with psychiatric disorders, proving their central role in psychiatric genetics. Common variants present multilayered challenges to functional interrogation due to their correlation structure, enrichment in the noncoding

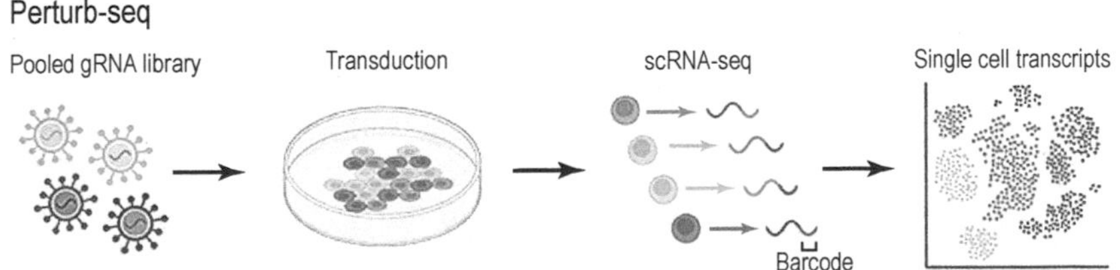

Figure 10.3 Perturb-seq merges a pooled CRISPR screen and scRNA sequencing for high-throughput identification of perturbation effects by cell type.

genome, and polygenic architecture. Such problems warrant tailored solutions for thorough investigation of polygenic disease etiology. One critical challenge lies in identifying causal variants and interrogating variant function, which can be advanced by high-throughput experimental strategies such as MPRA and CRISPR screens. However, the field needs to reach a consensus on how to define causal variants. Another critical challenge is to link variants to targetable genes. Population-scale molecular assays such as eQTLs have been playing a central role, whereas emerging evidence suggests that currently available eQTL resources alone may not lead to the complete understanding of GWAS. Here, we discussed complementary genomic resources to fill this gap (e.g., QTL resources that span multiple molecular assays, developmental stages, and cell types; multi-omic data sets that combine chromatin accessibility and interactions in a cell type-specific fashion). Finally, variant function needs to be extended to biological underpinnings that go beyond cataloging a new gene list. In linking variants to biology, we need to profile joint effects of the variants rather than characterizing individual variant effects to truly embrace the polygenic architecture of psychiatric disorders.

11

Contextualizing Convergent Common Variant Mechanisms through Systems Biology

Michael J. Gandal

Abstract

Psychiatric disorders are highly polygenic, with estimated contributions from hundreds to thousands of causal variants, across the allelic spectrum. Interpretation of such a widely distributed genetic risk architecture is a daunting challenge, as no single locus can explain disease etiology, yet it is also critical for mechanistic understanding and clinical translation. Systems biology can begin to contextualize genetic risk variation within our understanding of the hierarchical organization of the human brain, encompassing its cognate underlying cellular pathways and gene regulatory networks, cell types and states, cell–cell interactions, circuit-level function, and ultimately behavior. This chapter provides an overview of how high-throughput molecular "omic" profiling coupled with network-level inference can provide a framework for biological contextualization of established genetic risk factors to elucidate convergent disease mechanisms. Successes are highlighted leveraging systems biology to prioritize synaptic and chromatin complex genes, and next steps are enumerated to further the translational utility of these approaches.

Introduction

Large-scale genetic and genomic studies have now successfully identified hundreds of genetic loci robustly associated with risk for neuropsychiatric disorders. In schizophrenia (SCZ) and autism spectrum disorder (ASD), there are now well-established genome-wide significant contributions from common variants, recurrent large copy number variants (CNVs), and genes harboring rare protein-disrupting variants (Gandal et al. 2016; Marshall et al. 2017; Satterstrom et al. 2020; Singh et al. 2022; Trubetskoy et al. 2022). As gene discovery continues to move at a rapid pace, fueled by increasing cohort size and decreasing genotyping costs, the slow translation of associated variation into concrete molecular mechanisms—and ultimately therapeutic targets—remains a critical obstacle. This is particularly challenging in the context of daunting levels of polygenicity and incomplete penetrance, in which two unique affected individuals likely harbor distinct risk variant profiles. Consequently, it becomes imperative to decipher the convergent biological impact of multiple risk variants, both at the population level, to understand genetic pathophysiology more broadly, as well as within a given affected individual, to achieve the promise of "precision" medicine (Gandal et al. 2016).

Here, we address these challenges in the context of two major neuropsychiatric disorders—ASD and SCZ—which have similar estimates of heritability (~70%) and have been relatively well studied in terms of genetic risk architecture, functional genomics, and transcriptomics. Among neuropsychiatric disorders, ASD is the most advanced in terms of rare variant discovery from whole-exome sequencing (WES), whereas SCZ has the most well-powered genome-wide association study (GWAS), and both have well-established associations with recurrent CNVs (Gandal et al. 2016; Sullivan and Geschwind 2019). The principles described here are applicable for interpretation of genetic risk in other disorders, as gene discovery efforts catch up. Finally, discussion is limited to human genetics and functional genomics, as other chapters in this volume are devoted to approaches involving experimental and model systems.

State of Convergence

How can we begin to disentangle the relationship between hundreds to thousands of unique variants on complex brain-level cognitive and behavioral phenotypes? A key insight comes from the observation that for complex polygenic disorders, risk genes and molecules, although dispersed throughout the genome, often coalesce within specific "core" molecular pathways and cellular networks (Gilman et al. 2012; Parikshak et al. 2015). For psychiatric disorders, some of the first such glimpses were observed among rare syndromic forms of ASD, which appeared to converge at the synapse (Zoghbi 2003). As additional high-confidence ASD risk variants were subsequently uncovered through copy number variant profiling and WES, other pathways were implicated, including chromatin remodeling and gene regulation, in addition to synapse formation, neuronal cell adhesion, ubiquitination pathways, and targets of Fragile X mental retardation protein (FMRP), among others (De Rubeis et al. 2014; Glessner et al. 2009; Iossifov et al. 2014; Pinto et al. 2010; Sanders et al. 2015; Satterstrom et al. 2020). In SCZ, although the overall contribution of rare loss-of-function variation is smaller, similar convergence has been observed among synaptic and chromatin gene sets (Figure 11.1), as well as glutamate signaling, and FMRP targets, in particular (Fromer et al. 2014; Purcell et al. 2014; Singh et al. 2022).

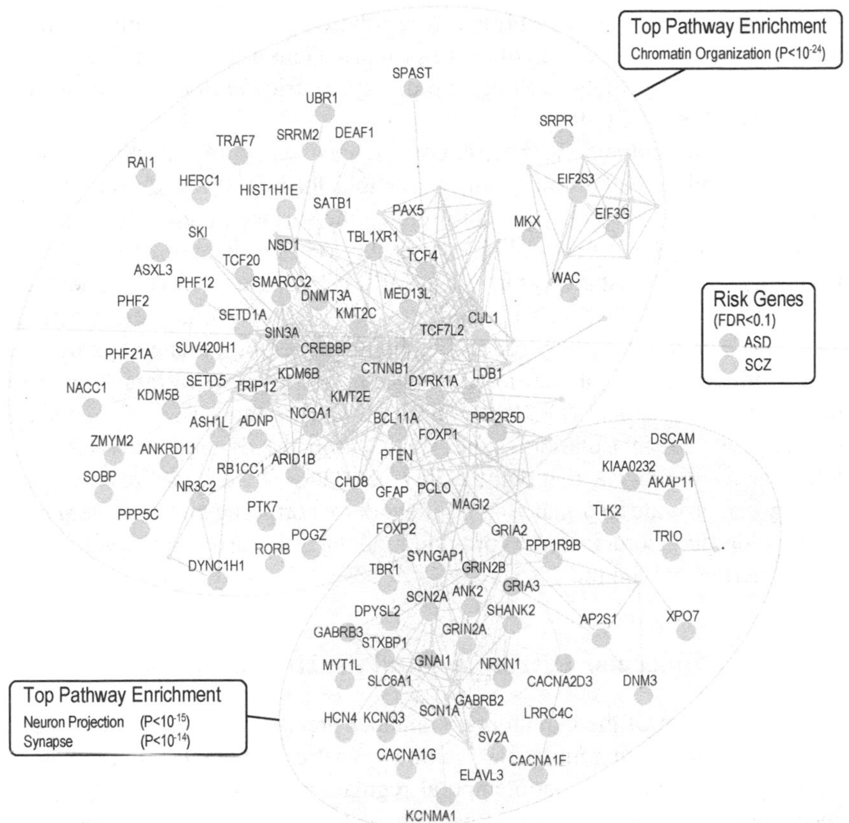

Figure 11.1 An interactome network of autism spectrum disorder (ASD) and schizophrenia (SCZ) risk genes highlights chromatin complex and synaptic gene clusters. A protein–protein interaction network seeded with rare variant implicated risk genes for ASD (n = 102 at FDR < 0.1; Satterstrom et al. 2020) and SCZ (n = 34 at FDR < 0.1; Singh et al. 2022) was built using StringDB (Szklarczyk et al. 2021). Two highly connected subclusters of the interactome network show distinct enrichments for chromatin organization and synapse pathways, as previously identified by (Sanders et al. 2015).

On the common variant side, the use of psychiatric GWAS to perform heritability enrichments (Finucane et al. 2015) and functional/proximity mapping (Watanabe et al. 2017) largely implicates similar pathways. Psychiatric GWASs are predominately enriched for brain tissues as well as neuronal cell types (Finucane et al. 2018; Gandal et al. 2018a; Skene et al. 2018; Xu et al. 2014). The most recent SCZ GWAS, which has the greatest power of any individual psychiatric GWAS, showed enrichment for gene sets that were largely synaptic and relatively nonspecific, such as "postsynaptic specialization" and "ion channel complex" (Trubetskoy et al. 2022). Cross-disorder psychiatric GWAS analyses further implicate synaptic, immune, and histone gene sets, as well as chromatin regulation in the developing human brain (Cross-Disorder Group of the Psychiatric Genomics Consortium 2019; Network Pathway Analysis Subgroup of Psychiatric Genomics Consortium 2015; Schork et al. 2019).

While these findings of "genetic convergence" provide a starting context for understanding pathobiology and a foothold for hypothesis-driven experimental dissection, they only begin to scratch the surface in terms of pinpointing overarching biological risk mechanisms with any degree of specificity. Convergence is almost always investigated at the population level, rather than within an individual where such findings are potentially much more actionable. These gene sets largely reflect manually curated or annotated pathways, often defined outside of the nervous system, although many are known to have distinct functional roles in the brain. Finally, gene set enrichments are typically viewed in isolation, rather than within the dynamic, diverse, and interconnected network that defines the CNS. Here, we discuss how systems biology can provide an organizing framework to interpret genetic convergence for psychiatric disorders and to provide modular, data-driven annotations for gene functions within the CNS.

Molecular Hierarchies and the Human Brain

The development of the human brain is under precise molecular genetic control, and the underlying molecular, cellular, genetic, and epigenetic regulatory landscape exhibits tight spatiotemporal regulation (Silbereis et al. 2016). As such, characterizing the dynamic patterns of gene expression and epigenetic changes in the brain throughout development can provide insights into the underlying regulatory logic defining neuronal cell types, states, as well as their maturation into functional neural circuits (Kang et al. 2011; Li et al. 2018). Along these lines, spurred by the rapid advent of high-throughput multi-omic profiling technologies, consortium-level efforts have been successful in mapping the whole-tissue transcriptome, epigenome, and proteome across developmental stages, brain regions, and sexes in neurotypical and psychiatric disease samples (Carlyle et al. 2017; Fromer et al. 2016; Gandal et al. 2018b; GTEx Consortium 2020; Hawrylycz et al. 2012; Jaffe et al. 2016, 2018; Kang et al. 2011; Li et al. 2018; Miller et al. 2014; Wang et al. 2018); see Figure 11.2.

The human brain has been most extensively genomically profiled at the level of the transcriptome, first with microarrays followed by bulk RNA sequencing and now with single-cell and spatial transcriptomic technologies. Initial seminal work from BrainSpan used microarrays to map gene expression trajectories across 1,340 tissue samples spanning 16 brain regions and 15 developmental timepoints, from 6 weeks postconception to 82 years (Kang et al. 2011). Later extended with RNA sequencing as part of PsychENCODE, these data

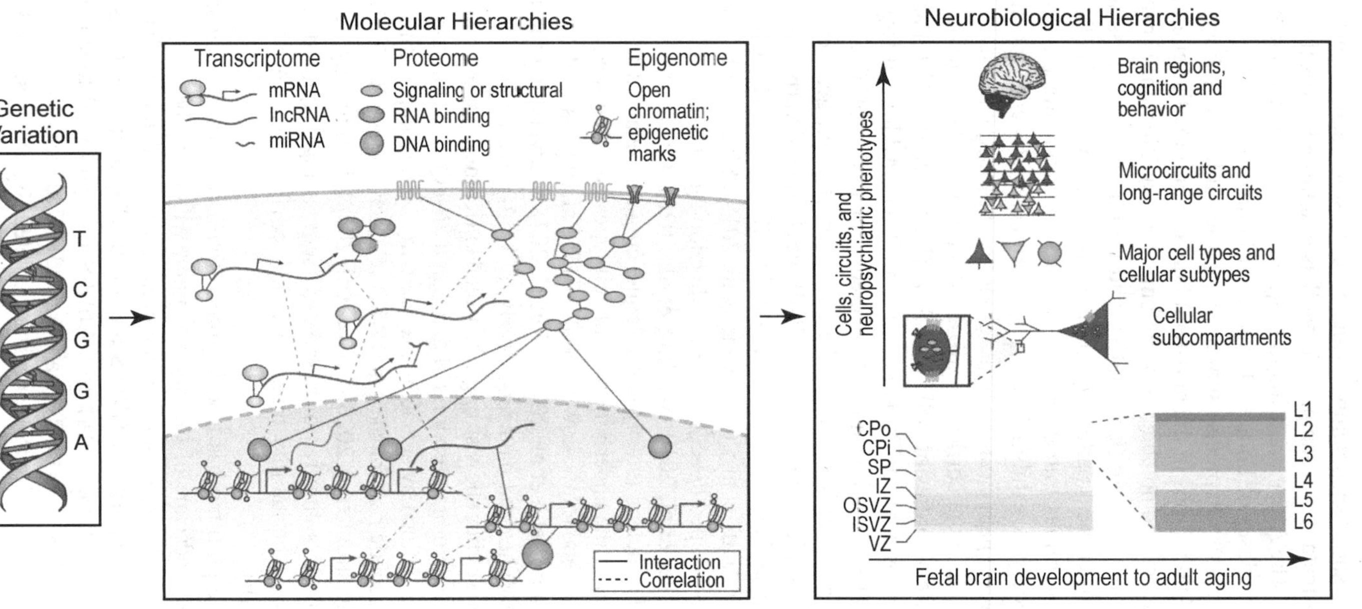

Figure 11.2 Molecular hierarchies and the human brain. Large-scale multi-omic profiling of human brain tissue samples has been undertaken to connect single nucleotide polymorphism-level genetic variation with transcriptomic, epigenomic, and proteomic changes. Reproduced with permission from Parikshak et al. (2015).

highlighted substantial spatiotemporal gene expression changes distinguishing pre- and postnatal brain samples, as well as a notable late-fetal transition (Li et al. 2018). The Allen Brain Institute generated comprehensive regional gene expression atlases of both adult and fetal brains. Gene expression was characterized across ~900 precise subregions in the adult brain (Hawrylycz et al. 2012) and ~300 regions in the mid-fetal human brain (Miller et al. 2014). The fetal atlas identified notable transcriptomic laminar differences capturing cellular maturation between proliferative and postmitotic layers, as well as clear gradients in cortical patterning along a frontotemporal axis. The adult atlas captured enormous transcriptomic variation by anatomic location, and although the neocortex exhibited relatively homogeneous transcriptomic signatures, there were again clear gradients along frontal-occipital axes. Notably, these typical gradients in cortical arealization have been shown to be attenuated in postmortem studies of ASD and SCZ (Haney et al. 2020; Parikshak et al. 2016; Roussos et al. 2012; Voineagu et al. 2011). Additional large-scale efforts from GTEx, CommonMind, BrainSeq, and PsychENCODE consortia, among others, have been undertaken to connect brain gene expression with single nucleotide polymorphism (SNP)-level genetic variation through *cis*-expression quantitative trait loci (*cis*-eQTL) (Fromer et al. 2016; GTEx Consortium 2020; Jaffe et al. 2018; Wang et al. 2018). Similar, albeit smaller, efforts have also mapped *cis*-eQTLs in the developing human brain (O'Brien et al. 2018; Walker et al. 2019; Werling et al. 2020). Finally, the advent of single-cell/single nucleus (sc/sn) RNA sequencing has enabled the bottom-up categorization of the underlying neural cell types and their developmental trajectories in the fetal (Nowakowski et al. 2017; Polioudakis et al. 2019) and adult human brain (Lake et al. 2018; Li et al. 2018). Leveraging these transcriptomic approaches and data sets, nearly all well-powered psychiatric genetic association studies show strong functional enrichment for brain genomic annotations, including brain-expressed genes and *cis*-eQTLs, with enrichment among cell types defined by sc/snRNA sequencing largely implicating neuronal lineages in genetic risk for SCZ and ASD (Calderon et al. 2017; Finucane et al. 2018; Satterstrom et al. 2020; Skene et al. 2018). Intriguingly, cell types defined by open chromatin regions (scATAC sequencing) captured substantially more disease heritability than those defined from scRNA sequencing (Kim et al. 2021b).

Genome-wide profiling has also begun to illuminate the molecularly defined epigenetic landscape of the human brain, which has been particularly critical for functional interpretation of the noncoding, regulatory regions of the genome where the majority of GWAS hits occur (PsychEncode Consortium et al. 2015). Girdhar et al. (2018) used ChIP-Seq to profile histone marks of active promoters (H3K4me3) and enhancers (H3K27ac) across two cortical regions from 157 neuronal (NeuN+), neuron-depleted (NeuN–), and bulk-tissue samples. Neuronal enhancers from the adult brain showed the strongest enrichment for SCZ GWAS signal, more so than bulk tissue or nonneurons. DNA methylation is another epigenetic signature exhibiting dynamic patterns in the human brain across development, regions, and cell types (Hannon et al. 2016; Jaffe et al. 2016; Rizzardi et al. 2019). Patterns of CpG methylation—particularly those that varied across brain regions, in neuronal (vs. nonneuronal) cell types, and fetal developmental periods—overlap substantially with GWAS loci for SCZ and other psychiatric disorders. Neuronal CpG sites exhibiting brain regionally variable methylation patterns captured the greatest degree of psychiatric heritability, but overlapped substantially with other measures of neuron-specific epigenetic regulation (Rizzardi et al. 2019). As discussed further below, these types of direct head-to-head comparisons between distinct molecular readouts are critical to build an integrative understanding of their biological interrelationships as well as to distill nonredundant insights into underlying genetic risk mechanisms.

Analyses of the alternative splicing landscape in the brain, which is particularly extensive compared with other tissues (Garrido-Martín et al. 2021; GTEx Consortium 2020), point to a strong contribution of genetic risk variants to splicing dysregulation, relatively orthogonal to effects on gene expression (Gandal et al. 2018b; Li et al. 2016; Takata et al. 2017). RNA-binding proteins coordinate many aspects of posttranscriptional regulation, including splicing, as well as subcellular localization, RNA stabilization and translational control, which are particularly important in neurons where transcripts are trafficked for long distances (Darnell 2013). Indeed, a number of RNA-binding proteins are themselves strong neurodevelopmental disorder risk genes, including *FMR1*, *RBFOX1*, *CHD8*, and *CELF4*, and their experimentally defined targets (Van Nostrand et al. 2020) exhibit strong enrichment for psychiatric GWAS signals (Park et al. 2021).

Advances in mass spectrometry have now begun to enable high-throughput proteomic profiling, although the sensitivity and dynamic range remains relatively limited compared with other genomic readouts. Large-scale, bottom-up proteomic profiling has been conducted across regions and postnatal timepoints in the human brain (Carlyle et al. 2017), as well as in SCZ case/control cohorts (MacDonald et al. 2020). Indeed, profiling of the synaptic proteome in auditory cortex from individuals with SCZ and controls (n = 48/group) identified significant alterations in >100 synaptosomal and homogenate protein levels, with a weak—but significant—correlation in effect size compared with transcriptomic changes observed in SCZ cortex (MacDonald et al. 2020). Further, "target capture"-based proteomics can be used to identify protein–protein interactions (PPIs), uncovering, for example, specific macromolecular complexes and interacting sub-networks among high-confidence ASD risk genes in cultured human neurons (Li et al. 2015; Pintacuda et al. 2021). While less scalable, such approaches complement existing PPI databases, which generally lack cell type and tissue (especially brain) specificity. Finally, although the genetic control of the human brain proteome has only recently begun to be elucidated through pQTL profiling (Robins et al. 2021), it has recently been integrated with psychiatric GWAS, for example prioritizing novel candidate risk proteins underlying depression GWAS loci, several of which were not captured at the transcriptome level (Wingo et al. 2021).

Finally, single-cell and cell type-specific genomic profiling are now feasible at a cost and scale necessary for capturing population-level allelic effects. Jaffe et al. (2020) profiled the granule-cell layer of the dentate gyrus, along with bulk hippocampal tissue, from 263 postmortem donors to generate cell type-specific QTL maps. Cell type-specific QTLs, a substantial fraction (15%) of which were not detectable in bulk tissue profiled from the same individuals, were used to prioritize *GRM3* and *CACNA1C* as risk genes within SCZ GWAS loci. Similar approaches, now being undertaken using snRNA sequencing from human brain samples, are beginning to uncover context-specific gene regulation across a wider range of cell types, with SCZ colocalization observed most substantially in excitatory neurons (Bryois et al. 2022).

Network-Level Inference

Given that so many features and layers of molecular regulation in the human brain contribute to psychiatric risk, how can we organize and integrate them into a coherent and interpretable set of functional units? Here, systems-level network biology provides a powerful organizing framework, which has been extensively leveraged particularly for brain transcriptomic data sets, as well as for protein interactomes (McGillivray et al. 2018; Parikshak et al. 2015). Network models are ubiquitous in biology, depicting connections between nodes (e.g., genes, proteins, regulatory elements) with edges defined by biologically measured or inferred relationships (e.g., co-expression or co-regulation, physical binding). Network topology can subsequently be characterized by patterns of connectivity and modularity. For example, many biological networks, including gene co-expression, exhibit scale-free topology, in which there are a few highly interconnected "hub" genes and many genes/nodes with few connections. Within this framework, nodes can be clustered into a small, discrete set of interconnected modules capturing the major axes of variation. Within each module, the most interconnected "hub" genes can be used to infer biological function, characterized based on enrichment for known cell types, gene ontology pathways, protein complexes, transcription factor binding sites, or other types of regulatory relationships (Kuleshov et al. 2016).

To date, network approaches have been most extensively leveraged in the context of large, bulk-tissue gene expression compendia, using techniques like Weighted Gene Correlation Network Analysis (WGCNA) and others (Langfelder and Horvath 2008). These approaches have revealed a robust, hierarchical organization to the human brain transcriptome, with co-expression modules recapitulating the unique cell types, subcellular organelles, and region-, sex-, and developmentally regulated processes (Gandal et al. 2018a, b;

Hawrylycz et al. 2012; Kang et al. 2011; Oldham et al. 2008). Co-expression networks provide a natural, data-driven means for organizing long lists of observed differentially expressed genes into modules, with presumed shared biological regulation and/or function. Indeed, co-expression modules built from large, human bulk brain data sets have been shown to capture all major CNS cell classes, with hub genes consisting of well-established cell type markers (Gandal et al. 2018a; Kelley et al. 2018). In practice, this enables *in silico* dissection of cell type-specific expression and/or cell proportion changes across conditions, as discussed further below. As proteomic profiling catches up with next-generation sequencing technologies, in terms of sensitivity and dynamic range, network-based analyses of the human brain proteome will provide important additional biological layers. Indeed, protein co-regulation networks from SCZ and control brain samples identified SCZ-downregulated modules representing synaptic mitochondria, very similar to what was observed at the gene expression level.

PPI-based networks, which define the interaction between two proteins (nodes) with binary edges representing physical binding interactions, have also been extensively characterized and leveraged in genomic analyses. These networks generally leverage literature-curated PPI databases, which compile results from experiments like yeast two-hybrid screens and immunoprecipitation followed by proteomics. As such, these networks can be sparse and incomplete, with established biases toward well-studied proteins, and generally lack tissue (e.g., brain) specificity (Corominas et al. 2014). Nevertheless, PPI networks more directly define macromolecular complexes than the guilt-by-association framework of co-expression. In addition, networks defined by PPIs show significantly increased co-expression (and vice versa), indicating concordance (Gandal et al. 2018a; Parikshak et al. 2015; Sakai et al. 2011).

Finally, gene regulatory networks are directional networks that map connecting genes and their regulators. Typically, gene regulatory networks integrate hierarchical relationships to predict gene expression by linking transcription factors to target *cis*-regulatory elements (e.g., enhancers and promoters) and target genes through experimentally defined binding site motifs. Typically, gene regulatory networks leverage the tissue and/or cell type specificity of such interactions, which can be inferred from comprehensive databases of epigenomic annotations (Marbach et al. 2016). In a comparison with PPI and gene co-expression networks, tissue-specific gene regulatory networks captured greater enrichment for SCZ and cross-disorder psychiatric GWAS signal, which most strongly implicated striatal and cortical tissues (Marbach et al. 2016). More recently as part of PsychENCODE, Wang et al. (2018) developed a comprehensive regulatory network for the human brain, linking 42,681 enhancers to target genes via eQTL and 3D chromatin conformation contacts. Approximately 43,000 transcription factor to target gene connections were then incorporated based on transcription factor binding site compatibility and regularized (elastic net) regression, which related transcription factor expression with that of the predicted target gene. Integrating this gene regulatory network with SCZ GWAS results prioritized specific transcription factors in disease risk, including *SOX7*, and further implicated excitatory neurons. Building true cell type-specific gene regulatory networks (Aibar et al. 2017) to leverage the wealth of emerging snRNA sequencing and multi-omic data from the human brain will be critical as these regulatory relationships are known to be highly context specific.

What Has Systems Biology Taught Us about Psychiatric Genetics?

Cellular-Spatial-Temporal Context

Leveraging the emerging wealth of data-driven functional annotations for the human brain coupled with network-based contextualization, several early papers demonstrated the promise of such "convergent" approaches to localizing the context in which diverse risk genes overlap. To pinpoint convergence at a molecular level, early exome-sequencing studies in ASD integrated results within protein interactome networks, identifying highly connected clusters including specific chromatin remodeling complexes (De Rubeis et al. 2014; Li et al. 2015; O'Roak et al. 2012b), WNT/β-catenin signaling (O'Roak et al. 2012b), synaptic genes (De Rubeis et al. 2014), and FMRP targets (De Rubeis et al. 2014; Iossifov et al. 2012). Further, given that many individual high-confidence ASD risk genes (e.g., *CHD8*) encode transcriptional regulators, gene regulatory networks built from the experimentally defined genomic targets for 26 such ASD-associated regulatory proteins showed strong, convergent enrichment for additional genetic signal (Satterstrom et al. 2020). Of note, while these direct (e.g., *cis*) regulatory targets implicate additional risk genes, stronger enrichments have been observed among the indirect (e.g., *trans*) targets—those genes that are downregulated upon *CHD8* knockdown but which are not direct targets of *CHD8* (Sugathan et al. 2014).

To place risk genes within a relevant spatiotemporal context, several studies leveraged BrainSpan (Kang et al. 2011) to build gene co-expression networks from neurotypical brains spanning early developmental epochs, finding that high-confidence ASD risk genes showed convergence within mid-fetal, prefrontal cortex networks and glutamatergic neurons (Ben-David and Shifman 2013; Parikshak et al. 2013; Willsey et al. 2018). Such findings were replicated using larger, updated high-confidence rare variant-implicated ASD risk genes, and, with the incorporation of scRNA sequencing data from the developing human brain, now have resolution to detect strongest enrichment among both early excitatory neuron and striatal interneuron lineages, among others (Li et al. 2018; Satterstrom et al. 2020). Similar findings were initially reported in SCZ, linking rare *de novo* variants to co-expression networks in the mid-fetal prefrontal cortex (Gulsuner et al. 2013). The more recent SCZ rare variant sequencing study from SCHEMA, however, did not observe a prenatal expression bias for the ten high-confidence SCZ risk genes (Singh et al. 2022).

Several tools have been developed to characterize GWAS enrichment patterns among specific cell types, tissues, brain regions, developmental time points, and co-expressed gene sets (Calderon et al. 2017; Finucane et al. 2018; Pers et al. 2015; Skene et al. 2018; Watanabe et al. 2017, 2019b; Xu et al. 2014). For both ASD and SCZ, there is evidence implicating GWAS signal within developmental—particularly mid-fetal—timepoints, although some genetic risk factors clearly also act postnatally, and the current largest ASD GWAS remains relatively underpowered to detect strong enrichments (Calderon et al. 2017; Grove et al. 2019; Parikshak et al. 2013; Walker et al. 2019). Spatially, genetic risk for these disorders appears to be distributed brain-wide, including across the cortex and cerebellum, rather than exhibiting any strong regional specificity (Haney et al. 2020; Hartl et al. 2021; Krishnan et al. 2016). Cell type-specific enrichment patterns for SCZ largely parallel those seen with rare variants in ASD, with clear enrichment for neuronal lineages but limited specificity beyond that (Skene et al. 2018). Intriguingly, greater specificity will likely be achieved with more detailed cell type specifications leveraging single-cell multi-omic profiling, which highlights a more prominent contribution to bipolar disorder GWAS risk from deep layer excitatory neurons (Luo et al. 2022).

Network-Informed Discovery and Interpretation of Risk Genes

Prioritizing candidate psychiatric risk genes from both WES and GWAS remains, in many cases, a major challenge. Index SNPs from GWAS typically fall within noncoding regions of the genome and often tag large haplotype blocks, obscuring both the identity of the true "causal" variant(s) as well as their target gene. In WES, interpreting the pathogenicity of identified variants, in particular missense variants which comprise the majority of coding mutations, remains difficult. In both cases, network-based approaches that incorporate functional genomic annotations have been successfully leveraged to improve prioritization and contextualization of disease-associated mutations as well as to increase power (Leiserson et al. 2013).

Among the most powerful demonstrations of network-informed risk gene discovery is the DAWN framework, which uses hidden Markov random fields to prioritize disease-associated gene clusters that exhibit strong patterns of co-expression in a relevant disease context (Liu et al. 2014). Leveraging the established convergence of ASD genetic risk within mid-fetal cortex gene networks, DAWN substantially boosts power in rare variant-sequencing studies of ASD, prioritizing dozens of additional risk genes (De Rubeis et al. 2014), many of which have since been replicated in subsequent, larger sequencing studies

(Satterstrom et al. 2020). Along similar lines, Krishnan et al. (2016) showed that incorporating machine learning with a brain-specific Bayesian gene-interaction network (comprised of gene expression, PPI, and regulatory-sequence based data sets) enhanced prediction of ASD risk genes as well as subsequent functional characterization of associated pathways. The strongest enrichments were observed for postsynaptic density genes and FMRP targets, and clustering further implicated pathways underlying genetic risk for ASD, including chromatin remodeling, WNT/β-catenin signaling and mRNA splicing, among others. Finally, Chen et al. (2018) leveraged an interactome network-based approach to facilitate interpretation of ASD-associated missense mutations, the pathogenicity of which can be difficult to decipher, by prioritizing mutations that affect the binding interfaces of hub proteins within a PPI network. These missense mutations further clustered with previously identified genes harboring *de novo* protein-truncating variants in ASD as well as with other relevant gene sets, including FMRP targets, chromatin modifiers, genes in the PSD, and genes expressed early in development.

Defining Molecular Pathology

Network-based approaches have proved a useful organizing framework to interpret results from molecular profiling studies of case/control cohorts. Although psychiatric disorders lack a clearly defined neuroanatomic or cellular pathology—in contrast with many neurologic conditions—large-scale, genome-wide transcriptomic profiling has now established a characteristic brain-level molecular pathology for several psychiatric disorders, including ASD and SCZ (Fromer et al. 2016; Gandal et al. 2018a; Parikshak et al. 2016; Voineagu et al. 2011). Initial postmortem human gene expression profiling studies of psychiatric case/control cohorts were small and often reported variable results, particularly at the individual gene level; this was likely due to cohort heterogeneity, analytic or methodologic differences, or statistical noise (Hernandez et al. 2021). Nevertheless, several key findings emerged that have since been extensively replicated in larger mega- and meta-analytic studies, including a downregulation of synaptic, interneuron, and mitochondrial related genes in SCZ and ASD cortices as well as a concordant upregulation of neural-immune and inflammatory gene expression signatures (Gandal et al. 2018a, b; Horváth and Mirnics 2015; Parikshak et al. 2016; Voineagu et al. 2011). Furthermore, ASD cases showed similar, but more extreme changes, in these gene expression patterns compared with SCZ. Importantly, these early studies paved the way for large-scale consortium-level efforts including BrainSeq (Collado-Torres et al. 2019; Jaffe et al. 2018), CommonMind (Fromer et al. 2016), and PsychENCODE (Gandal et al. 2018b; Li et al. 2018; Wang et al. 2018) to perform transcriptome profiling at sufficient scale to generate reproducible results.

Network-based approaches, like WGCNA, have yielded important insights into the molecular pathology of these disorders. For example, in our cross-disorder paper which reported on 700 postmortem human brain samples, including from subjects with ASD, SCZ, and bipolar disorder (Figure 11.3), co-expression modules clearly captured major CNS cell types, with hub genes consisting of canonical cell type markers, enabling an *in silico* dissection (Gandal et al. 2018a). Modules representing gene expression patterns within neurons (and synaptic mitochondria) were downregulated across the three disorders, whereas reciprocal upregulation was observed for gene expression signatures of astrocytes. Notably, a microglial module was specifically upregulated only in ASD. It remains unclear whether such findings reflect changes in underlying cell proportion and/or cell type-specific gene expression patterns, although emerging analyses using snRNA sequencing seem to indicate subtle, at best, cell fraction shifts in ASD (Velmeshev et al. 2019).

Postmortem brain transcriptomics characterize the current, reactive state of a biological sample and therefore cannot differentiate causal from reactive or compensatory effects. Integration of transcriptomic results with directional genetic anchors, through GWAS and rare variant enrichments, can provide orthogonal evidence for pathophysiological versus compensatory or reactive changes. For example, the CommonMind paper built unsigned co-expression networks from bulk RNA sequencing profiling of >500 prefrontal cortex brain samples and identified a module (M2c; 1411 genes) that captured genes differentially expressed in SCZ as well as were enriched for multiple classes of genetic risk variation, including signals from GWAS, recurrent CNVs, and rare variants (Fromer et al. 2016). This module was enriched for neuronal markers and relevant pathways including ARC and NMDA-receptor signaling, PSD genes, and FMRP targets. Further, module hub genes included the NMDAR subunit *GRIN2A* and the GABA-B receptors *GAB BR2*, both of which have subsequently been prioritized by the latest GWAS and rare variant-sequencing studies in SCZ (Singh et al. 2022; Trubetskoy et al. 2022). Similarly, in the cross-disorder paper described above, the neuron/synaptic module (CD1) downregulated in ASD and SCZ showed convergent enrichment for GWAS signal, non-synonymous *de novo* variation, and recurrent psychiatric CNVs (Gandal et al. 2018b). Finally, we expanded this approach in the PsychENCODE data set of >1,300 samples across the lifespan to build co-expression modules using transcript-isoform (along with gene-level) expression measures. Isoform-level networks captured the same processes as gene networks but added biological specificity and showed greater genetic enrichments overall. Here, an isoform-level module comprised of oligodendrocyte markers and neuron projection pathways exhibited the greatest overall GWAS enrichment for SCZ and was downregulated in ASD and SCZ (Gandal et al. 2018b).

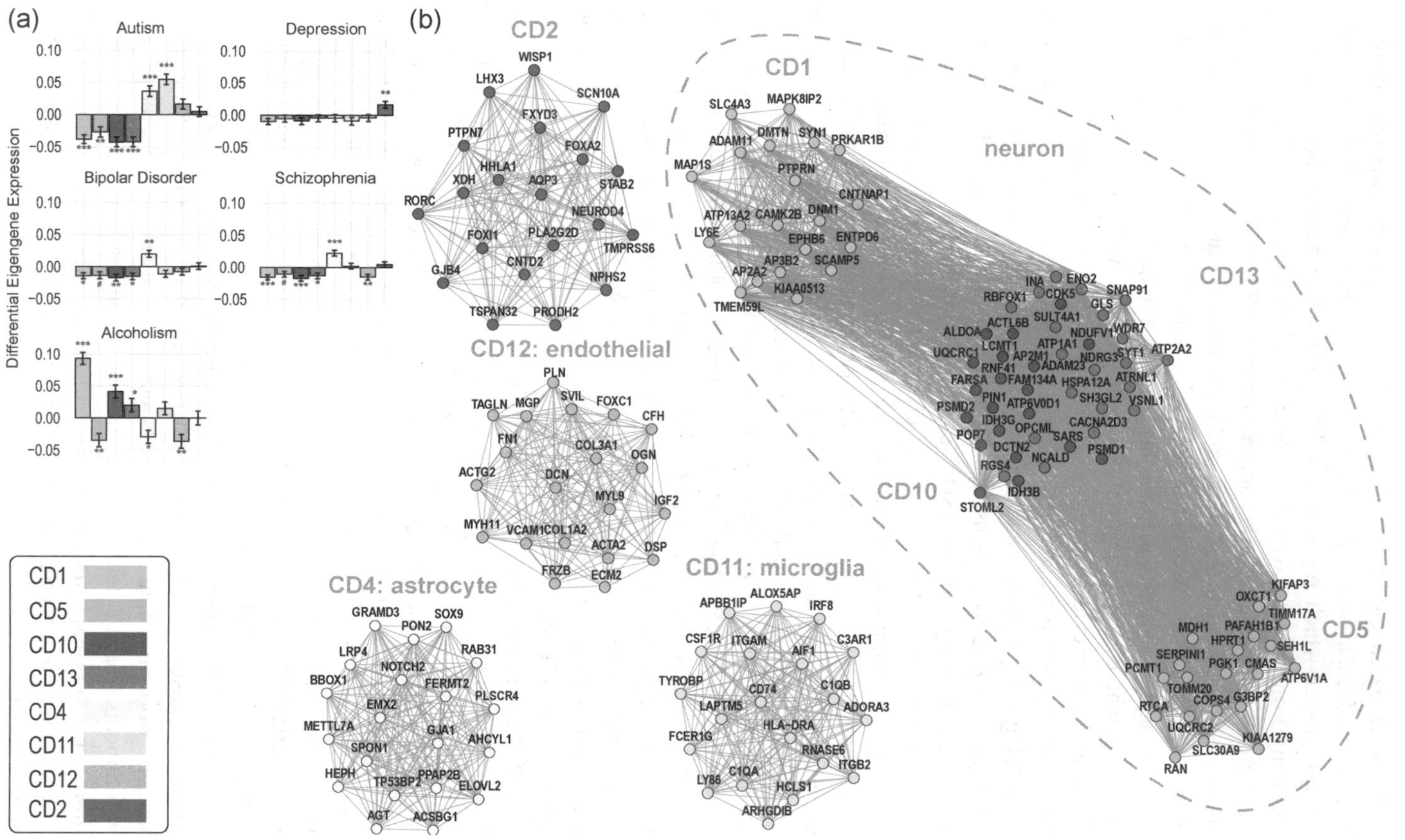
(a)
Differential Eigengene Expression
Autism
Depression
Bipolar Disorder
Schizophrenia
Alcoholism
0.10
0.05
0.00
−0.05
(b)
CD2
WISP1
LHX3
SCN10A
FXYD3
PTPN7
FOXA2
HHLA1
XDH
AQP3
STAB2
RORC
NEUROD4
PLA2G2D
FOXI1
TMPRSS6
CNTD2
GJB4
NPHS2
TSPAN32
PRODH2
CD12: endothelial
PLN
TAGLN
MGP
SVIL
FOXC1
CFH
FN1
COL3A1
OGN
ACTG2
DCN
MYL9
IGF2
MYH11
VCAM1
COL1A2
ACTA2
DSP
FRZB
ECM2
CD4: astrocyte
GRAMD3
PON2
SOX9
LRP4
NOTCH2
RAB31
BBOX1
FERMT2
PLSCR4
EMX2
METTL7A
GJA1
AHCYL1
SPON1
HEPH
PPAP2B
TP53BP2
ELOVL2
AGT
ACSBG1
CD11: microglia
APBB1IP
ALOX5AP
IRF8
CSF1R
ITGAM
AIF1
C3AR1
TYROBP
CD74
C1QB
LAPTM5
ADORA3
HLA-DRA
FCER1G
RNASE6
C1QA
ITGB2
LY86
HCLS1
ARHGDIB
CD1
neuron
CD13
CD10
CD5
SLC4A3
MAPK8IP2
ADAM11
DMTN
SYN1
PRKAR1B
MAP1S
PTPRN
CNTNAP1
ATP13A2
CAMK2B
DNM1
LY6E
EPHB6
ENTPD6
AP3B2
SCAMP5
AP2A2
KIAA0513
TMEM59L
INA
ENO2
RBFOX1
CDK5
SNAP91
GLS
ACTL6B
SULT4A1
ALDOA
NDUFV1
WDR7
UQCRC1
LCMT1
ATP1A1
AP2M1
NDRG3
SYT1
ATP2A2
RNF41
ADAM23
FARSA
FAM134A
HSPA12A
ATRNL1
PIN1
ATP6V0D1
SH3GL2
VSNL1
PSMD2
IDH3G
OPCML
CACNA2D3
POP7
SARS
DCTN2
PSMD1
NCALD
RGS4
IDH3B
STOML2
KIFAP3
OXCT1
TIMM17A
MDH1
PAFAH1B1
HPRT1
SEH1L
SERPINI1
PGK1
CMAS
PCMT1
ATP6V1A
TOMM20
COPS4
G3BP2
RTCA
UQCRC2
KIAA1279
SLC30A9
RAN
CD1
CD5
CD10
CD13
CD4
CD11
CD12
CD2

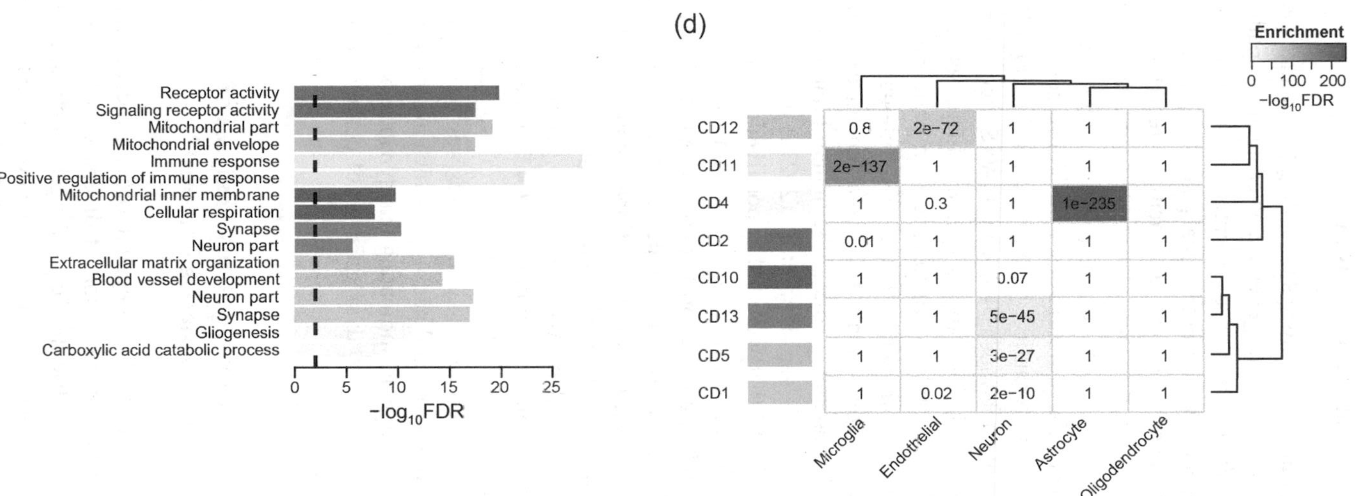

Figure 11.3 Network-level contextualization of the transcriptomic molecular pathology across major psychiatric disorders. Co-expression networks generated from 700 human brain samples enabled *in silico* dissection of shared and distinct cell type-specific gene expression alterations across disorders, with downregulation of neuronal and synaptic gene expression profiles across ASD, SCZ, and BD. The downregulated neuronal CD1 module exhibited significant, convergent enrichment for disease-associated common and rare genetic variation. Adapted from Gandal et al. (2018a).

Improved Annotation of Brain-Level Pathways

A deep understanding of the key pathways mediating psychiatric genetic risk necessitates a clear definition of the genes involved in these pathways and their interrelationships. While a number of essential expert- and literature-curated databases organize genes within ontological pathways, existing resources largely fail to capture the complexity and specificity of gene functions within the nervous system. To address this gap, data-driven network approaches can leverage guilt-by-association to generate improved functional genomic and pathway annotations, particularly for tissues with highly complex and less well-characterized regulatory dynamics, such as the human brain (Parikshak et al. 2015). As an example, the most significant GWAS signal for SCZ lies within the major histocompatibility complex region, which was subsequently fine mapped to the *C4* locus and shown to reflect, in part, increased copy number and upregulation of *C4A* (Sekar et al. 2016). Although *C4A* has been well characterized as a key component of the complement cascade and the innate immune system, its functional role in the human brain remains much less understood. To address this gap, Kim et al. (2021a) characterized brain co-expression partners of *C4A* that were either positively or negatively correlated with *C4A* expression across varying *C4A* genomic copy numbers, annotating their cell type and pathway contributions as well as their relation to established SCZ genetic risk factors. This type of "seeded" network or top-down approach can provide an unbiased functional annotation for a poorly understood gene by capturing coherent biological processes that covary across samples (Parikshak et al. 2015). This work identified a putative transcriptomic signature of *C4A*-mediated synaptic pruning, reinforcing the idea that overpruning likely contributes to SCZ pathogenesis and/or progression (Feinberg 1982). Further, this study found that negatively co-expressed genes with *C4A* are overrepresented for synapse-related pathways, which in turn were enriched for convergent SCZ genetic signals, indicating that synaptic pathways are the key biological link between genetic dysregulation of complement signaling and SCZ pathophysiology.

How Do We Move Systems Analyses of Psychiatric Genetics Forward?

As detailed above, network biology has begun to provide a coherent, organizing framework for functional interpretation of diverse genetic and genomic changes associated with psychiatric disorders. As genomic associations continue to multiply, however, much more needs to be done to enhance specificity and to move toward mechanistic insight and therapeutic target prediction within an individual. Here, I outline some critical next steps.

Connecting Major Findings

Among the most striking unanswered questions that have arisen from network-level insights is what relationship, if any, exists between risk genes that cluster within the two most enriched psychiatric risk pathways (chromatin complex and synaptic gene sets)? These are among the most strongly and broadly implicated pathways, yet it remains unclear whether these reflect distinct disease subtypes or have an underlying biological connection. They exhibit subtle but distinct functional differences: chromatin complex genes exhibit earlier developmental expression patterns and synaptic genes peak more postnatally (Satterstrom et al. 2020). One proposed hypothesis is that chromatin modifiers somehow regulate the later expression of synaptic genes. However, when empirically tested, Satterstrom et al. (2020) failed to find significant overlap in terms of PPIs, co-expression networks, or known regulatory targets of chromatin complex (e.g., "GER") and synaptic (e.g., "NC") genes. Likewise, understanding how FMRP targets connect with other observed pathways and levels of convergence remains an open question (Clifton et al. 2020). Here, there are more potential direct connections, as FMRP is known to regulate the translation of long, brain-expressed genes, which include many known synaptic proteins, in an activity-dependent manner (Clifton et al. 2020).

Integration across Functional Hierarchies

More broadly, integrative efforts need to better connect distinct levels across the molecular hierarchy. While each omic measurement offers a unique snapshot of a complex system, molecular layers are often highly interdependent and reflect a common, latent underlying biological process. Although multiomic integration has been an active area of research for some time, particularly in the cancer field (Huang et al. 2017; Ritchie et al. 2015), substantial methodological challenges remain in terms of analysis and visualization, which are further complicated by the scarcity of human brain tissue available for profiling. Among the unsupervised methods, similarity network fusion performs sample level clustering on each molecular feature independently and then fuses resulting similarity networks to identify subclusters with shared changes across multiple axes of molecular readouts (Wang et al. 2014). Ramaswami et al. (2020) leveraged this approach to integrate gene and microRNA expression (and co-expression), along with DNA methylation and histone acetylation changes across ASD and control brain samples and found convergent patterns of dysregulation across the transcriptome and epigenome. The predicted model based on these results suggested that ASD genetic risk factors were acting to downregulate neuronal gene expression, with DNA methylation and some histone acetylation changes acting in a secondary or compensatory fashion. As demonstrated, this integrative approach can be powerful and interpretable but requires relatively large numbers of samples with shared measurements.

Supervised and semi-supervised methods leverage *a priori* knowledge about sample identities and biological relationships between features to build connections. A notable example comes from PsychENCODE, in which Wang et al. (2018) implemented a multilevel, generative deep learning model called a Deep Structured Phenotype Network (DSPN). This DSPN model linked common genetic variation (input) with psychiatric phenotypes (output), through a series of visible layers comprised of gene regulatory linkages, cell fractions, and co-expression modules, as well as a series of intermediate hidden layers. Interrogation of the latent nodes within this framework prioritized key contributory pathways—including synaptic activity, splicing, immune response and chromatin modification, among others—as well as the "best" positive paths connecting these nodes with both SNP genotypes and psychiatric traits. A major advantage of generative models centers on the ability to interrogate these hidden layers; however, far too often, integrative efforts to connect multiple molecular profiles have a "black box" feel, without the ability to visualize or directly interpret such connections. The utility of integrative models will ultimately rest on (a) whether the key underlying predicted biological connections can lead to new experimentally testable insights into disease mechanisms, and/or (b) whether these models can lead to biologically informative individual-level predictions in independent clinical populations.

Finally, it is important to note that recent large-scale integrative effects connecting functional genomic readouts with common variation (e.g., GTEx, PsychENCODE) to build maps of expression and splicing QTLs have largely focused on regulation within individual loci (e.g., *cis* effects) to maximize power. Moving forward, efforts to connect genetics directly with network-defined phenotypes (e.g., *trans*-regulatory effects) will almost certainly uncover relevant biology, particularly in the context of environmental stimulation (Kolberg et al. 2020).

Improved Specificity of Gene Annotations, Particularly at the Synapse

Given the strong convergence of neuropsychiatric risk genes at the "synapse," and the observation that synaptic dysfunction is strongly implicated in nearly all such disorders, we must gain more comprehensive and specific insights into the genetic underpinnings of synaptic architecture and diversity. The human brain is estimated to comprise hundreds of distinct synaptic types, with diverse structural and functional properties, including neurotransmitter specialization, neuromodulatory activity, and release probability (Südhof 2018). Yet, it remains unclear whether some of these are more predominantly impacted in specific disorders or by specific genetic risk profiles, which could provide important insights as to which specific circuits may be affected. For example, it is tantalizing to speculate that the recent identification of glutamate receptors *GRIN2A* and *GRIA3*—two of the top ten rare variant-associated

SCZ risk genes (Singh et al. 2022)—provides credence to the decades-old NMDA-receptor hypofunction model (Olney et al. 1999). Yet, to address this question rigorously, we need a much more comprehensive understanding and catalog of the molecular machinery underlying diverse synaptic architectures. Historically, proteomic profiling, in combination with biochemical techniques such as subcellular fractionation and/or immunoprecipitation, has been a critical tool for high-throughput interrogation of molecular complexes at the synapse. To provide an organizing framework for these types of data, the SynGO consortium built an online knowledge base of expert-curated annotations for 1,112 synaptic genes with respect to protein locations and synaptic functions (Koopmans et al. 2019). While this is an important start, the resulting synaptic ontologies remain sparse, limited perhaps by the substantial efforts required for manual curation. Technological advances in high-throughput single-cell and spatial transcriptomic profiling coupled with viral tracing or barcoding strategies (Muñoz-Castañeda et al. 2021), as well as approaches that integrate molecular and physiological readouts within single cells (e.g., Patch-seq; Cadwell et al. 2016), have the potential to expand our understanding of such synaptic ontologies greatly. Further, the recent advent of proximity ligation-based approaches now enables proteomic profiling of synaptic structures with exquisite temporal and spatial resolution, including those difficult to isolate biochemically (Loh et al. 2016; Uezu et al. 2016). Altogether, integration of such high-throughput readouts across a wide array of cellular connections, developmental timepoints, and disease-relevant genetic perturbations is likely to greatly facilitate future systems-level dissection of psychiatric genetic risk mechanisms.

Synaptic genes are 2.6-fold longer with 1.7-fold more transcript-isoforms than nonsynaptic brain-expressed genes, indicative of a substantially expanded capacity and complexity of alternative splicing (Koopmans et al. 2019). Furthermore, isoform-level quantifications have been shown to capture greater differential expression effect sizes and GWAS enrichments than at the gene level in SCZ, particularly with neurons (Gandal et al. 2018b). As such, one approach that will very likely improve the specificity of our understanding of synaptic gene ontologies is to incorporate specific transcript-isoforms into these annotations, particularly as such data becomes increasingly available with long-read sequencing technologies. For example, the presynaptic cell adhesion molecular and high-confidence psychiatric risk gene *NRXN1* has now been shown to encode thousands of unique isoforms, many of which are regulated independently and thought to mediate diverse functions at the synapse (Treutlein et al. 2014). Furthermore, patient-specific *NRXN1* mutations have been shown to disrupt splicing, resulting in mutant isoforms that themselves are capable of disrupting neuronal activity in culture (Flaherty et al. 2019). Finally, Corominas et al. (2014) developed a novel protein interaction network by experimentally cataloging interactions between brain-expressed alternatively spliced isoforms of ASD risk genes, many of which localize to the synapse. The resulting “autism spliceform interaction network” showed that splicing altered ~50% of detected interactions and uncovered a substantial proportion of new PPIs. Altogether, these results highlight the potential added benefit of an isoform-centric approach for enhancing our understanding of synaptic architecture, particularly as it relates to psychiatric genetics.

Moving Beyond Enrichment

Although measures of population-level genetic convergence have gotten us this far, we must begin to now pivot toward interpretation—and *prediction*—of convergent risk within an individual. Personalized gene regulatory networks have been proposed as one approach to integrate distinct risk profiles within an individual and move toward precision medicine (van der Wijst et al. 2018). Polygenic risk scores will become more impactful as they incorporate multiple classes of genetic variation (SNPs, CNVs, and rare variants) along with improved identification of the underlying causal variant(s) across populations. As polygenic risk scores become more powerful, this will create new opportunities to incorporate network biology and pathway-level knowledge. For example, do affected individuals with synaptic risk gene profiles show distinct phenotypic trajectories or outcomes from those with risk variants affecting chromatin biology? Could targeted interventions be tailored to these distinct underlying risk profiles? Such predictions will require rigorous statistical validation in independent data sets to avoid overfitting.

Conclusions

The highly complex risk factors contributing to psychiatric disorders like ASD and SCZ, with polygenic contributions from variants across the genome, indicate that no simple parsimonious model will likely ever be able to fully explain mechanistic etiopathogenesis with any degree of generalizability. However, network-level embedding of complex genetic risk variation can begin to elucidate key underlying cellular and molecular pathways, providing a tractable framework for future experimental dissection, biological contextualization, and the potential for enhanced predictive modeling.

Acknowledgments

I would like to thank members of the Gandal Lab for helpful discussions and feedback for this chapter, especially Minsoo Kim, Leanna Hernandez, Pan Zhang, Michael Margolis, and Connor Jops.

Clinical Considerations

12

Maximizing Near-Term Clinical Opportunities for Psychiatric Genetics

Lea K. Davis, Paul S. Appelbaum, Jehannine C. Austin, Franziska Degenhardt, Sébastien Jacquemont, Brenda W. J. H. Penninx, Jordan W. Smoller, Fabian Streit, and Cathryn M. Lewis

Abstract

Over the past two decades, genomics research has been enormously successful in identifying specific genes, pathways, and mechanisms that play a role in the development of psychiatric and neurodevelopmental disorders. The translation of these findings into the clinical setting has been slow but steady. Current clinical advances range from identifying genetic etiologies for neurodevelopmental disorders to pharmacogenomic dosing guidelines for psychiatric medications. Many more advances can be anticipated, given the paradigm-shifting knowledge produced by the field. Principally, genomics research has produced neurobiological hypotheses that are likely to yield therapeutic advances only in the long term. Nonetheless, opportunities to improve clinical care also exist in the near term. This chapter evaluates and prioritizes these opportunities in terms of their feasibility and potential impact. Barriers to the successful translation of these findings are identified and areas for research highlighted to support their translation into clinical settings.

Introduction

This chapter is the result of an extended discussion between a group of psychiatrists, ethicists, medical geneticists, research geneticists, and genetic counselors, all of whom have extensive experience in their respective field. Our discussion was grounded on a common understanding that psychiatric genetic research, embedded in a human rights framework, can positively impact medical care, societal treatment, and quality of life for people with psychiatric illness and neurodevelopmental disorders. While our discourse was rooted in this shared perspective, it was also informed by our unique experiences, including lived experiences. As expected, consensus was reached on many themes, but for some issues, opinions diverged. In producing this report, we aim to represent the gestalt of our discussions fairly, including the diversity of perspectives. As such, the style of this chapter emphasizes the fluid nature of our discussions at the Forum. We are deeply indebted to the Ernst Strüngmann Forum for providing space for this debate and believe that there are multiple, exciting near-term clinical opportunities for psychiatric genetics.

We consider three layers of genetic information and will describe, for each, the status of clinical provision, the research gaps, and the potential for future implementation to improve clinical care and patient outcomes. We begin with a look at the potential return of rare variant genetic diagnoses for indications beyond childhood intellectual disability and autism spectrum disorder, for which a consensus already exists regarding clinical utility. Next, we look further ahead to the potential use of polygenic scores in clinical practice, identifying both the endpoints likely to have most utility and the substantial research gaps that need to be filled. We then consider the role of genetic counseling in the absence of testing and discuss provision of genetic education in the general population. Next, we discuss barriers to the application of genetics in clinical practice. Finally, throughout our discussions, themes of equity, diversity, and community engagement arose frequently. These themes are, therefore, presented as guiding principles for all future research and implementation.

Near-Term Opportunities and Challenges for Rare Copy Number and Sequence Variants

Currently, clinical care and access models for genetic testing and genetic counseling in psychiatric disorders are provided by medical genetic and genetic counseling professional organizations. In terms of clinical genetic testing, an established consensus exists to support the genetic testing of minors with intellectual disabilities and autism. The current best practice in the United States, Canada, and several European countries is to return an interpretation of rare and clinically relevant copy number variants (CNVs) identified through whole-exome sequencing or array-based technologies. We anticipate that whole-genome sequencing technologies will eventually replace whole-exome sequencing and array-based methods. Existing guidelines typically recommend clinical genetic counseling to occur at the point of care when genetic test results are returned. As of the writing of this chapter, we are unaware of any professional association guidelines that stipulate which patients who receive a psychiatric diagnosis, in the absence of intellectual disability or global developmental delay, should be offered genetic testing.

Accordingly, we discussed what research would be needed to identify who else would benefit from clinical genetic testing, and the circumstances that would facilitate such a benefit.

Currently Available Genetic Testing in Clinical Psychiatry

Currently, most medical genetics professional societies provide guidelines and recommendations for offering exome sequencing or chromosome microarray to children diagnosed with global developmental delay (GDD), autism spectrum disorder, major malformations, or epilepsy (Finucane et al. 2021, 2022). The diagnosis of GDD requires a delay in reaching at least two early childhood developmental milestones, including fine or gross motor skills (e.g., delayed walking), cognitive development (e.g., intellectual disability), and social or communication (e.g., shared attention, speech, and language) milestones. GDD is common and is diagnosed in approximately 1–3% of children younger than five years of age (Bélanger and Caron 2018). Currently, an underlying genetic etiology can be discovered in approximately 40% of children with a diagnosis of moderate to severe GDD (Savatt and Myers 2021; Wortmann et al. 2022) and 24–45% of children with epilepsy (Sánchez Fernández et al. 2019). While current guidelines for offering CNV testing in children with GDD, epilepsy, and major malformations are appropriate, the uptake and implementation of these guidelines for minors who meet these criteria are inconsistent across healthcare systems and individual clinicians. For example, in the Netherlands, any clinician can request clinical testing, but reimbursement only occurs when the request is filed by a medical specialist in a hospital or a general practitioner. In the United States, clinical diagnostic genetic testing for patients with congenital anomalies, developmental delay, or intellectual disability is recommended by the American College of Medical Genetics and Genomics and the American Academy of Pediatrics. However, implementation varies greatly across states and institutions (Manickam et al. 2021; Miller et al. 2010), and many children who meet criteria are never tested. While many factors can contribute to this inconsistency (e.g., insurance status, access to clinical geneticists, reimbursement), one major barrier is that primary care providers may not be familiar with the guidelines for care and referral (Tremblay et al. 2018; Truong et al. 2021). Thus, the shift from clinical guidelines to a true standard of care is still ongoing and should be supported by research in implementation science.

Providing Clinical Genetic Testing Services to Adults with Developmental Delay and Intellectual Disability

As described above, consensus recommendations from professional societies and expert groups are available for the diagnostic workup of children with neurodevelopmental delay (Manickam et al. 2021; Sabo et al. 2020; Thygesen et al. 2018). Nonetheless, many children who meet the criteria are never offered genetic testing, and the technologies required for such a workup are relatively young. Together, these factors contribute to a substantial population of adults who would have met current criteria for genetic testing in their childhood but were never offered genetic testing, either because it did not exist when they were children or because the technology and counseling were not available to them. There is a growing body of evidence that the diagnostic yield in adult patients with intellectual disability is comparable to the pediatric population with intellectual disability; however, similar guidelines on clinical genetic testing for adults have been slow to emerge (Finucane et al. 2020).

Given the guidelines currently in place for children with GDD, should genetic testing also be offered to adults with GDD? Two primary reasons support this action. First, ethical principles regarding justice dictate that adults who would have met criteria for genetic testing as children have a right to the standard of care offered to children today. Second, early studies have found that carriers of CNVs associated with neurodevelopmental disorders, regardless of the level of neurodevelopmental delay, demonstrate increased rates of age-related disease (e.g., diabetes, hypertension, obesity, renal failure, and early mortality) and that carriers were twice as likely to seek hospital emergency services (Auwerx et al. 2022; Finucane et al. 2022). These studies highlight the importance of specific genotype-phenotype research across the lifespan for CNV carriers to inform continuing clinical management. Little is known about the long-term clinical management of patients who carry a neurodevelopmental CNV or other high-impact rare variant. We believe that this should be a priority area of research—one that could be filled by engaging adults who experienced GDD early in life and now choose to investigate the underlying genetic etiology as adults.

Given that existing studies have focused almost exclusively on children, additional work is needed to characterize the diagnostic yield from genetic testing in an adult population. These data are important for the continual development of clinical guidelines, as there will be populations of adults who may benefit from genetic testing for many years to come. In addition, it is critically important to understand the potential positive and negative psychosocial impacts of receiving a genetic diagnosis in adulthood. Ethical questions also arise. For example, a relative who serves as guardian for an adult, who experienced GDD as a child, may also be personally impacted by the decision to pursue (or not) genetic testing. In that situation, the potential exists for a guardian to make a choice based on the guardian's own interests rather than those of the ward. In this case, it would be important to include genetic counselors in the process to work with the family unit on understanding the potential risks and benefits of pursuing genetic testing (Morris et al. 2022). An evidence base should be built to maximize improved psychosocial and clinical outcomes in adults with GDD. Finally, studies should be prioritized to determine the impact of genetic testing on the clinical and health economics management of adult patients with qualifying disabilities.

Childhood, Early-Onset, and Adult Psychosis

Guidelines for genetic testing in individuals with intellectual disability are well established, yet no clinical guidelines exist for genetic testing in other early-onset psychiatric disorders. Emerging evidence suggests that children with early-onset psychosis benefit from a clinical genetics evaluation. For example, a recent study showed that the yield of chromosome microarray testing was identical in autism spectrum disorder and psychosis in children and adolescents younger than 18 years (Brownstein et al. 2022), and ethical analysis suggests equivalent benefits (Morris et al. 2022).

Key pieces of information are lacking in the population with early-onset psychosis, including the genetic testing yield by age at onset, level of premorbid cognitive functioning, and the additional clinical or family history modifiers that might increase the yield. For example, it is currently unclear whether children with early-onset psychosis and no history of GDD, but who have a sibling with epilepsy or autism, are more likely to have a positive genetic test than a child without these additional family history modifiers. In this population it is critical to assess yield, its clinical and family history modifiers, and whether there are any other factors (e.g., severity, chronicity, comorbidity) that could increase yield and trigger the offer of testing.

Finally, in adult-onset psychosis (≥ age 18) without a history of GDD, research is needed to determine whether there are clinical features (e.g., severity, chronicity, treatment resistance) that can serve as indicators for a rare genetic cause underlying the psychiatric disorder. Currently, no clinical guidelines exist for this population despite significant evidence that genetic counseling (even in the absence of genetic testing) increases empowerment and improves outcomes (Semaka and Austin 2019).

Additional Themes

Several themes emerged throughout our discussions. Preeminent among these was the need to increase representation of diverse genetic ancestries, as this will improve the interpretation of genetic testing results. Prior studies demonstrate that lack of diversity can result in a bias in which patients with increasing non-European ancestry are more likely to receive "variants of unknown significance" from high-throughput sequencing screens. This knowledge gap, in terms of clinical significance of some genomic variation, is an artifact of the limited investment in genomes from diverse ancestries over the past decades. Additional themes that emerged included the need for more systematic study of (a) the impact of genetic testing on subsequent clinical management of patients and (b) the impact of genetic counseling (with or without genetic testing) on the psychosocial well-being of patients. There was strong consensus that research should proceed under a community engagement framework that increases the presence of patient representatives and advocates at all levels of research. These issues are key translational areas in which linkages with clinical implementation science should be initiated early.

Near-Term Opportunities and Challenges for Polygenic Scores

Polygenic risk scores (PRSs) are per-person estimates of the cumulative genetic risk conferred by common single nucleotide polymorphisms, as opposed to rare genetic events. PRSs are estimated with respect to an index phenotype (e.g., depression, schizophrenia, externalizing behavior) that has been measured and tested for genetic association in large independent samples. They demonstrate imperfect, but measurable, average differences between groups of individuals with and without these index traits. While PRSs are not ready for clinical implementation in a psychiatry setting today (Araújo and Wheeler 2022; Lewis et al. 2022; Pereira et al. 2022), there is promise for their near-term use in certain identified contexts (e.g., differential diagnosis, screening, and prevention) (see Smoller, this volume). We recognize that PRSs are, *de facto*, already available to the public through direct-to-consumer genetic testing companies and third-party services (Peck et al. 2022). For certain cancers, PRSs are being utilized in some oncology genetic counseling clinics, and psychiatric PRSs may soon be included in genetic testing reports for psychiatric indications. These issues sparked a great deal of discussion on the type of research that could be instructive to implement PRS testing in clinical practice. We considered three classifications of patients: (a) genetically defined high-risk individuals, (b) phenotypically defined high-risk individuals, and (c) the general population. The research needed to determine PRS utility in each group is considered below.

Use of Polygenic Risk Scores in "Genetically Defined" High-Risk Populations

Individuals who are positive for clinical genetic screens (e.g., 22q11.2) may be at high-risk of developing a later psychiatric diagnosis. It is possible that a PRS for the "highest risk" psychiatric diagnosis may provide additional clinical utility. For example, in a child who has received a positive CNV test result but does not yet have a psychiatric disorder (e.g., a 22q11.2 deletion but no psychosis), the addition of a PRS for schizophrenia may meaningfully increase the positive predictive value of the initial genetic finding. Inherent in this hypothesis are two critically important issues. The first is whether the risk index is increased with addition of the PRS. The second is whether the increase is "clinically meaningful." We note, however, that there is little consensus on what constitutes a "clinically meaningful" increase in risk. We concluded that a "clinically meaningful" improvement in positive predictive value should impact at least one of the following domains: the time to diagnosis, clinical management, early intervention, surveillance and monitoring, or treatment selection. Either way, evidence shows that for families of individuals with the 22q11.2 deletion, genetic counseling regarding the chance for psychiatric manifestations can be helpful (Carrion et al. 2022).

The addition of PRS to CNV results could meet at least some of the clinically meaningful criteria. For example, a recent study found that among individuals with a 22q11.2 deletion, the rate of schizophrenia diagnosis (and thus the positive predictive value) increased from 20% (95% CI = 0.16, 0.24) at or below the 50th PRS percentile to 33% (95% CI = 0.222, 0.428) at or above the 90th PRS percentile. The 50th percentile represents the sample median PRS (also the mean for z-score scaled distributions). Equally important, the rate of schizophrenia diagnosis decreased from 20% to 9% in the lowest 10th percentile of PRS among 22q11.2 deletion carriers (Davies et al. 2020). This study, therefore, suggests that the risk for developing schizophrenia, relative to the "average PRS risk" given a 22q11.2 deletion, could be refined for patients at both ends of the schizophrenia PRS distribution. Similarly, much larger-scale studies have shown that PRS significantly improves the positive predictive value yield for breast cancer in individuals at high risk due to rare variants in *BRCA1/2* (Kuchenbaecker et al. 2017; Wray et al. 2021). Further research is needed, however, to replicate and test the generalizability of these findings. The additional benefits of genetic counseling required to understand the contribution from polygenic risk alongside rare variant risk (e.g., in CNV carriers) should also be evaluated. Finally, it is unclear whether clinical psychiatric management or surveillance recommendations would differ for those patients at the highest versus lowest decile of risk, nor have the potential negative consequences for patients and their treatment been explored systemically. These remain high-priority areas of future research.

Use of Polygenic Risk Scores in "Phenotypically Defined" High-Risk Populations

Patients who are "phenotypically defined" as high risk for a psychiatric disorder may be in a prodromal phase or may already have one or more conditions that increase their risk of developing a later psychiatric disorder. While there is clear evidence of the positive impact of genetic counseling and psychoeducation in helping patients adapt to a diagnosis already received (Ryan et al. 2015), there are fewer data on the best approach for helping patients adapt to genetic risk for a mental illness in the absence of that diagnosis (Carrion et al. 2022; Gerrard et al. 2020). In the case of a patient who is phenotypically defined at high risk for a major mental illness, there are additional ethical and practical considerations for communicating risk in a way that optimizes positive outcomes, patient autonomy, and patient-provider relationships, while minimizing negative consequences such as self-stigma, demoralization, therapeutic nihilism, and discrimination (Ryan et al. 2015). The group identified this as a critical area of genetic counseling research and elaborates on this subject below in the genetic counseling section of this chapter.

Use of Polygenic Risk Scores in the General Population

While a well-powered PRS for a highly heritable psychiatric disorder can index increased relative risk for developing a given disorder, the absolute risk in the general population remains low for disorders with a low prevalence (e.g., schizophrenia or Tourette syndrome). This reduces the predictive value of these tests. For example, the relative risk of developing schizophrenia for an individual with a PRS in the highest 1% of the distribution is 5.6 (compared to all others in the population), but the absolute risk is approximately 5% (Lewis and Vassos 2022; Trubetskoy et al. 2022). The utility of this knowledge for early diagnosis, prevention, or enhanced surveillance has yet to be determined. For common psychiatric disorders (e.g., depression, anxiety), the prevalence is higher but the heritability of the disorder is lower. The PRS explains less of the phenotypic variability between people, but given higher prevalence, absolute risks may be high.

We discussed the potential for PRS to be part of a tiered screening system aimed at promoting resilience and positive health behaviors. Given the potential for the PRS to influence *perceptions* of risk, the communication of the uncertainty inherent in PRS interpretation is critical to ensure the beneficial integration of genomic knowledge into the patient's view of their current and future mental health. Thus, research is needed to identify the most effective approaches to delivering the information given the clinical context of PRS screening. Understanding the psychosocial impacts of receiving such a score, and the role that clinical genetic counseling could play in mitigating any negative impacts, could further improve the benefit-to-risk ratio. Additional research is needed to determine which determinants of health (e.g., clinical, family history, social) increase risk and should thus be considered when prioritizing patients for screening. This will also inform the process of providing feedback to patients about their PRS.

Use of Polygenic Scores in Treatment Selection

Existing PRSs have primarily been trained on case/control labels for DSM constructs (e.g., major depression or schizophrenia). Thus, there is a need for further discovery research to guide treatment selection and predict treatment response (including presence of side effects). Existing genome-wide association studies (GWASs) of treatment response remain limited by sample size, outcome measurement, and design approaches. For example, treatment response phenotypes are often limited to "response versus nonresponse" of a single medication. A more valuable clinical use for PRS would be to distinguish which medication out of the many existing options might yield the best response.

Identifying the polygenic component to treatment response is challenging, and more robust polygenic predictors of treatment response are needed. As with GWAS of diagnostic labels, large sample sizes are key to success, but sample sizes for treatment response studies are currently low compared to case-control GWAS. Further studies focused on specific drugs or drug classes are needed to build relevant PRSs aimed at facilitating the prescription of decisions for a patient. Expanding the data sources with high-quality, individual-level response to treatment will be crucial to performing well-powered studies needed to identify genetic predictors of response to treatment. Limitations include lack of access to data from clinical trials (particularly from pharmaceutical companies), difficulties in determining response in real-world data, and confusion that arises from polypharmacy.

An open question is the extent to which genomic predictors for disorder risk are also predictive of treatment response. Current studies in depression show only modest overlap (Pain et al. 2022b), but confusion may exist since GWAS finds that people with high PRS are more likely to have severe, recurrent, or chronic disorder; this alone may account for poorer treatment response. There is an urgent need to develop novel data sources for treatment response, or surrogate measures, with validation of the measure and understanding of the biases, strengths, and weaknesses of each data source. Possibilities include:

- Exploiting electronic health record data using natural language processing to extract measures of treatment response.
- Using treatment-resistant cases, with the assumption that change of drug after a suitable prescribing period indicates a lack of response.
- Seeking innovative data sources, such as passive data collection from wearable devices or phone apps that can capture indicators of treatment response.

Equity in the Use of Polygenic Scores

As discussed above, we recognize that equitable translation of PRS is a barrier to current implementation. The Eurocentric history of GWAS discovery research has resulted in PRSs that are primarily tuned for performance in European-ancestry populations and which underperform in non-European ancestries. Clinical translation prior to equitable performance of such genomic tools will exacerbate health disparities. Thus, representation and equity must be a primary emphasis in any new discovery GWAS.

The Impact of Genetic Counseling with and without Genetic Testing on the Clinical Management of Mental Illness

As defined by the National Society of Genetic Counselors, "genetic counseling is the process of helping people understand and adapt to the medical, psychological and familial implications of genetic contributions to disease" (Resta et al. 2006). Genetic counselors provide genetic risk estimation, support decision making in relation to genetic testing, and obtain patient consent. They are involved in the interpretation and management of test results. Furthermore, they assist the patient in adapting to the genetic information and in managing the resulting psychosocial consequences (Patch and Middleton 2018). We believe that genetic counseling should be considered in two contexts: (a) counseling that accompanies genetic testing and (b) counseling in the absence of genetic testing.

Counseling that accompanies clinically recommended genetic testing, which can be ordered and interpreted by clinical geneticists or genetic counselors, aims to help people understand the results of their specific genetic test and the implications of those results. There was consensus in our group that clinical genetics services traditionally focus on rare disorders with Mendelian inheritance patterns. However, the genetic architecture of mental health disorders is complex and genetic testing is not routinely recommended. Hence, only a subset of those who might benefit from genetic *counseling* are referred to clinical genetic services for genetic *testing*.

Patients who do receive a genetic test result indicating the presence of an underlying genetic syndrome might experience changes in clinical management. Here, genetic counselors and/or medical geneticists can help patients and families adapt to these new healthcare needs. For example, young children with a 22q11.2 deletion will be referred to other areas of medicine (including cardiology to assess associated cardiac anomalies) and may benefit from referral to psychiatry services for surveillance for early psychosis symptoms. The positive predictive value of some rare genetic variants, especially when combined with additional genetic factors (i.e., PRSs), has the potential to provide increased clinical value (i.e., additional referrals or targeted surveillance). Information about underlying genetic causes can be beneficial for the planning of appropriate educational interventions, family support, and advocacy. In these contexts, genetic counselors and/or medical geneticists may also work with family members who seek family planning services or other recommendations (Butler et al. 2022). Early involvement and close collaboration of primary care, clinical genetics, and developmental pediatrics with child, adolescent, and adult psychiatry may help provide clinical care that can optimize outcomes.

Genetic testing may be absent in the counseling process when a patient has been offered genetic testing but declines or when genetic testing is not available. The latter is true in most cases. We agreed that patients with a psychiatric disorder would benefit from receiving general information on the genetic contribution to their disorder. However, we could not agree on how this intervention—in the absence of available genetic testing—should be delivered or what it should be called. Some argued that this falls under the umbrella of genetic counseling while others felt that the intervention was best described as psychoeducation.

In support of this first position, we reviewed the large body of evidence that supports the position that helping people understand the genetic contributions to disease has a positive impact on patients' lives, even in the absence of genetic testing (Morris et al. 2021; see also Austin, this volume). Genetic counseling provides a better understanding of how genes and environment contribute to the development of illness. This is particularly helpful to clinical management, as dispelling misperceptions related to etiology increases patient autonomy, reduces stigma, shame, blame, and guilt, and empowers patients to adopt healthy lifestyle changes that can reduce the chances of a psychiatric episode (Morris et al. 2021). For example, patients could work with a genetic counselor to understand how their genetic risk interacts with environmental risk and to identify factors that contribute to their own resilience (e.g., through sleep, physical activity, and medication adherence).

Acknowledging the limited resources available to provide genetic counseling, an alternative view is that this more specialized type of counseling should be reserved for patients who fulfill the criteria for being offered genetic testing or who specifically request genetic counseling for other reasons (e.g., questions about family planning or adoptions in the presence of family history of mental illness). Throughout our discussion, there was significant debate on the nomenclature used to describe genetic counseling in the absence of genetic testing. As previously indicated, there are currently no guidelines for psychiatric genetic counseling despite robust evidence of the positive and lasting impact that genetic counseling can have in helping patients change their beliefs about the origin of their psychiatric illness and their degree of control over their future. An alternative approach to prioritizing patients to be referred for genetic counseling was proposed, based on patient need. For example, in addition to those eligible for genetic testing, patients who have the lowest levels of empowerment could be prioritized for referral to a genetic counselor. Research suggests that this group benefited greatly after receiving genetic counseling in terms of increases in empowerment (Gerrard et al. 2020).

In terms of challenges related to the workforce, there is a general lack of education in psychiatric genetics among psychiatrists, psychologists, social workers, and other mental health professionals as well as a lack of interdisciplinary work among all relevant stakeholders. In some parts of the world, there are training programs for psychiatric counselors; however, opportunities to practice are limited as the creation of positions has not kept up with the supply of trained counselors (Dillon et al. 2022). The creation of genetic counseling positions is driven by demand for genetic counseling, as indicated by physician referrals, yet these tend to be driven by the availability of genetic testing (Chanouha 2022). In other parts of the world, there are few or no training programs for psychiatric genetic counselors. This has led to a workforce shortage and a reliance on clinical geneticists, psychiatrists, and primary care physicians to provide genetic information to patients.

The Impact of Genetic Education on Public Discourse Regarding Mental Illness

Genomic information is often perceived by the public as deterministic and immutable, which can lead to increased stigma and decreased sense of autonomy and control when an individual is diagnosed with a psychiatric condition. We identified the inclusion of information about the etiology of psychiatric conditions (including genomics) in public mental health campaigns as a priority area in public education. Key concepts that should be communicated to the public in awareness campaigns include the probabilistic nature of genetic variation, the spectrum nature of genetic risk (and phenotypes), and the complex interaction between genetics and environment throughout the lifespan (e.g., Ke et al. 2015). In addition, we recommend genomics education be included in schools alongside mental health education. Anticipating and addressing misconceptions is important when developing this type of awareness campaign, as is measuring outcomes to assess understanding and remaining gaps. Thus, partnering with patient representatives, mental health advocacy groups, national mental health institutes, and public mental health forums could provide avenues for these types of engagement and awareness campaigns.

Barriers to the Application of Genetics in Clinical Mental Health Practice

Multiple and diverse barriers inhibit adequate implementation of clinical genetics in clinical mental health practice at several levels: societal, healthcare organization, clinician, family, and patient. The specific issues experienced may vary, but the general barriers are similar regardless of the specific clinical genetic intervention under discussion. Table 12.1 lists barriers which cut across three forms of clinical genetic interventions: (a) clinical genetic testing and counseling, (b) genetic counseling in the absence of testing, and (c) increasing health literacy and genetic knowledge of psychiatric conditions.

Further barriers that cut across all classifications include institutional obstacles to implementation, poor diversity and representation, psychiatry-specific challenges to the use of genetic testing, and the potential for excessive medical conservatism. In terms of implementation, the lack of electronic health record support inhibits the integration of genetic information into the health record, needed to facilitate clinical management and inform (not confuse) clinicians and patients. Regardless of the type of clinical information being returned,

Table 12.1 Barriers to the availability of clinical genetic services.

Societal	• Limited knowledge of genetics and misperception of genetic determinism • Fear that genetic explanations of mental illness will increase stigma • Disparities in access to clinical genetic services
Healthcare systems	• Inconsistent payment structures that sometimes disincentivize services • Limited human resources (e.g., clinical psychologists, psychiatrists, and psychiatric genetic counselors) • Limited workforce education on the role of genetics in psychiatry
Clinician	• Historical disconnect between psychiatry and clinical genetics • Failure to recognize the role of genetics in the context of complex psychiatric disorders, resulting in neglect of genetics in psychoeducation • Disagreement regarding role of genetic counselors in the absence of genetic testing
Family and individual	• Overestimation of absolute and relative risk • Concerns over genetic privacy and discrimination • Fears of eugenic motivations regarding clinical genetic services

patients from non-European ancestries are disadvantaged by the lack of ancestral diversity in existing genetic databases. Patients from non-European genetic backgrounds who meet criteria today for clinical testing are more likely to have variants that are currently of unknown significance. Additionally, PRS that are trained on genetic data collected from European-ancestry populations are not portable to non-European populations. Some of the barriers identified were unique to psychiatry, including the fact that psychiatric diagnoses remain stigmatized and that fears of the eugenic use of psychiatric genetic information are substantial.

Guiding Principles for Future Research and Implementation

Throughout our discussions, the need to improve education (clinical and public) was viewed as crucial. To aid progress, we propose a strategy that would build on existing pathways of information sharing and create a two-pronged awareness campaign aimed at both general and clinical audiences (see Figure 12.1). This campaign would utilize the World Health Organization and other groups to distribute educational materials developed by the International Society for Psychiatric Genetics (ISPG). Professional organizations, including the American (APA), European (EPA), and/or World (WPA) psychiatric associations could utilize these materials to educate professionals in training and practice, and potentially to develop clinical consensuses and practice guidelines. Other groups, preferably those with existing public awareness

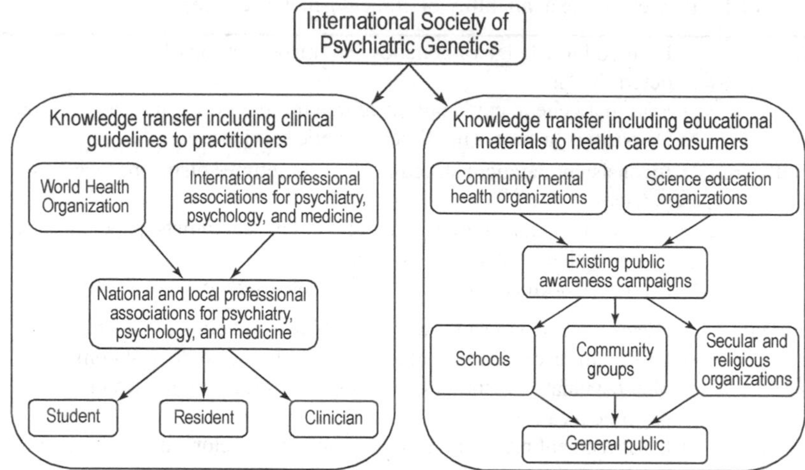

Figure 12.1 Strategy for psychiatric genetic awareness campaign.

campaigns, could use these materials to dissemination information on genetic risk and resilience to the general population, perhaps through schools and other community and faith-based organizations.

To support and optimize the near-term clinical opportunities for innovative psychiatric genetics, there are significant future research needs. In addition to innovation, future research must aim to remove existing barriers and be conducted according to the following principles. First, diversity in genetic data sets is paramount to facilitate equitable clinical use of genetic information. As described by Ronald et al. (this volume), capacity building must be a first principle of global diversity in psychiatric genomics, and we argue that capacity building for genetic research should not ignore the eventual goal of clinical implementation for the communities in which a research program is being established. Second, patient representatives must be meaningfully engaged at every level of research from discovery to research aimed at clinically oriented outcomes. This is both an ethical imperative and an essential design aspect of sustainable and relevant research programs. Third, experts in the field of implementation sciences and health economics should be consulted and ideally embedded in research teams that confront the challenges of psychiatric genetics translation described here. Finally, scientific communication experts, such as genetic counselors, are essential to the field, as they can advise on how to communicate effectively. This does not, however, absolve the psychiatric genetics community of the responsibility to learn how to communicate their own work to the public effectively. Further high-priority areas include:

1. Critical needs in translational psychiatric genomics: (a) Evaluation of clinical genetic testing in psychiatric disorders, including evaluation of the use of PRSs. Currently, it is unclear how much the incremental

increase in risk provided by additional genetic information in the form of PRS might change clinical management. (b) Both existing and future data collections are needed to address the paucity of large-scale genomic studies of treatment response, further articulated below. (c) Studies aimed at assessing and positively impacting psychosocial consequences of genetic testing and risk stratification are needed, as the delivery of information can influence health behaviors in both positive and negative ways. Thus, best practice guidelines for delivery of genomic information related to mental health are essential.

2. Evaluating clinical genetic testing in general psychiatry: Studies are needed to identify the added value of genetic testing in psychiatric disorders for which there are currently no recommendations for testing (e.g., adult-onset psychosis). For example, the first episode of psychosis may initiate a battery of tests ranging from cognitive assessments to brain imaging, yet it is still unclear whether the addition of genetic data to those batteries can decrease the time to diagnosis or guide clinical management in situations with poor diagnostic specificity. Clinical trials are needed to determine whether diagnostic delay can be shortened and treatment selection improved. Importantly, these studies need not be limited to genomic data but may instead evaluate decisions based on risk or response calculators that incorporate genetic and nongenetic factors. Although risk calculators may be most useful when addressing questions of differential diagnosis, response calculators could be helpful in guiding management decisions.
3. Research on the clinical use of genetic testing to encompass patient-oriented outcomes and experiences: Treatment decisions are often made before a clear diagnosis has emerged. Thus, best practices are needed to guide interventions for at-risk patients. This could include interventions that promote positive attitudes toward mental health and avoid stigmatizing children and families. Indeed, the very definition of successful risk reduction is itself an active area of research. How should risk reduction be measured? Is there a role for genetic counseling and/or psychoeducation in risk-reduction strategies? Outcome studies are needed to determine whether individuals with positive genetic test results would benefit from additional genetic information in the form of PRS. These studies should assess the positive and negative predictive values of the addition of the PRS to the knowledge already conferred by the presence of the rare variant. In each case, patient engagement is critical to identify outcomes that are most important. For example, it may be a higher priority for families to learn whether the incorporation of the PRS can aid in treatment decisions and avoid diagnostic prognostication.
4. Improving genomic studies of treatment response: Genomic studies of treatment response for psychiatric conditions are lacking, in part due to

limited collections in which genotype and treatment response are both measured at scale. Existing large-scale samples of genotyped patients with longitudinal treatment response data should be available within electronic health records; however, these data are rarely standardized and are often embedded as textual descriptions in the clinical notes of the care provider. Thus, developing tools in the electronic health record for efficiently recording treatment responses to psychiatric medications should be a priority for learning healthcare systems, as these data could inform a myriad of studies. Furthermore, new data collection efforts should consider the ethical application of innovative approaches to the collection of treatment response data that allow for both active (ecological momentary assessment) data collected (e.g., from mobile phones) and passive monitoring (e.g., of activity, sleep levels, voice modulation) from wearables. This could provide richer context for genetic studies of treatment response.

5. Large GWAS of treatment response to generate PRS: This may be more informative in guiding treatment selections than PRS which primarily measure genomic predisposition to develop particular psychiatric conditions. Again, clinical data from electronic health records coupled with large-scale biobanking efforts could be extremely useful; however, they are not without problems (e.g., polypharmacy, formulary differences, and variation in medication adherence), all of which can complicate interpretation of outcome data. Thus, it is important that clinical trials also include the collection of genetic data from participants, and that these data are shared with researchers under precompetitive research agreements. Again, inclusion of diverse patient populations at every step of the research process will be critical in guiding decisions on identifying multiple outcomes, all of which constitute important responses to treatment.
6. Best practices for delivery of genomic information in a psychiatry setting: More studies are needed that aim at assessing and positively impacting psychosocial consequences of genetic testing. These studies should identify contextual modifiers (i.e., social determinants) and develop best practices to enhance positive effects and reduce negative effects of genetic testing. As mentioned, though PRS interpretation is not currently supported in clinical workflows, many patients have access to their PRS through direct-to-consumer products, and patients are beginning to bring these genetic test results to their providers for interpretation. Thus, despite the lack of clinical guidelines on genetic testing in general patient populations, best practice recommendations are needed for clinicians to counsel patients effectively on existing PRS results brought into the clinical setting. This includes referral guidelines, approaches to genomic education, and guidelines on *how* and *who* should counsel patients to help them understand their PRS

(NSGC, in press). Best practice guidelines are likely to differ based on the patient population.

Conclusion

Psychiatric genetics holds promise for improving prediction and diagnosis of psychiatric conditions, as well as the selection and implementation of effective treatment. In the short term, utilization is likely to remain focused on children and adults with neurodevelopmental disorders and might extend to children and adolescents with early-onset psychosis. Fulfilling the promise of psychiatric genetics for other disorders awaits the development of a more robust research foundation for the use of genetic information (including PRS) in clinical settings, including studies aimed at assessing their added value for clinical decision making. Of key importance is the development of ancestry-diverse databases for the interpretation of genetic findings, necessary for the equitable use of genetic testing, and the provision of enhanced training for mental health professionals in psychiatric genetics. An understanding of one's diagnosis (including the potential genetic contribution) should include psychoeducation and/or genetic counseling. Thus, it is important that all providers be trained to deliver high-quality information to patients and families. Finally, public education on genetics, including the genetics of psychiatric disorders, is essential to improve understanding of genetic test results and to reduce such negative consequences as stigma and discrimination.

13

The Use of Polygenic Risk Scores in Clinical Psychiatry

Opportunities and Obstacles

Jordan W. Smoller

Abstract

Large-scale genome-wide association studies have demonstrated that psychiatric phenotypes are highly polygenic, involving thousands of loci of individually small effect. Polygenic risk scores (PRSs), which sum these effects, can provide a composite index of an individual's genetic vulnerability. There has been growing interest in the potential use of PRS for clinical applications and advancing precision psychiatry. Here, I summarize the prospects for implementing PRSs in a range of potential use cases including predicting disease risk, reducing diagnostic uncertainty, forecasting prognosis, guiding treatment selection, informing genetic counseling, and validating prevention strategies. PRSs represent one of the most robust biomarkers in psychiatry, but as reviewed here, several important challenges remain before they can be used in clinical practice. Future work will need to address the limited predictive value of current scores, the Eurocentric bias of available data, the need to optimize the integration of PRS with other risk factors, and the validation of actionable risk-stratified interventions. Efforts to translate PRS to real-world applications will also require research using an implementation science framework. Nevertheless, the potential value of PRS for improving clinical care in psychiatry justifies investments in research and implementation strategies to overcome these challenges.

Introduction

Genetic research in psychiatry has proceeded, broadly speaking, with two related goals in mind. The first goal is to leverage genetic findings to uncover the biological underpinnings of psychopathology. By linking specific genes and pathways to psychiatric phenotypes, we hope to unravel the etiology and pathogenesis of psychiatric disorders. The second goal is to find ways of translating genetic discoveries to improve clinical practice, for example, by identifying new therapeutic targets or identifying risk profiles that could predict or guide diagnosis, treatment, or prevention. Over the past two decades, the advent of large-scale genome-wide association studies (GWASs) of common and rare variation has enabled substantial progress toward the first goal. Genomic studies have illuminated the genetic architecture of psychiatric disorders and hundreds of genetic variations and genes have been convincingly associated with a range of psychiatric disorders. Functional genomic follow-on studies have linked these loci to molecular pathways and neural circuits. In contrast, progress toward the second goal—clinical translation—has been less dramatic. The highly polygenic nature of psychiatric disorders and the modest effects of individual common variants have complicated the clinical application of genetic findings. At the same time, this polygenicity has spurred great interest in leveraging polygenic risk scores (PRSs) for clinical use. Polygenic scores capture substantial genetic vulnerability in a single index by aggregating a large number of individual genetic signals. In this chapter, I review the status of efforts to apply PRSs to address clinically relevant questions.

The details of developing and validating PRSs have been described elsewhere (Choi et al. 2020c). In brief, determining PRSs begins by estimating effects of single nucleotide polymorphisms (SNPs) in a GWAS of a given phenotype. Polygenic scores can then be calculated for individuals in an independent sample by multiplying the number of risk alleles (0, 1, or 2) at each SNP by its effect size (e.g., logarithm of the odds ratio) derived from the discovery sample and then summing these values across all SNPs included in the PRS. This is appealing in part because PRSs provide a single index of common variant genetic loading and can be calculated from a single biospecimen collection at any time. They have been calculated for a broad range of psychiatric and behavioral phenotypes and are arguably the best validated biomarker of risk in psychiatry. At the same time, PRSs have well-recognized limitations. First, the trait variance they capture is bounded by the heritability of the trait. This upper bound, however, will never be reached because PRSs reflect only the genetic component attributable to common SNPs. Most investigators regard PRSs by themselves as insufficiently informative for clinical use in predicting psychiatric outcomes. In addition, most available PRSs have been derived from GWAS of individuals of European ancestry, and PRS performance in those of other ancestries can be markedly attenuated, particularly for those of African ancestry (Mars et al. 2022; Martin et al. 2019b). A variety of strategies have been developed to enhance PRS performance. In particular, methods that use a Bayesian framework and incorporate genetic architecture have shown superior results (Ni et al. 2021).

Despite their limitations, there has been great interest in exploiting PRS for clinical applications (Murray et al. 2021; Wray et al. 2021). In the following sections, I will briefly summarize a range of use cases in which there has been interest in using PRSs for clinical applications in psychiatry.

Use Case I: Predicting Risk of Psychiatric Disorder

A large body of research—from twin studies to genomic analyses—has convincingly documented the important role of genetic variation in risk of psychiatric illness. GWASs have established that psychiatric disorders are highly polygenic and that common variation accounts for the largest share of their genetic architecture (though to varying degrees depending on the specific disorder). Polygenic scores for numerous disorders have shown highly statistically significant associations with risk of the disorders for which they were derived. As such, PRSs could provide an attractive opportunity as a tool for risk prediction. As noted earlier, the magnitude of PRS effects is inherently limited by disorder heritability, and, to date, available PRSs fall far short of reaching this theoretical upper limit. The ever-expanding sample size of psychiatric GWAS will help narrow this gap, but at present the predictive performance of PRSs remains relatively modest. In the realm of psychiatry, the most powerful PRSs thus far have been developed for schizophrenia (SCZ). In the largest GWAS of SCZ (Trubetskoy et al. 2022), PRSs explained 7.3% of the variance in disorder risk, with 5.6-fold increased odds of SCZ among those in the top 1% compared to all others. These results, of course, were derived from cohorts that were ascertained for research purposes (after meeting a range of inclusion/exclusion criteria) and often relied on semi-structured diagnostic assessments. Different results might be obtained in samples derived from real-world clinical practice. Indeed, in a study by the PsycheMERGE Consortium using diagnoses derived from real-world electronic health record data across four large U.S. health systems, patients in the top decile versus all others had a more modest 2.3-fold increased odds of SCZ (Zheutlin et al. 2019). Still, that magnitude of effect is comparable to those seen with risk factors we commonly use in clinical assessment of risk for other disorders. For example, the hazard ratio associated with smoking in the Framingham Risk Score for cardiovascular disease risk is less than 2.0 (D'Agostino et al. 2008).

However, relative risks are not necessarily of greatest interest to patients and clinicians. If I wish to know my risk of a disease, I would be more interested in my *absolute* risk (over some time period), and this will be strongly influenced by the base rate of the disorder. Given that the lifetime risk of SCZ is approximately 1% or less, even a 5.6-fold increased risk would imply less than a 6% absolute risk (and thus a 94% probability of not developing the disorder). Could this be clinically useful? That seems unlikely, although not inconceivable. For example, widely accepted recommendations for primary prevention of heart disease suggest that initiating statin therapy is appropriate for individuals with a 10-year absolute risk of atherosclerotic cardiovascular disease of $\geq$7.5% (Arnett et al. 2019). Guidelines for breast cancer screening recommend initiating annual mammography for women aged 35–39 whose 5-year risk is $\geq$1.7% (Lewis et al. 2021). Ultimately, the appropriateness of a given absolute risk threshold is a judgment that will depend in part on whether there are actionable interventions for prevention. In the case of coronary heart disease, such interventions are well established and include medication (e.g., statins) and lifestyle changes. For SCZ and most other psychiatric disorders, risk modification and preventive strategies are limited to date. However, some actionable interventions have been validated, even for primary prevention. These include school-based anti-bullying programs, avoidance of substance abuse, and certain lifestyle changes (Arango et al. 2018). In the case of major depressive disorder, clinical and epidemiologic studies have documented the preventive effect of social connection and physical activity (Gariepy et al. 2016; Pearce et al. 2022). Recent analyses have demonstrated that these factors lower the risk of incident depression even among those with higher levels of PRS for depression (Choi et al. 2019, 2020a, b). Thus, while PRSs for major depressive disorder have smaller effect size compared with PRSs for SCZ, an argument could be made for using PRSs to help target higher risk individuals for these relatively low burden interventions.

Most studies that have examined PRS prediction in psychiatry have reported effect estimates (e.g., beta coefficients or odds ratios) and p-values for statistical association. While these metrics have established PRS as a risk factor for complex disorders, they are not sufficient to validate clinically relevant predictive performance. There are a range of established metrics for evaluating the performance of a prediction model (for a review, see Steyerberg et al. 2010). These include sensitivity and specificity (the proportion of cases and non-cases that are correctly classified, respectively), and measures of discrimination—most commonly the area under the receiver operator curve (AUC), which reflects the ability of the model to discriminate those with and without the outcome. AUC values range from 0.5 (no better than chance) to 1.0 (perfect discrimination), and values of 0.80 or above are considered good to excellent. When they have been reported, AUCs reported for psychiatric PRSs have been moderate, in the range of 0.65–0.75 for SCZ (Trubetskoy et al. 2022), bipolar disorder (So and Sham 2017), and alcohol use disorder (Ksinan et al. 2022), and lower for major depression (Privé et al. 2019; So and Sham 2017). Perhaps more clinically relevant are the positive and negative predictive values (PPV, NPV). The PPV gives the probability that those who "test positive" (i.e., exceed a threshold probability) actually have or will have the target disease whereas the NPV represents the probability that those who test negative will not have the disease. These predictive values, which correspond to absolute risks, have typically not been reported.

Two approaches have been examined for enhancing the predictive utility of PRSs. The first is to apply PRSs in groups with a higher probability of illness. For a test with given sensitivity and specificity, the PPV (again, the absolute risk of disease among those who "test positive") depends on the base rate of the disease. Applying the test (here, PRS) in a population with an elevated base rate should enhance its predictive value. Davies et al. (2020) examined a SCZ PRS in a cohort of patients with 22q11 deletion syndrome, a genomic disorder known to confer substantially increased risk of psychotic illness. Among those in the top decile of SCZ PRS, the PPV was 33%—more than 30-fold higher than the risk seen for individuals in the top PRS decile in healthcare system biobanks (Zheutlin et al. 2019). These findings suggest that PRS may have a defensible role in predicting outcomes among individuals with a known high prior probability of the target outcome. This is also consistent with a growing literature demonstrating that PRS modifies the penetrance of rare structural or monogenic disease mutations (Bergen et al. 2019; Fahed et al. 2020; Niemi et al. 2018; Oetjens et al. 2019).

Apart from those at high risk due to carrying large-effect copy number variants (CNVs) or Mendelian mutations, there are several other clinically relevant scenarios in which predicting disorder among high-risk patients would be useful. For example, individuals with prodromal features of psychosis or "clinical high risk" have been reported to have a 20–35% risk of converting to a full-blown psychotic disorder within two years (Fusar-Poli et al. 2013). Perkins et al. (2020) examined the association between SCZ PRS and conversion among clinical high risk (N = 764) and unaffected individuals (N = 279) who were followed for two years. In high-risk individuals, PRS values were significantly but modestly higher among those who converted to psychotic illness compared to those who did not, though only among those of European ancestry. The AUC was relatively modest with a maximum of 0.65 among clinical high-risk patients of European ancestry. In another smaller longitudinal cohort (N = 97) of 22q11 deletion carriers followed for an average of 3.8 years, a SCZ PRS was associated with negative symptoms of SCZ, cognitive decline, and decreased hippocampal volumes (Alver et al. 2022).

A second strategy for improving prediction has been the addition of PRS to established (or novel) clinical risk models. To date, this strategy has been more extensively studied in other areas of medicine. For example, several studies have examined the addition of PRS to clinical risk models such as the widely used pooled cohort equations in heart disease. While some of these studies found significant improvement in model performance (e.g., AUC), the effects have often been modest (Elliott et al. 2020; Mosley et al. 2020; Petrazzini et al. 2022; Sun et al. 2021), even though PRS appears to be largely uncorrelated with risk predicted by pooled cohort equation risk factors (Hindy et al. 2020). A recent review of these studies found that adding the PRS to clinical risk models resulted in a negligible to modest improvement in AUC and net reclassification index, leading the authors to conclude that coronary heart disease PRSs are not useful at present for improving clinical decision making (Groenendyk et al. 2022). On the other hand, a recent overview and scientific statement from the American Heart Association struck a more optimistic tone regarding the potential clinical utility of PRS, in combination with clinical risk factors, for improving risk prediction for a range of cardiovascular conditions (O'Sullivan et al. 2022).

In a study of nearly 8,000 children at high risk for type I diabetes based on HLA genotype who were followed from birth to age 9, a combined risk score comprising a type I diabetes PRS, autoantibodies, and family history achieved AUCs > 0.90 and doubled the efficiency of population-based newborn screening to prevent ketoacidosis (Ferrat et al. 2020). Addition of PRS to clinical risk models has also resulted in improved prediction performance and net reclassification in a range of other conditions including breast and prostate cancers, type II diabetes, and atrial fibrillation (Hurson et al. 2022; Lee et al. 2019a; Mars et al. 2020).

In the realm of psychiatric disorders, however, few examples have been reported to date. In the Perkins et al. (2020) study of individuals with clinical high risk for psychosis, addition of the PRS to an established risk calculator based on clinical variables did not result in a significant improvement in prediction.

Overall, then, the evidence that PRSs on their own are sufficiently predictive to warrant clinical implementation to predict illness onset is weak. Nevertheless, PRSs represent one of the few well-validated biomarkers of risk and may well provide clinical value in combination with other risk factors. Studies examining the incorporation of PRSs into multivariable risk models are scant, however, and should be prioritized. In addition, PRSs could be useful in a multistage screening workflow in which those at elevated risk on the basis of PRSs could be targeted for further evaluation. For example, an elevated PRS has been reported to improve the PPV of PSA screening for prostate cancer (Byrne and Toland 2021; Seibert et al. 2018). Again, however, there has been little work done to evaluate the utility of such stepwise screening for psychiatric applications.

Future studies of using PRSs for prediction of psychiatric outcomes will need to address a series of challenges. First, a major challenge to the clinical application of PRSs is the lack of genetic diversity in most data sets from which PRSs have been trained and validated. By far, most such data sets comprise individuals of European ancestry, and generalizability of effect estimates is poor across ancestries (Mars et al. 2022; Martin et al. 2019a, b). As such, predictions based on available PRSs are unlikely to be valid for individuals of non-European descent. Clinical use of existing PRSs could thus exacerbate the already substantial health disparities that such individuals may already experience. Even if data were available to derive ancestry-specific PRSs, their clinical implementation would be problematic as this would require defining groups either based on self-reported race or ancestry (which are imprecise and socially constructed categories) or defining genetic ancestry prior to the return of results. A more defensible approach would be to derive multi-ancestry PRSs for which a growing number of methods have been developed (Ruan et al. 2022; Wang et al. 2022; Weissbrod et al. 2022). As a prelude to studying the prospective return of PRS risk reports to individuals in clinical settings, the eMERGE network has been developing and validating several muti-ancestry

PRSs with promising results (Ge et al. 2021; Khan et al. 2022; Namjou et al. 2022). For example, Ge et al. (2021) developed a trans-ancestry PRS for type II diabetes using a Bayesian PRS modeling method (PRS-CSx) and GWAS data from European, African American, and East Asian populations. When applied to several muti-ethnic cohorts, those in the top 2% of the PRS distribution were found to have a 2.5- to 4.5-fold increased risk of the disorder relative to those below this threshold across all ancestries studied.

It should be noted that the impact of ancestry differences on PRS performance is one instance of a larger challenge. That is, any difference in the characteristics of samples in which PRS risk estimates are derived (e.g., research cohorts) and those in which they are applied for clinical use could impact prediction accuracy. Mostafavi et al. (2020) have shown that even *within* ancestry groups, mismatch in sex, age, or socioeconomic status distributions between training and target data sets can substantially alter prediction performance. Similar effects could be expected for differences in environmental exposures, ascertainment, disease comorbidities, and other factors. The extent of such threats to PRS portability remains to be defined.

Another issue, alluded to earlier, is that the clinical utility of psychiatric PRS remains almost entirely unexplored. Demonstrating this utility will require more than establishing robust association between PRSs and a given disease outcome. Even beyond determining prediction model metrics of discrimination, predictive value, and calibration, clinical implementation may require consideration of net reclassification, number-needed-to-test, and net benefit, which captures the trade-off between benefit and harm for implementation of a predictive model (Steyerberg et al. 2010; Vickers et al. 2016). Relatedly, the predictive value of a PRS may depend on a variety of other factors. For example, a PRS for risk of SCZ, like most other known risk factors for the disease, would be less useful for patients whose age is beyond the usual period of risk.

Clinical implementation of PRS could, of course, raise a number of ethical issues as well (reviewed by Appelbaum, this volume). For many psychiatric conditions—including psychotic disorders, bipolar disorder, anorexia nervosa, and others—evidence-based strategies for prevention or early intervention are limited. Given the regrettable but persistent stigma attached to mental illness, identifying individuals as "high risk" without offering the benefit of clear options to address that risk could simply result in anxiety or concerns about labeling without improving outcomes. For conditions where the baseline risk is relatively low, this could be compounded by the fact that most individuals with high PRS values are unlikely to develop the condition (i.e., there would be a high false positive rate). A recent controversy has arisen around the potential use of PRSs for embryo selection aimed at primary prevention of complex disorders, including SCZ. The controversy arose after several private companies began to market this service. In response, several commentaries and quantitative evaluations have appeared highlighting the substantial ethical challenges such a practice would raise and demonstrating that the expected gain in risk reduction would be far lower than clinicians and consumers might assume (Lázaro-Muñoz et al. 2021; Lencz et al. 2021; Turley et al. 2021).

Use Case II: Reducing Diagnostic Uncertainty

Psychiatric diagnosis is a notoriously complex process that relies on patient self-report, behavioral observation, and clinician judgment. The dominant classification frameworks (DSM and ICD) define psychiatric conditions as syndromes whose signs and symptoms often overlap. Except in rare cases, the relevance of diagnostic tests, such as laboratory blood tests or imaging, has been limited. The costs of diagnostic uncertainty, both personal and economic, can be substantial. For example, the mean delay between onset of bipolar disorder and appropriate diagnosis is typically 6–10 years (Dagani et al. 2017; McIntyre et al. 2020). For most individuals with bipolar disorder, illness onset begins with a depressive episode, commonly leading to a misdiagnosis of major depressive disorder. Treatment of underlying bipolar disorder with antidepressants in the absence of mood stabilizing medication can result in worsened outcomes, apparent "treatment resistant depression," and even iatrogenic triggering of manic or rapid cycling episodes (Singh and Rajput 2006).

As noted, PRSs offer one of the few established biomarkers of psychiatric disorder liability. As such, the possibility of using PRSs to reduce diagnostic uncertainty is appealing. Clearly an elevated PRS will never be necessary or sufficient for establishing or excluding a psychiatric diagnosis. There are no pathognomonic features of common psychiatric disorders, and PRS will not qualify as one. In the ultimately Bayesian process of diagnosis, however, it is conceivable that PRS could play a role as one piece of evidence in differential diagnosis.

Along these lines, Knevel et al. (2020) developed GPROB (genetic probability tool) to calculate the probability of different diseases for a given patient using PRS and applied it to differential diagnosis of inflammatory arthritides. Like many psychiatric disorders, these conditions (rheumatoid arthritis, systemic lupus erythematosus, spondyloarthropathy, psoriatic arthritis, and gout) present with similar findings and can be difficult to distinguish at an initial evaluation. GPROB uses multiple disease PRSs to calculate an individual's probability of having each of the target diseases, assuming that the patient has one of the diseases. In validation cohorts, the method appeared to improve differential diagnosis at a patient's first visit relative to clinician diagnosis alone. Whether this or similar methods could improve diagnosis in psychiatry remains to be seen.

A recent cross-sectional analysis (Liebers et al. 2021) compared bipolar disorder and SCZ PRS distributions between 843 individuals with bipolar disorder and 930 with major depressive disorder. Although both bipolar disorder and SCZ PRS were associated with bipolar disorder versus major depressive disorder, discrimination was modest (AUC = 0.64) compared to that seen with a model based on symptoms and clinical factors (AUC = 0.85). Addition of PRS to the clinical model did not improve discrimination. A larger, longitudinal analysis (Musliner et al. 2020) examined the association between PRS (bipolar disorder, major depressive disorder, SCZ) and progression to bipolar disorder or psychotic disorder diagnoses among nearly 17,000 individuals initially diagnosed with major depressive disorder in the Danish iPSYCH study. The association between bipolar disorder PRS and progression to bipolar disorder was statistically significant though modest (HR = 1.11; 95% CI, 1.03–1.21), and substantially lower than that seen for parental history of bipolar disorder, even after adjusting for PRS (HR = 5.02; 95% CI, 3.53–7.14). Thus, the potential value of PRS to inform differential diagnosis, while conceptually appealing, remains unclear and understudied.

Use Case III: Predicting Prognosis

Even when diagnosis is established, clinicians and patients face uncertainty about the course of illness an individual will experience, complicating treatment planning. The severity and chronicity of illness is central to the burden faced by individual patients and families in terms of both personal suffering and potential socioeconomic consequences. Here again, the availability of a validated biomarker that could help predict clinical course of illness would be a welcome advance. A challenge here is that most existing PRSs have been trained on labels of lifetime occurrence of disorder rather than longitudinal course. There is no *a priori* reason to think that a PRS derived from a case-control GWAS of disease would be strongly associated with course among those already affected with the disease. Perhaps, not surprisingly, then, recent efforts to explore PRS for prognosis prediction in psychiatry have shown very modest effects. In a longitudinal analysis of 249 patients followed for twenty years after a first admission for psychosis, a SCZ PRS was associated with higher ratings of avolition at baseline that remained over follow-up (Jonas et al. 2019). The PRS was not associated with symptom or severity changes over time, though higher SCZ PRS was associated with diagnostic shift to nonaffective psychosis among those originally diagnosed with affective psychosis (reported AUC = 0.62). A larger analysis of patients with psychotic disorders from multiple cohorts found no benefit of adding SCZ PRS to clinical features in predicting poor clinical outcomes (Landi et al. 2021). An analysis in the Danish iPSYCH cohort (Musliner et al. 2021) examined whether a major depression PRS could predict recurrence of depressive episodes (8 weeks or more) following an initial episode of depression. In a model adjusted for sex and PRS for bipolar disorder and SCZ, a modest increased risk of recurrent depression (HR per standard deviation of major depression PRS = 1.07; 95%

CI, 1.04–1.10) was observed. The increase in absolute risk associated with high PRS was also modest but increased over time: at twenty years of follow-up, 46% of those with PRS two standard deviations above the mean vs. 34% for those two standard deviations below the mean. The impact of treatment was not reported and outcomes were based on the documentation of a single ICD code. Finally, a PRS derived from GWAS of alcohol consumption was associated with alcohol-related morbidity and mortality in a longitudinal study of several Finnish cohorts (Kiiskinen et al. 2020). In a fully adjusted model that included baseline alcohol consumption, those in the top PRS quintile had a 58% relative increased risk of alcohol-related morbidity compared to those in the bottom quintile. The study also reported prediction metrics and found that adding PRS to the model improved the C index (comparable to AUC) by 0.02 and significantly improved the net reclassification index and integrated discrimination index. These performance improvements were lost, however, when baseline alcohol consumption was entered into the model. The performance of PRS for prognosis might be improved with training on disease course variables themselves. Studies in other areas of medicine have had some success with that approach (Aittokallio et al. 2022; Tremblay et al. 2021), but this remains largely unstudied in psychiatric conditions.

Use Case IV: Stratification to Enhance Treatment Selection

Psychiatric treatment remains largely a one-size-fits-all, trial-and-error process. Despite decades of research aimed at identifying predictors of treatment response, clinicians have few demographic, clinical, or biological factors that can reliably guide treatment selection. The potential value of such a predictor is clear. With antidepressant or other psychopharmacologic treatments, therapeutic response may be unclear for weeks or months. Each cycle in the trial-and-error process can mean months of prolonged suffering, disability, and adverse social and financial consequences for patients. As one example, data from the STAR*D study—a large prospective study of sequential treatment strategies for depression—only about 30% of patients achieved remission after 14 weeks of SSRI treatment and one-third of patients did not achieve remission even after four rounds of sequential treatment options that included alternative antidepressants or cognitive therapy (Gaynes et al. 2009). The notion of using genetic information to guide therapy is not a new one, and pharmacogenetic tests (primarily based on polymorphisms in drug metabolizing enzymes) are already available for psychotropic and other classes of medication in both clinical and direct-to-consumer offerings. The clinical utility of existing pharmacogenetic tests has been controversial in part due to open questions about their clinical benefit and cost-effectiveness (Milosavljevic et al. 2021; Murphy et al. 2022; Pardiñas et al. 2021; Zeier et al. 2018). The prospect of using PRS to guide treatment selection is supported in part by

GWAS analyses demonstrating statistically significant SNP-based heritability estimates for psychotropic treatment response, though conflicting findings have also appeared (Li et al. 2020; Tansey et al. 2013). Given the limited availability of predictors or treatment-relevant outcomes, a polygenic score could be highly useful even if it only moderately altered the prior probabilities of therapeutic response, tolerability, or adverse drug effects. To date, however, robust findings for psychotropic drug treatment are lacking. Statistically significant but modest associations have been reported between various polygenic scores and response to antipsychotic medication treatment of psychosis (Zhang et al. 2019), lithium treatment in bipolar disorder (Intl. Consortium on Lithium Genetics et al. 2018), antidepressant treatment of depression (Fanelli et al. 2022; Meerman et al. 2022; Ward et al. 2018), and electroconvulsive therapy for depression (Sigström et al. 2022). In a cohort of patients who presented with first-episode psychosis, PRS for cholesterol-related traits were associated with metabolic dysregulation after antipsychotic treatment (Segura et al. 2022). In one of the few efforts to combine PRSs with clinical predictors, Cearns et al. (2022) conducted treatment response modeling in a pooled analysis of 1,034 bipolar disorder patients treated with lithium. Polygenic scores for major depressive disorder and SCZ were both associated with lithium response, although they explained less variance than models based on clinical predictors. The best performance, explaining 13.7% of variance in lithium response, was seen with clinical models trained after first stratifying patients into the top versus bottom PRS quartiles.

Almost all studies of PRS prediction of psychotropic treatment response have been restricted to patients of European ancestry and effect sizes have been small. Most of these studies have also relied on PRS for disease risk rather than on polygenic scores trained specifically on treatment response. In addition, studies examining associations with treatment response have typically compared responders (by varying definitions) to non-responders. However, the clinically relevant question for clinicians is not whether a patient is more likely than not to respond, but rather which of the available treatment options is more likely to be effective. In sum, with respect to use of PRSs for treatment stratification, there is great potential to enhance clinical care, but the evidence base for utility in psychiatric practice is lacking.

Polygenic scores may also inform clinical trials of medication treatment. For example, a range of analyses in cardiovascular medicine has demonstrated that polygenic scores can be used to identify and enrich trials for patients more likely to respond to treatments for primary or secondary prevention of heart disease (Fahed et al. 2022). In principle, this strategy holds similar promise for trials of psychotropic agents and might facilitate the development of more targeted therapies.

Other Potential Clinical Uses

There are several additional scenarios in which PRS might inform clinical care, some related to the issues addressed above. First, PRS might be valuable as a component of *genetic counseling*. At present, genetic counseling typically focuses on the impact of moderate- to high-penetrance structural variants (e.g., rare CNVs, triplet repeats) and Mendelian disease mutations, as well as family history. In a widely cited analysis of data from the UK Biobank, Khera et al. (2018) showed that high PRS for coronary artery disease confers risk of the disease that is comparable in magnitude to that seen with Mendelian mutations causing familial hypercholesterolemia while identifying a substantially larger fraction of at-risk individuals. Notably, the risk of coronary artery disease associated with high PRS is largely independent of risk associated with family history or clinical variables (Aragam et al. 2020). There is growing interest in the possible utility of incorporating PRS into genetic counseling in complex diseases, including cardiovascular disease (Reid et al. 2021) and breast cancer (Gregory et al. 2022). Promisingly, a randomized trial that disclosed genetic risk scores for patients at intermediate risk for coronary artery disease found a significant reduction in LDL at six months. Those randomized to receive genetic risk score results, in addition to conventional risk scores, had lower LDL levels at six months compared to those who received conventional risk scores alone. The reduced LDL was attributable to increased statin initiation among those receiving the genetic risk scores, while physical activity levels and dietary fat intake were unchanged (Kullo et al. 2016).

For common psychiatric disorders, genetic counseling regarding disease risk has largely focused on family history, with the notable exception of neurodevelopmental disorders, where pathogenic genetic mutations and CNVs have become an accepted part of diagnostic evaluation (Schaefer et al. 2013; Srivastava et al. 2019). There is increasing evidence that genetic testing for CNVs such as 22q11del may be useful for routine evaluation of patients with SCZ, especially in the presence of intellectual disability or other syndromic features (Lowther et al. 2017). One recent study (Alkelai et al. 2022) examined the diagnostic yield of whole-genome sequencing in 251 families with at least one offspring with psychotic illness and their parents. Pathogenic mutations or CNVs were identified in 6.4% of probands but SCZ PRS was also significantly elevated among affected individuals compared with unaffected family members. In addition, as noted earlier, the penetrance of pathogenic rare variants can vary with background polygenic risk, suggesting that PRSs may prove useful in refining and individualizing penetrance estimates for neurodevelopmental disorders (Cleynen et al. 2021; Niemi et al. 2018; Oetjens et al. 2019). However, the role of PRS as an adjunct to psychiatric genetic counseling is largely unexplored and requires careful consideration.

Contextualizing the probabilistic implications of polygenic risk will require a substantial process of education for both counselors and clients as well as an awareness of the limitations inherent in PRS interpretation, as discussed above (Polygenic Risk Score Task Force of the Intl. Common Disease Alliance 2021). In addition, the substantial genetic overlap among psychiatric disorders means that PRS may confer risk beyond a single disorder, and this possibility may need to be incorporated into genetic counseling (Lee et al. 2021). Nevertheless, interest in this information on the part of patients and consumers might be substantial. In a recent analysis of users of a direct-to-consumer tool for calculating personalized PRS (impute.me), psychiatric disorders were among the most commonly explored (Folkersen et al. 2020). Among those who obtained PRS results, more than 60% reported experiencing a negative reaction, and such reactions were more common among those with poorer understanding of the implications of PRS (Peck et al. 2022). At this point, most experts, including the International Society of Psychiatric Genetics, have held that return of PRS information to patients and families is premature.

Polygenic scores might also be useful in *validating* or *targeting prevention strategies*. For example, those with a high PRS for coronary artery disease also appear to benefit more than those at lower genetic risk from statin therapy, for primary prevention, and PCSK9 inhibition, for secondary prevention of coronary artery disease (Damask et al. 2020; Mega et al. 2015; Natarajan et al. 2017). Among individuals with high PRS for coronary artery disease, Khera et al. (2017) demonstrated that healthy lifestyle behaviors were associated with a nearly 50% lower relative risk of coronary artery disease. Healthy lifestyle has also been associated with lower risk of incident dementia among cognitively healthy adults with elevated Alzheimer disease PRS (Lourida et al. 2019). Similar analyses have shown that healthy lifestyle, physical activity, and increased social connectedness are associated with substantial reductions in risk of incident depression among those with high polygenic risk (Cao et al. 2021; Choi et al. 2020a, b, c). There is also some evidence that risk of psychotic symptoms is greater among cannabis users at higher levels of polygenic risk for SCZ (Wainberg et al. 2021). If PRSs do become available in clinical settings, validating actionable risk reduction strategies for those at high polygenic risk could inform genetic counseling and improve outcomes.

Conclusions and Remaining Challenges

Clearly, PRSs hold promise for the evolution of precision psychiatry toward improved prevention, diagnosis, and treatment of mental disorders. They represent one of the few established biomarkers of disease risk for a growing number of psychiatric disorders and can be calculated at any point during an individual's lifetime. There is compelling evidence from other areas of medicine, especially cardiology and oncology, that incorporation of PRS in clinical risk assessment could have value in primary prevention of disease. In the field of psychiatry, given the general lack of actionable predictors of disease risk, objective indicators for differential diagnosis, and evidence-based tools for optimizing treatment selection, even modest improvements in information conferred by PRS could enhance clinical decision making. However, as noted throughout this review, a number of key challenges remain before PRS can be implemented in clinical practice. I summarize these below and discuss potential solutions.

Limited Power and Precision

The predictive value of PRS is inherently limited by the heritability of the target trait or disease as well as by the fact that PRSs index only the common variant contribution to heritability. In addition, a recent analysis of UK Biobank data (Ding et al. 2022) demonstrated that individual PRS risk estimates can be quite imprecise: less than 1% of those with point estimates in the top decile of PRS risk across 13 traits had 95% credible intervals that were fully within that decile. Thus, assigning risk status based on thresholds of PRS quantiles may lead to misclassification. Larger GWASs should improve the precision and power of PRS effect estimates, but at present, they remain limited.

Lack of Ancestral Diversity

The Eurocentric bias of existing GWASs and PRSs creates a substantial obstacle to clinical implementation. Most available PRSs are mis-calibrated for individuals of non-European ancestry who comprise the global population. Their use in clinical practice would require extensive caveats about their diminished utility and could exacerbate health disparities. For reasons described earlier, the use of ancestry-specific scores, even if they were available, is problematic. Addressing this gap will require a major expansion of the ancestral composition of GWAS cohorts and the development and application of methods to optimize and validate trans-ancestry PRSs. Emerging efforts to broaden the diversity of genetic studies (such as the U.S. National Institute of Health *All of Us* Research Program, H3Africa, and the growth of Asian biobanks) and to develop improved PRS methods (e.g., the Polygenic Risk Methods in Diverse Populations, PRIMED, Consortium) should help deliver on this promise.

Need for Expanded Reporting of PRS Performance Metrics

To date, the performance of PRS models, especially in psychiatry, has largely evaluated a limited range of metrics such as variance explained, relative effect estimates (e.g., odds ratios), and, in some cases, measures of discrimination (e.g., AUC). Such metrics provide little insight regarding clinical utility. Greater attention should be paid to metrics that are well established in the evaluation of clinical risk models, such as PPVs and NPVs, model calibration, net reclassification, and net benefit analysis (Cook 2018; Steyerberg et al.

2010). In addition, studies have commonly reported PRS effect estimates that compare tails of the PRS distribution (e.g., highest vs. lowest decile). This approach maximizes the apparent effect size but is uninformative for real-world clinical implementation where patients' scores span the full distribution of possible values. More useful effect estimates would compare those above a given threshold to those below the threshold or those around the median of the PRS distribution. In general, clinical risk reporting should include absolute risks, which tend to be more clinically interpretable than relative risks. Tools are available to convert PRS effects to the absolute risk scale (Pain et al. 2022). It is important to recall that statistical association is not the same as prediction, and detecting a significant association between PRS and a given outcome, in multivariable models, does not imply practically useful prediction (Bzdok et al. 2021). The lack of attention to clinical utility in psychiatric prediction modeling is hardly unique to studies of PRS. A recent systematic review of 308 prediction models for psychiatric outcomes found only two that had formally assessed clinical utility and 94.5% of models examined had high risk of bias and overfitting (Meehan et al. 2022).

Limited Integration of PRS and Other Risk Factors

Polygenic scores alone are unlikely to provide sufficient predictive value for most clinical use cases. However, combining PRSs with other risk factors could enhance their performance and clinical utility, as demonstrated in other areas of medicine. For example, the widely used BOADICEA model for breast cancer risk incorporates clinical, family history, reproductive factors, pathogenic mutations and PRS, which has been shown to enhance model discrimination (Carver et al. 2021; Lee et al. 2019a; Li et al. 2021d). Unfortunately, few nongenetic risk models have been well-validated in psychiatry (Meehan et al. 2022), and studies evaluating the predictive utility of integrating PRS with nongenetic risk models are even more rare.

Need to Expand Data Resources for Prediction of Treatment Response and Prognosis

Given the lack of validated predictors of treatment response, the use of PRS to inform treatment selection would seem to be "low-hanging fruit." Two related challenges exist, however. First, there is a need for larger studies of treatment outcomes to enhance the power of PRS-stratified models. Data from industry-driven clinical trials could be an important component, though data sharing restrictions have been an obstacle. Second, most PRS studies of treatment response have relied on PRS trained on cases and controls defined by lifetime disorder status. It seems likely that improvements in predictive value could be achieved if PRSs were trained on actual treatment response itself. The same issues pertain to models of illness course and prognosis.

Need to Validate Actionable Risk-Stratified Interventions

The clinical value of risk stratification depends strongly on the availability of actionable strategies for risk mitigation and prevention. In their absence, labeling individuals as high risk may simply leave patients with added anxiety and stigmatization and clinicians with a sense of helplessness and added burden. As reviewed above, such strategies have been identified for some psychiatric disorders (e.g., avoiding substance abuse, enhancing social support, increasing physical activity), but there is a lack of well-validated options. The use of antipsychotics to prevent conversion to psychotic illness among patients at "clinical high risk of psychosis" is highly controversial and may even be harmful, though it is reportedly common in China (Zhang et al. 2020a). More generally, the low PPV of all available PRS prediction models would translate to a high rate of false positive misclassification, risking unnecessary costs and iatrogenic harm from poorly validated interventions. A greater emphasis on establishing effective strategies for primary, secondary, and tertiary prevention will be essential if PRSs are to be considered for clinical use.

Importance of an Implementation Science Framework

Even if optimized PRS models and actionable interventions are established, the integration of PRS into clinical practice will require a great deal of additional work. The so-called "last mile" of translating prediction models into clinical decision support tools can be arduous and complex. Studies of psychiatric PRS have largely ignored the realities involved in this process, for which an implementation science framework will be essential. The field of implementation science encompasses a broad range of issues and study designs that focus on the uptake of clinical innovations into real-world clinical care (Bauer and Kirchner 2020; McGinty and Eisenberg 2022). These include efforts to identify and enhance facilitators and overcome barriers to implementation. Relevant elements of this approach involve stakeholder engagement, cost-effectiveness analyses, and effectiveness-implementation hybrid studies that simultaneously assess outcomes and feasibility of implementing clinical innovations (Curran et al. 2012; Eisman et al. 2020; Landes et al. 2019) and enable us to address questions such as:

- How will patients and clinicians respond to PRS information?
- Does return of PRS information improve real-world clinical outcomes at a systems level?
- Where are the incentives and barriers to integration into busy clinical workflows?
- Should PRS be sequenced as an initial stratification or screening tool followed by more extensive work-up?

- How will risk assessments be integrated into electronic health record systems?
- What unforeseen costs and harms may occur and how can they be mitigated?

Without addressing these issues, the development and validation of PRS modeling risks being nothing more than an academic exercise. To some extent, we might learn from the developing experience with the return of highly penetrant mutations and CNVs in healthcare settings (e.g., Blout Zawatsky et al. 2021; Orlando et al. 2019; Sperber et al. 2021; Williams 2019; Williams et al. 2019; Zebrowski et al. 2019). In addition, the eMERGE network's ongoing pragmatic trials of integrating PRS for ten complex diseases into clinical care across diverse healthcare systems will provide essential information about the risks and benefits of implementation. These efforts highlight the complexity of integrating genomic medicine in clinical settings, providing effective provider and patient education, and facilitating health system adoption of evidence-based clinical decision support. Nevertheless, the potential value of PRS for improving clinical care in psychiatry justifies investments in research and implementation strategies to overcome these challenges.

14

Ethical Challenges Associated with Advances in Genetic Prediction of Neuropsychiatric Disorders

Paul S. Appelbaum

Abstract

From the earliest days of predictive genetic testing, concerns have been expressed about the potential negative consequences of informing people of their genetic risks. Most studies to date have suggested that the impact of genetic testing is generally benign, albeit with some variation across individuals. There is, however, little evidence about the effects of predictive testing in neuropsychiatric disorders, especially for the major syndromes. As polygenic approaches to the prediction of genetic risk are refined and considered for introduction to the clinic, it will be important to consider potential adverse effects, including stigmatization, demoralization, therapeutic nihilism, and self-fulfilling prophecies. Prior to adopting polygenic prediction of vulnerability to neuropsychiatric disorders, response to treatment, and negative outcomes such as side effects and suicidality, careful evaluation of the risks and benefits of such technologies is required.

Introduction

With the growing use of genetic and genomic testing in psychiatry has come a diverse set of ethical concerns. Their salience for psychiatrists and patients cannot be separated from the unhappy history of the abuse of genetic concepts of neuropsychiatric disorders for eugenic purposes. During the first three-quarters of the twentieth century in the United States, roughly 65,000 people who were thought to manifest "feeblemindedness" or "insanity" were involuntarily sterilized on eugenic grounds (Bashford and Levine 2010). Under the Nazi regime's eugenics program in the twentieth century, more than 350,000 people—primarily persons with schizophrenia, intellectual disability, and alcoholism—were involuntarily sterilized. Approximately 70,000 psychiatric patients were later put to death as part of the Aktion T4 program, and another 200,000–300,000 psychiatric patients were killed during World War II, sometimes to free hospital beds for war casualties (Meyer 1988). This brutal history shapes contemporary concerns about the potential misuse of neuropsychiatric genetic information—especially among disenfranchised groups—compelling a focus on whether genetics is more likely to help or harm people with neuropsychiatric conditions; that is, whether it comports with clinicians' obligations to benefit patients (beneficence) and avoid needless harm (non-maleficence).

Previous reviews of the ethical issues in neuropsychiatric genetics have identified a range of issues broader than can be covered thoroughly in this paper, many of which are applicable to genomic medicine more broadly. Such topics include the challenges of obtaining informed consent for genetic testing; the stigmatizing impact of genetic diagnoses; the potential for discrimination on the basis of genetic information in schooling, employment, insurance, and other areas; and responsibilities for the disclosure of genetic information to patients' family members, when the genetic results may have implications for their health. Readers are referred to previous reviews for more extensive coverage of these important issues (Appelbaum and Benston 2017; Hoge and Appelbaum 2012). Here, however, I focus on a set of issues that reflect ethical concerns emanating from advances in genomic technologies that open new areas for prediction and intervention.

Psychosocial Impact of Neuropsychiatric Genetic Testing

From the earliest days of genetic testing in neuropsychiatry, there have been concerns that genetic results would have adverse impacts on the persons being tested and their family members. Reports of suicides following the introduction of genetic testing for Huntington disease only reinforced these concerns. Early surveys of patients and families, when the availability of genetic testing for common psychiatric disorders was largely hypothetical, showed that strong interest in obtaining genetic test results was accompanied by a range of concerns about their impact. For example, 62% of unaffected persons in a genetic research study of depression expressed concern that a positive test result could make people feel stressed, depressed, or vulnerable (Wilhelm et al. 2009). Other studies similarly found worries that results indicating a genetic predisposition to psychiatric disorders might induce negative self-perceptions or fatalistic views, creating a self-fulfilling prophecy of failure in life (Lebowitz and Appelbaum 2019). Concerns that children might also be at higher risk for psychiatric disorders could preoccupy parents, to the detriment of their child-rearing obligations.

Experimental studies indicate some basis for these concerns. One notable study, for example, demonstrated decrements in both perceived memory and memory test performance of persons who learned that they carry a risk allele for Alzheimer disease, when compared with other carriers of the allele who were not told their test results (Lineweaver et al. 2014). Participants in a second study told randomly that they carried a gene indicating a propensity for risk taking were subsequently found to be making more risky choices, compared with a control group (Wheat et al. 2022). In another study, participants who were randomly selected to be informed that they carried a genetic predisposition to depression expressed significantly lower confidence in their ability to cope with depressive symptoms than those who did not receive this information (Lebowitz and Ahn 2018). Diagnostic genetic testing can raise similar issues, given evidence that labeling a psychiatric, neurologic, and behavioral condition as "genetic" can negatively affect people's views of its prognosis and treatability (Lebowitz et al. 2013), which in turn could affect their optimism about their lives and their behavior. For example, the more that people who are overweight attribute their condition to biological causes such as genes, the less changeable they believe their body weight to be (Pearl and Lebowitz 2014). Indeed, mere exposure to genetic explanations for lower levels of physical activity among inactive people reduced perceived self-efficacy in overcoming barriers to exercise, as well as decreasing expressed intentions to exercise (Beauchamp et al. 2011). Similarly, exposure to genetic explanations of obesity increased food intake (Dar-Nimrod et al. 2014).

Studies of people who have received actual genetic results, though, have tended to be more reassuring. Most notably in neuropsychiatry, the REVEAL study, which disclosed the results of ApoE4 testing to participants from families with histories of Alzheimer disease, identified only minor and transient reactions to telling people that they carried alleles that would increase their risk for the disorder (Green et al. 2009). This finding has been echoed in recent, as yet unpublished, work conducted by our group at Columbia University, which has looked at the impact of diagnostic genetic testing of children with autism. Parents of children for whom a diagnostic genetic finding was identified showed on most measures of identity, responsibility, and life-planning no significant differences from parents for whom no causative variants were identified. In other areas of medicine as well, similar results have been reported, even when risk genes for serious and potentially fatal conditions such as cancer are found (Hamilton and Robson 2019).

Several caveats are warranted, however, before we conclude that all concerns about the psychosocial impact of genetic testing for neuropsychiatric disorders were overblown. First, studies of moderate risk genes for Alzheimer disease or diagnostic testing in autism may not generalize to other neuropsychiatric disorders, such as schizophrenia, bipolar disorder, or depression, where data on responses to predictive or diagnostic testing are lacking, given the absence until recently of applicable genetic tests. Predictions about conditions with onset earlier in life than dementia may affect people in very different ways. Second, the context in which testing takes place can make a difference in how people react to the results. An expectant parent being told that a fetus is at high risk for autism or another neurodevelopmental or neuropsychiatric disorder may have very different responses than a parent receiving confirmatory genetic testing in autism when the diagnosis is already known. Finally, existing data, especially from qualitative studies that look in depth at individual participants, suggest considerable variability in response, such as in the context of prenatal and newborn screening (Grob 2019). Even if most people react with equanimity or only transient anxiety to findings that indicate a propensity for neuropsychiatric illness, some may have profound negative reactions. An ability to identify that group in advance, so as to prepare them for the possible results of testing and have supportive interventions available post-disclosure would be desirable.

Ethical Concerns about Advances in Genetic Prediction of Neuropsychiatric Disorders

As is evident from the discussion above, prediction of future disease onset has always been a goal of neuropsychiatric genetic testing. However, the first generation of approaches to clinical prediction of neuropsychiatric conditions was limited to monogenic conditions with complete penetrance (e.g., Huntington disease). Even more recent efforts focused on autism or neurodevelopmental disorders in the clinical realm have relied on single-gene or copy-number variant effects with high penetrance. That has left most common psychiatric disorders, with their complex genetics and environmental contributions to causation, outside the scope of clinical genetic testing. However, the technical advances that permitted large-scale genome-wide association studies (GWASs) have led to the development of polygenic risk scores (PRSs) for a wide variety of medical, including neuropsychiatric, conditions. Although most PRSs still account for only a small proportion of the variance in the development of neuropsychiatric disorders, and there are certain intrinsic limits to the specificity of their predictions (i.e., due to pleiotropic effects of many variants related to psychiatric disorders and environmental influences on disease onset), the general expectation in the field is that the proportion of the variance accounted for by PRS will continue to grow. Similarly, though the data sets on which most PRSs have been generated to date have largely been drawn from groups of European ancestry, limiting the applicability of the resulting PRSs to other populations, large-scale efforts to diversify data sets and generate PRSs that are valid across ancestry groups are currently underway. Moreover, as machine learning/artificial intelligence approaches are introduced, allowing predictions to be based on combinations of clinical, historical, environmental, and genetic factors, predictive models may further improve (Murray et al. 2021).

Prediction has the potential to benefit persons at risk by enabling them to monitor the early appearance of symptoms and seek treatment promptly; to avoid behaviors and situations that might increase the risk of disease onset (e.g., use of cannabis among people at elevated risk for schizophrenia or prolonged sleep disruption among people at increased risk of bipolar disorder); and to participate in potentially helpful research. As an example, work with our collaborators at Columbia University—using results of hypothetical testing for a genetic variant associated with greater risk of developing schizophrenia on exposure to cannabis—suggests that genetic test results indicating that marijuana use will increase one's schizophrenia risk may incentivize abstinence, especially for those with prior marijuana use (Lebowitz et al. 2021).

Moreover, multiple studies that ask people if they would seek predictive testing, should it become available, have shown strong interest. In a survey of 162 parents who had at least one child with autism, earlier evaluation/intervention, closer monitoring, and reduced anxiety levels were reasons cited for seeking predictive testing if it were available for a younger sibling, and 80% indicated they would pursue genetic testing if it could identify the risk in a younger sibling. Interest in genetic testing appears to be affected to some degree by the utility of the resulting information for prevention or treatment, as well as the conclusiveness of the results (Narcisa et al. 2013). Laegsgaard et al. (2009) reported that many Danish patients would undergo genetic testing if treatment or prophylaxis were available: 35% of anxiety patients, 28% of bipolar patients, 46% of schizophrenia patients, and 51% of depression patients. But many others would opt for testing notwithstanding treatment possibilities: anxiety 41%, bipolar 55%, schizophrenia 31%, and depression 36%. Other studies indicate that interest is often associated with the degree of certainty a test offers. A survey by Meiser et al. (2007) of bipolar depressed or schizoaffective patients and unaffected family members, all enrolled in genetic research, showed that if a positive test would indicate a 25% lifetime risk, 75% of patients and 79% of family members were probably or definitely interested; those figures increase to 91% of patients and 92% of family members for a 100% lifetime risk.

Learning about a potential genetic cause before any symptoms emerge could help parents avoid self-blame and feel less vulnerable to stigma, as genetic explanations can supplant stigmatizing explanatory frameworks, such as those that attribute neuropsychiatric disorders to poor parenting. Indeed, preliminary data from our current study of diagnostic genetic testing for children with autism demonstrate this reduction in stigma and self-blame. Moreover, learning of a potential genetic cause of a child's condition may allow parents to seek support from advocacy groups specific to the genetic syndrome in question, though it is uncertain whether the same benefit will occur in a context like prediction of neuropsychiatric disorders, where the specific diagnostic and prognostic implications of the genetic information returned to parents may not always be clear. Other potential benefits of early identification, especially in children, include the ability to monitor for the occurrence of comorbid conditions, such as epilepsy in autism.

Notwithstanding the generally reassuring literature on the impact of predictive genetic testing referred to above, there are reasons to suspect that predictive testing for psychiatric disorders, especially when conducted during childhood or early adolescence, may be somewhat less benign in its psychosocial impact. Negative effects on parents could include increased anxiety or feelings of hopelessness about their child's future (as genes are often perceived to operate in a deterministic and immutable fashion); self-stigma, if parents interpret the results as an indication that their child, and therefore they, are "defective"; or, in the case of inherited variants, guilt about having caused or passed down a pathogenic genetic variant to the child. Parents who learn about a child's genetic risk could also demonstrate behavioral effects, such as hypervigilant monitoring of their child's development, altering their reproductive or life-planning decisions to accommodate possible future impairment, or avoiding the possibility of having a second child at elevated risk for a serious neuropsychiatric disorder.

Moreover, if newborn genomic screening becomes a widespread practice, as some experts have advocated and as is currently being tested (Holm et al. 2018), the added impact of disclosures in the newborn period needs to be anticipated. The period immediately following the birth of a child can be joyful but is also inherently stressful for parents, who are typically sleep-deprived, given the frequent feedings and short sleep cycles of newborns. The anxiety associated with pregnancy has given way to worry over attending to the needs of a newborn, especially among first-time parents. Mothers may experience a decrease in mood—the so-called "baby blues"—and in some cases more serious depression or other postpartum psychiatric disorders. Fathers, too, can experience depressed mood in the newborn period, and both parents may worry about their ability to bond appropriately with their baby. As the critical process of bonding unfolds, parents may be uncertain whether their child's responses are "normal." Receiving genetic test results during the first six weeks of life that indicate a child's increased risk for a significant neuropsychiatric disorder—with its uncertain likelihood, manifestations, and implications for the child's development and future—could be highly upsetting to new parents, whose coping abilities may already be stretched to their limits by the stress of dealing with their infant. Hence, the generally reassuring findings from studies of the psychosocial consequences of predictive genetic testing may not apply to newborn screening for neuropsychiatric conditions (Grob 2019).

Even later in life, there may be concerns about the potential negative impacts of predictive information. Although genetic and other biomedical explanations of mental disorders can reduce individual blame by casting symptoms as outside of individual control, as suggested by classical attribution theory, they can simultaneously evoke stigmatizing attitudes and prognostic pessimism, through the mechanism of genetic essentialism (Lebowitz and Appelbaum 2019). Indeed, for neuropsychiatric disorders, which implicate mental and behavioral domains deeply associated with selfhood, genetic and other biomedical causal explanations have been linked to decreased blame as well as to assumptions of reduced treatability and poor prognosis (i.e., the view that a disorder, because it has a genetic basis, will be permanent). Compounding those concerns is the degree to which a person's negative perceptions of their own propensities and capabilities may create a self-fulfilling prophecy in which they assume a fatalistic posture that reduces their motivation to achieve what would otherwise be their life goals (e.g., "Why bother doing well in school or even going to college if I'm just going to be a schizophrenic for the rest of my life?"). One might expect this to be a particular issue during adolescence, a time when predictive testing for psychotic and bipolar disorders might have special utility, but also a period of consolidation of identity and formulation of life goals. In some ethnic and religious communities in which marriages are arranged, especially when there is an assumption that known predispositions to disease will be disclosed as part of the matchmaking process, the marriage prospects of a person at elevated risk of a neuropsychiatric condition may be markedly diminished. Additionally, information about a person's genetic risk could induce "courtesy stigma"—a form of stigma in which negative attitudes about a person "spill over" to impact unaffected individuals, such as genetically related family members (Alareeki et al. 2019)—even when the causal variants arise *de novo*.

Another challenge for people receiving predictive information about a heightened risk for a neuropsychiatric disorder will be the need to cope with the inherent uncertainty of their (or their child's) prognosis. Although the genetic contribution to many neuropsychiatric conditions is high, the less-than-perfect concordance in identical twins for these conditions suggests that other, nongenetic factors play a role during critical periods of development and, as noted, current approaches to prediction using PRS account for relatively small proportions of the variance. It is unclear how environmental and genetic factors interact to cause neuropsychiatric disorders. Thus, in almost all cases, it will not be possible to say with certainty whether a person will develop a disorder for which their risk is elevated, and studies suggest that uncertain genetic information presents the greatest challenges to individuals' coping skills (Werner-Lin et al. 2019). An additional complicating factor in interpreting the implications of genetic test results is that many genes associated with neuropsychiatric conditions are pleiotropic in their effects (i.e., they are associated with multiple psychiatric disorders and in some cases with neurological disorders such as epilepsy). Hence, people at elevated risk and parents of children at increased risk will need to face the prospect of uncertainty as to whether any disorder will develop, which disorder it will be, and with what degrees of symptomatology or impairment it will be associated.

A different facet of uncertainty arises from the imbalance in representation of global populations in genetic data sets used to conduct GWAS and generate PRSs. Notwithstanding ongoing efforts to diversify the populations sampled, available data today are derived overwhelmingly from groups of European descent. As a result, PRSs in neuropsychiatry, and medicine more broadly, tend to be much less predictive of outcomes in non-European populations (Martin et al. 2019a). Until this imbalance is corrected and valid transethnic PRSs are generated, European ancestry groups, which are already relatively advantaged in many countries compared with populations originating elsewhere in the world, will most likely benefit disproportionately from advances in predictive approaches. Conversely, Eurocentric PRSs that are applied to other groups may be substantially misleading, heightening the risk of harm.

Finally, mention needs to be made of the controversial use of prenatal genetic testing for predispositions to a variety of conditions, including neuropsychiatric disorders. Techniques are being perfected for prospective parents undergoing *in vitro* fertilization and eager to have the most perfect child possible, to conduct predictive testing of embryos for polygenic traits and disorders prior to implantation (Johnston and Matthews 2022). One suspects that such testing will become even more widely available if noninvasive prenatal testing technology ever progresses to the point of allowing it. At this point in time, though, given the relatively small percentages of variance in the occurrence of neuropsychiatric conditions accounted for by PRSs and the reality that parents selecting against some conditions are inevitably selecting embryos with predispositions for other conditions, there is no basis at all to support such testing. Indeed, its use is likely to raise exactly the same eugenic concerns that have plagued neuropsychiatric genetics from its inception (Turley et al. 2021).

The concerns enumerated above are not reasons to abandon efforts to develop polygenic and other approaches to prediction of risk for neuropsychiatric disorders, given the potential benefits that such technologies can bring. They do, however, constitute reasons for caution in introducing such tests into clinical use. Prior to taking that step, the potential impact of genetic prediction should be examined in controlled research settings, among people who have knowledgeably consented to run the risks of such studies. Predictive testing might first be used in lower risk contexts (e.g., in later adolescence and adulthood) before being introduced for children and ultimately newborns. To the extent that negative consequences are identified in research use, efforts should be made both to ascertain whether predictors of adverse responses can be identified (e.g., elevated anxiety at baseline) and whether interventions to mitigate untoward effects can be developed. Although it is assumed that there will be benefits from predictive testing, this remains a hypothesis that needs to be confirmed—and a positive benefit/risk ratio demonstrated—before clinical use of predictive polygenic testing is warranted.

Ethical Challenges around Genetic Prediction of Other Outcomes: Treatment Response, Side Effects, and Suicide

Polygenic scores may have utility not only for prediction of the development of neuropsychiatric disorders, but also to anticipate treatment response. A recent review suggests that we do not yet have enough data from large-scale studies to know whether this will prove to be the case (Murray et al. 2021), although early studies have found a negative association between PRS for depression and response to treatment (e.g., Ward et al. 2018); a polygenic profile for response to antidepressants distinct from genetic risk for depression (Pain et al. 2022b); and indications that treatment response in schizophrenia may be inversely related to the PRS for that condition (e.g., Zhang et al. 2019). If this line of research ultimately supports the use of PRS to predict response to treatment, potential benefits for patients include avoidance of medication trials and medication side effects in situations in which the likelihood of a positive treatment response is small. Should it prove possible to distinguish among medications in terms of the likelihood of response, more selective psychopharmacology would become possible.

There are, however, potential risks to patients that need to be taken into account when deciding whether attempts to predict treatment response are an appropriate use for PRSs. First, it is unlikely that PRSs will ever be able to identify patients who are completely unlikely to respond to treatment. Rather, they may help clinicians sort patients into groups with higher and lower probabilities of responding to antidepressant or antipsychotic medications. Thus, even some patients who are in a group that is deemed less likely to have a positive response to medication will have a good response if exposed to the medication. Understanding that reality requires educating both clinicians and patients, which may run into inherent tendencies toward genetic determinism (i.e., the tendency to view genetic results as wholly determinative of future outcomes) (Lebowitz and Appelbaum 2019). Especially in the case of patients for whom other approaches have failed, it would be unfortunate if either psychiatrists or patients were dissuaded from trying appropriate medications by a misinterpretation of the implications of PRS-based prediction.

Other negative effects of using PRS to anticipate treatment response that will need to be anticipated include the induction of fatalism and hopelessness in clinicians and patients alike. As noted above, experimental studies have shown that when neuropsychiatric conditions are attributed to genetic and other biological causes, they are viewed as less likely to respond to any treatment and more permanent, and such findings can discourage efforts to ameliorate the condition. If those reactions are associated with results indicating a genetic predisposition to neuropsychiatric conditions, they may be even more likely to arise when the testing is said more directly to indicate a poor likelihood of response to treatment. The actual impact of such information should be carefully assessed prior to introducing genetic predictive models of treatment response into clinical practice.

Perhaps a more benign use of PRS would be to identify patients at increased risk of specific side effects from medication treatment. Campos et al. (2021), using PRS for depression, found that scores were associated with most side effects from antidepressants, in particular the emergence of suicidal thoughts and behavior. Whether suicidality can actually be attributed to the medication, being able to identify in advance patients who are likely to be at increased risk for suicide might allow closer monitoring and more rapid intervention—an issue addressed in more detail immediately below. An increased likelihood of developing side effects, which in Campos et al. (2021) was present across antidepressant medications, could also suggest the value of trying other forms of treatment (e.g., cognitive behavior therapy) before moving to medications. It might, of course, be anticipated that patients who are told that they are at higher risk of side effects will be more likely to develop them, a phenomenon often referred to as the "nocebo effect" (Colloca and Barsky 2020). Additionally, both clinicians and patients may misinterpret the association with PRS to mean a certainty rather than a possibility of developing adverse effects from the medication, leading to an unwillingness even to try the medication when it could be the most helpful option.

Another area of active research involving the use of PRSs involves suicidal behaviors, which have been known for some time to have a genetic component. Beginning in the early 1950s, twin studies found increased concordance for suicide in monogenic versus dizygotic twins, with familial clustering confirmed in later, population-based research. Estimates of heritability have approached 50%. Recent GWAS have identified single nucleotide polymorphisms associated with suicide attempts and suicide deaths, although replication has been a challenge. PRSs generated from GWAS, however, have been shown to have significant predictive power, to be associated with familial risk for suicide, and to be moderated by psychosocial variables (Mullins et al. 2022).

The impetus to develop PRSs for suicide derives from the public health impact of suicide attempts and deaths and the challenges in predicting suicidal behaviors. Data from the Centers for Disease Control and Prevention (2022) show that "in 2020, an estimated 12.2 million American adults seriously thought about suicide, 3.2 million planned a suicide attempt, and 1.2 million attempted suicide," with 45,979 of those attempts leading to death. Many of the attempts that do not result in death lead to serious and sometimes permanent injury. Clinicians have been stymied in their efforts to reduce the toll of deaths from suicide by the limitations of current predictive approaches. A recent meta-analysis found no improvement in low levels of predictive accuracy over fifty years of research (Franklin et al. 2017). Even an incremental improvement associated with PRS, therefore, could potentially save many lives, as enhanced predictive power allows more effective intervention (e.g., initiation of psychotherapy or medication; hospitalization) to reduce the current toll of suicide deaths.

Given the imperative to improve prediction of suicide risk, but uncertainty about the clinical value of a suicide PRS, we are likely to see PRS begin to be tested in clinical settings. Before that occurs, careful consideration of potential negative effects is needed. People who are told that they are at higher genetic risk of suicide could experience hopelessness and an increased likelihood of self-harm. Knowledge of increased risk may contribute to perceptions that treatment is less likely to be useful and to a tendency to favor medication over psychosocial interventions that may be as or more effective. Clinicians who are told that their patient is at increased risk of suicide may experience reduced empathy and could overreact to minor increases in symptoms or the presence of fleeting suicidal ideation, resorting to intrusive interventions such as involuntary hospitalization. To date, there is only one empirical study on the anticipated effects of PRS for suicide, involving three focus groups with eight suicide survivors and 13 family members who identified both desirable and undesirable consequences (Kious et al. 2021). As with other uses of PRS for neuropsychiatric disorders, an increased systematic study of these issues is essential to anticipate the positive and negative effects of introducing suicide PRS into clinical practice and, if necessary, to identify approaches to reducing risks.

Conclusion

Predictive efforts using PRSs clearly hold the prospect of considerable value in identifying people at risk for neuropsychiatric disorders and their behavioral consequences so that preventive interventions and prompt treatment can occur, and in anticipating treatment response, including side effects. There is, however, also a potential for adverse consequences stemming from popular views of genetic essentialism and determinism. Hence, careful examination is needed of the positive and negative consequences of PRS use in psychiatry before these practices make their way into the clinic.

15

Psychiatric Genetic Counseling

Next Steps

Jehannine C. Austin

Abstract

The world's first specialist psychiatric genetic counseling clinic opened in 2012. Despite ample evidence that psychiatric genetic counseling produces excellent outcomes for patients, even in the absence of any genetic testing, this service is still not widely available clinically despite efforts to train practitioners in the delivery of this intervention. Patients could benefit *now* from the delivery of psychiatric genetic counseling (even in the absence of testing), and we have an ethical duty to consider how to ensure that the infrastructure is in place to ensure optimal outcomes for patients. This is particularly important as we move closer toward the clinical application of genetic testing in the context of psychiatric conditions. It is important to consider *how* such testing might be deployed and to ensure that any testing is delivered according to the established practices for psychiatric genetic counseling that produce the best patient outcomes. This chapter reviews evidence that patients benefit from psychiatric genetic counseling and discusses the barriers to its broader implementation.

Introduction

The potential for benefits to patients from psychiatric genetic counseling has been discussed in the literature for decades, and studies examining its application and outcomes have recently emerged. Without exception, these studies demonstrate positive, meaningful outcomes for patients after receiving this service. The world's first specialist psychiatric genetic counseling service opened its doors in February 2012 and has continued to examine patient outcomes of this service in a naturalistic setting. Such studies are important for examining the effects of an intervention in a real-world setting, rather than in the tightly controlled environment of a randomized controlled trial (RCT) or hypothetical scenarios. Data from the clinic continue to demonstrate positive, meaningful patient outcomes, including large effect size increases in empowerment, increases in self-efficacy (Inglis et al. 2015), knowledge, improvements in accuracy of risk perception (Hippman et al. 2016), and potential impacts on behavior change (Semaka and Austin 2019) and mental health outcomes (Morris et al. 2021).

Although there is as much (or more) data demonstrating the value of genetic counseling for psychiatric conditions as there is for many other types of genetic counseling already widely available, psychiatric genetic counseling is underutilized and not widely available to patients (Moldovan et al. 2019). This situation is problematic. Not only do we have data demonstrating that patients could benefit now from a service that already exists, we need to consider how to ensure that the infrastructure is in place to ensure optimal outcomes for patients. This is particularly important as we implement genetic testing in the context of psychiatric settings. Specifically, we need to consider not just if but *how* such testing might be deployed and to ensure that any testing is delivered according to the established practices for psychiatric genetic counseling that produce the best patient outcomes.

In this chapter, I present the concept of genetic counseling as it relates to psychiatric conditions. Thereafter, I discuss barriers to its widespread implementation in an effort to lay the groundwork for overcoming these impediments to patient benefit from this service.

Genetic Counseling: History, Models, and Theories

Genetic counseling emerged as a concept in the 1940s (Resta 1997) and as a specialist healthcare discipline in the 1960s. Initially, applied to situations involving family planning (e.g., genetic syndromes) and genetic testing (e.g., hereditary breast and/or ovarian cancer), genetic counseling aims to support people in making informed, autonomous decisions in line with their values, and it does not necessitate or require genetic testing or a family planning trigger. Genetic counseling is best conceptualized as "a process of helping people understand and adapt to the medical, psychological, and familial implications of genetic contributions to disease" (Resta et al. 2006). In the context of etiologically complex conditions like psychiatric conditions, genetic counseling involves holistic discussion of both the genetic and environmental contributors to the condition.

Today, in Canada, the United States, Australia, and the United Kingdom, genetic counselors are board-certified, MSc-level specialists (Resta 2006) who use a person-centered approach and a model of reciprocal engagement (Veach et al. 2007) to help people make meaning about the causes of a condition in a family, to understand chances for illness in relatives, and to consider options for intervention (Biesecker 2001; Resta 2006; Resta et al. 2006). Genetic counseling is neither a purely education/information-based nor counseling-based service; it is a hybrid (Austin et al. 2014) that seeks to increase empowerment

(McAllister et al. 2010) and facilitate behavioral change to improve health (Austin 2015; Zierhut et al. 2016). Genetic counseling is informed by the *common-sense model of illness representation*, which posits that people gather and integrate information from multiple sources to appraise and develop representations of health that inform self-management and coping (Diefenbach and Leventhal 2010).

Psychiatric Genetic Counseling

As a discipline, genetic counseling has existed for around sixty years, and its application in psychiatric contexts has been extensively discussed (Austin and Honer 2004; DeLisi and Bertisch 2006; Finn and Smoller 2006; Hodgkinson et al. 2001; Kumar 1968; Lyus 2007; Reveley 1985; Stancer and Wagener 1984). Still, it was not until the 2000s that empirical investigations began (Austin and Honer 2008). Since then, many studies on the utility of genetic counseling have been published (Costain et al. 2012, 2014), including RCTs (Hippman et al. 2016) along with qualitative (Semaka and Austin 2019), naturalistic (Bodnar and Wisner 2005; Gerrard et al. 2020; Inglis et al. 2015), and meta-analytic (Moldovan et al. 2017) studies.

Manuals for psychiatric genetic counseling have been developed (Austin 2019). Typically, counseling involves an initial 1–1.5 hour session (Uhlmann et al. 2010), followed by a check-in one month later; information is gathered from and provided to the patient, along with support (Austin et al. 2006, 2008; Peay and Austin 2011). The information-gathering component of psychiatric genetic counseling entails uncovering the patient's existing explanation for the cause of illness and eliciting and documenting a detailed family history. The information-provision component involves the following:

- Research-based information about the factors associated with the indicated condition are related to the participant's family history and their existing explanation for cause of illness—in lay language and with visual aids to facilitate comprehension.
- Information about factors that contribute to the development of illness is used as a framework to discuss evidence-based strategies for protecting mental health; for example, through sleep, nutrition, and exercise (Baglioni et al. 2011; Bodnar and Wisner 2005; Harvey et al. 2018; Lakhan and Vieira 2008).
- Family history and empiric data are used to discuss chance for self as well as chance for family members (e.g., children) to develop the indicated condition, if relevant and desired (Austin et al. 2006, 2008; Peay and Austin 2011).

The genetic counselor also works to uncover and address emotional ramifications (e.g., guilt, shame, stigma, fear) that may be evoked (Veach et al. 2007).

Psychiatric genetic counseling typically involves the provision of written material to patients related to the content of the sessions. For further details of this process and the visual aids, see Austin (2019).

Based on data showing that psychiatric genetic counseling improves patient outcomes, the world's first specialist psychiatric genetic counseling clinic was established, and outcomes continue to be studied (Borle et al. 2018; Gerrard et al. 2020; Inglis et al. 2015; Semaka and Austin 2019). In summary, data show that:

- Psychiatric genetic counseling increases empowerment and self-efficacy (Inglis et al. 2015), both of which are necessary for engaging people in behavioral change to reduce their risk for mental illness (Holloway and Watson 2002).
- People report changing their behavior after psychiatric genetic counseling (e.g., sleep, nutrition, exercise) to reduce their risk for mental illness (Semaka and Austin 2019).

Data accumulated thus far and new, unpublished work suggest a rationale for examining the impact of psychiatric genetic counseling on mental health outcomes. Both suggest that mental health outcomes might be positively influenced by the provision of psychiatric genetic counseling.

Even without any of the more distal outcomes of psychiatric genetic counseling, the proximal outcome of increasing empowerment is deeply meaningful. Empowerment has been conceptualized as the opposite of internalized stigma (Livingston and Boyd 2010), and internalized stigma is a profoundly important issue in the context of psychiatric conditions. For individuals with psychiatric conditions, such as schizophrenia, the effects of stigma can actually outweigh symptoms associated with the condition itself, even those that dramatically influence language, thought, affect, perception, and sense of self (Hinshaw and Stier 2008). Self-stigma, which arises from experiences and perceptions of discrimination (Livingston and Boyd 2010), has been postulated to be central to the psychological harm caused by stigma (Boyd Ritsher and Phelan 2005; Corrigan and Watson 2002; Livingston and Boyd 2010). Therefore, increasing empowerment through genetic counseling is a deeply meaningful outcome in its own right.

Genetic Testing for Psychiatric Conditions

Though they are not the same thing, genetic counseling and genetic testing are often conflated as concepts. As discussed above, there are meaningful and substantive benefits of genetic counseling for psychiatric conditions even in the absence of providing any genetic testing. Given that discourse in psychiatric genetics is increasingly considering the possibility of implementing genetic testing clinically, this issue deserves special consideration in relation to genetic counseling.

Psychiatric conditions are complex and heterogeneous, and currently there are no genetic tests with which to confirm, refine, or establish a psychiatric diagnosis. Both common variants of small effect (single nucleotide polymorphisms) and rare variants of larger effect (copy number variations, CNVs) can contribute to the etiology of these conditions.

Polygenic Risk Scores

To measure genetic risk, the collective risk due to the total of an individual's common variation can be summarized into a single variable: a polygenic risk score (PRS) (Wray et al. 2018a, 2021). Public interest in genetic information has led an increasing number of people to upload their raw data (e.g., from 23andme.com, ancestry.com) to third party websites (e.g., impute.me) and to generate their own PRS information (Janssens 2019).

Psychiatric conditions are among the conditions for which PRSs are most frequently sought on these platforms (Folkersen et al. 2020). Relatives of people with psychiatric illness worry about and are interested in understanding/mitigating their own risk for developing these conditions (Austin et al. 2006; DeLisi and Bertisch 2006; Erickson et al. 2014; Lyus 2007; Meiser et al. 2005, 2008; Quaid et al. 2001; Quinn et al. 2014; Wilhelm et al. 2009). Data show, however, that ~60% of people who access their own PRS for any complex condition online (where only information is provided, but no support) have some negative reaction (e.g., sad/anxious), and ~5% may even experience PTSD (Peck et al. 2022).

Copy Number Variations

For autism spectrum disorder, testing for CNVs is considered a first-tier test, yet there are important caveats concerning how the diagnostic criteria related to autism have evolved over time, as laid out by Morris et al. (2022).

While CNV testing is an established practice in pediatric settings when a patient experiences developmental delay or intellectual disabilities, its benefits are less clear when these features are not present, and its application in these circumstances is actually off-label under current FDA approval parameters. Many of the potential benefits and harms associated with CNV testing are detailed in relation to different contextual factors by Morris et al. (2022). CNV testing is *not* an established practice in psychiatric settings. Its consideration as a first-tier test in the context of autism has led to the proposal of justice-based arguments in support of CNV testing within psychiatric populations. Careful ethical analysis, however, reveals differences in the potential for benefits and harms associated with CNV testing in different populations (Morris et al. 2022). While many of the harms could potentially be mitigated through testing in the context of psychiatric genetic counseling, it is critical to consider the timing of testing in relation to whether there are immediate consequences for care delivery dependent on the test and the individual's capacity to consent. If there are no immediate care consequences dependent on the test results, testing should be delayed for children until they are able to consent (Botkin et al. 2015).

Insights into the Outcomes of Genetic Testing for Psychiatric Conditions

Though outcomes of other types of genetic testing in *non*-psychiatric contexts are generally benign (see Bloss et al. 2011; Collins et al. 2010; Green et al. 2009 but also Lineweaver et al. 2014; Turnwald et al. 2019), genetic risk testing for *psychiatric*-related conditions may have some negative outcomes. Especially for those whose results indicate higher risk, potential negative outcomes include increases in negative affect and distress up to three months after the test (Dar-Nimrod et al. 2012; Lebowitz and Ahn 2017; Wilhelm et al. 2009).

Although clinicians tend to focus almost exclusively on *what* information from genetic testing should be communicated, it is increasingly becoming clear that *how* this information is communicated matters at least as much. In sum, any genetic testing implemented clinically for psychiatric conditions should be delivered in the context of the current evidence-based gold standard intervention that exists to help people who are concerned about psychiatric risk, which is psychiatric genetic counseling.

Barriers to Adoption and Implementation of Psychiatric Genetic Counseling

Although studies have shown that large proportions of people with psychiatric conditions and their family members would like genetic counseling, less than 5% have received it (DeLisi and Bertisch 2006; Kalb et al. 2017; Lyus 2007; Michael et al. 2020; Quaid et al. 2001). Given the evidence of meaningful benefits of genetic counseling for people with psychiatric conditions, together with evidence of interest in genetic counseling within this population, it is important to examine the barriers to the more widespread adoption and implementation of psychiatric genetic counseling.

Conflation of Genetic Counseling with Genetic Testing

There is a tendency to think that meaningful and valuable genetic counseling is not possible without genetic testing. Those of us within the psychiatric and clinical genetics communities tend to have an implicit assumption that for our knowledge about the genetic contributions to conditions to be clinically useful, we need to have a very detailed and specific level of understanding and ideally a genetic test to offer. Accordingly, the value of genetic counseling is typically thought of as providing information about genetic testing. Therefore, since there is currently no genetic testing being routinely clinically implemented for psychiatric conditions, the perception is that there is no reason to consider providing genetic counseling yet. As discussed above, this is a misunderstanding: evidence shows that psychiatric genetic counseling can provide meaningful positive outcomes for people, even without the provision of genetic testing. Indeed, genetic counseling as a profession began at a time when there was very little to offer in terms of genetic testing for many conditions. Thus, the emphasis was on counseling to help people adapt to the condition or risk of condition in their families. Psychiatric genetic counseling is, in many ways, a return to the very well-established roots of the profession.

Counseling without Genetic Testing Is Not Valued

A closely related concept worth mentioning is the fact that in medical practice and healthcare research, the activity of counseling is at an axiological disadvantage relative to genetic testing. As a society, we place more value on information and technological solutions (e.g., genetic testing) than on care-based activities (e.g., counseling). Our focus tends to be on generating information that we might ultimately deliver (developing genetic testing) and thinking about what information to deliver, rather than on considering how to deliver it. At every level, this results in difficulties in advancing the psychiatric genetic counseling agenda: from securing funding for research to establish best practices and outcomes, to implementing new clinical services. This devaluing of care-based activities is at odds with data that demonstrate that if we want to reap the benefits of precision medicine, by helping people to change their behavior to reduce their risk of common complex conditions, then simply providing information is not enough (Marteau et al. 2010). *Counseling* about genetic information, however, holds the potential to help people change behavior. It overcomes some of the fundamental problems, such as addressing emotions that act as barriers to behavior change and connecting behaviors with genetic information in a coherent manner to provide people a sense of agency (Austin 2015).

Turf Wars over Who Should Deliver Psychiatric Genetic Counseling

If we consider psychiatric genetic counseling to be more about counseling than about genetic testing, then questions arise about who should provide psychiatric genetic counseling. Obvious candidates include genetic counselors and physicians, particularly psychiatrists and family practitioners. Psychiatrists tend to point out, quite rightly, that they have ongoing relationships with patients; thus, they are ideally positioned to provide psychiatric genetic counseling.

Given that psychiatric genetic counseling typically involves uncovering and addressing issues connected to feelings of guilt, shame, blame, fear, and stigma that accompany the explanations people have about their condition, psychiatrists refer (entirely appropriately) to their expertise in addressing these emotions. Family practitioners have similar long-standing relationships with their patients. Theoretically, as primary care providers, they would also be ideally placed to address these issues, at least from an accessibility standpoint. In reality, many physicians lack the time (due to being consumed with crisis intervention and medication management), the confidence, or the expertise in issues related to genetics (Finn et al. 2005; Hoop et al. 2008; Hoop and Salva 2010) to have these conversations with their patients. It is important to point out that psychiatric genetic counseling is *not* a brief or group-based intervention (like psychoeducation can often be). Therefore, simply using visual aids to explain to a patient "your condition is caused by genes and environment acting together" does not constitute useful psychiatric genetic counseling. To be effective, counseling must be personalized and involve a two-way exchange of information together with the provision of counseling support. According to research, a typical session takes ~90 minutes. Psychiatrists sometimes point out the similarities between psychiatric genetic counseling and *personalized* psychoeducation interventions. When the latter is available to patients, it may address the issues addressed by psychiatric genetic counseling. (Note: group-based psychoeducation is quite different and will not meet personalized needs in the same way). However, in practice, personalized psychoeducation is inconsistently provided at best.

Ultimately, although physicians may feel it is their role to provide psychiatric genetic counseling, in practice they are rarely able to deliver it, and if patients are not referred for genetic counseling, they will not benefit from what the intervention has to offer. Anyone with clinical expertise in both genetics and psychiatric conditions could reasonably provide psychiatric genetic counseling. In different jurisdictions, different types of healthcare professionals may be best placed to deliver psychiatric genetic counseling. Importantly, what matters is not *who* delivers psychiatric genetic counseling—or even whether it is called "individual psychoeducation" or psychiatric genetic counseling—but *how* it is delivered. It should be delivered in an evidence-based manner. It is obviously important to consider issues that impact cost: physicians' time is more expensive than that of genetic counselors, and there is a need for all healthcare practitioners to work to the top of their scope of practice (i.e., they should engage with tasks that only they can do, and that cannot be delegated to someone less senior). This highlights another barrier to psychiatric genetic counseling.

The Perceived Shortage of Genetic Counselors

There is no doubt that genetic counselors are in high demand. Although the popular assumption is that there are not enough genetic counselors, the profession has reacted to growing demand by developing, for example, practice models to aid healthcare professionals through genetic counseling assistants, use of decision aids, and chatbots to facilitate information provision. In North America, there has been a rapid expansion in the number of training programs and available positions within existing training programs (Hoskovec et al. 2018). In several European countries, where genetic counseling does not yet exist as a profession, efforts are underway to develop this specialty (Ormond et al. 2018). The number of genetic tests available is increasing with incredible speed. Given that genetic counseling is often considered to be something that becomes relevant once genetic testing is available, this creates a situation in which the creation of genetic counseling positions is prioritized according to demand, which in turn is typically driven by genetic testing. The genetic counseling service system constantly reacts to external pressures rather than proactively strategizing to create new positions. Therefore, because genetic counselors do not see referral pressure of patients with psychiatric conditions, positions in this specialty are not created (Chanouha et al. 2022). Referral demand creates genetic counseling position supply; if specialty positions in psychiatric genetic counseling were created, research shows that genetic counselors would want to fill them (Van den Adel et al. 2022).

Stigma Associated with Psychiatric Conditions and with Genetic Counseling

Stigma plays out in relation to psychiatric genetic counseling in different ways. First, psychiatric conditions themselves are, of course, stigmatized. Therefore, within the genetic counseling profession there is a degree of lack of comfort with serving this population (Booke et al. 2020). Interventions have been developed to decrease stigmatizing attitudes toward psychiatric conditions among genetic counselors (Anderson and Austin 2012). Specialized training workshops have been offered (Dillon et al. 2022) and found effective in increasing genetic counselors' comfort with delivering psychiatric genetic counseling. The lack of referrals for psychiatric genetic counseling services means, however, that those who have been through these workshops have little chance to practice their skills and very limited clinical exposure to counsel people with psychiatric conditions.

Second, the term genetic counseling seems to be associated with a degree of stigma from the perspective of psychiatrists. Specifically, when the first specialist psychiatric genetic counseling clinic was opened, psychiatrists who could potentially refer their patients expressed a level of discomfort associated with referring a patient to something called "genetic counseling." They explained that they were concerned that their patients might think that a referral to genetic counseling implied a perception that they should not have children. Although psychiatrists valued the psychiatric genetic counseling service and the outcomes they witnessed, they were reluctant to refer patients because of this fear. Through conversation and with their guidance, the decision was taken to rename the service to the "Adapt Clinic," and this was an effective remedy for this barrier.

The term genetic counseling can also inhibit referrals by physicians because of misperceptions that it only involves a discussion of the role of genetics in the etiology of the condition. If this were the case, this would indeed be problematic, as physicians appreciate and discuss the roles of stressors in contributing to the development of psychiatric conditions with their patients. Referring to a service that uses a different conceptual model of etiology would be difficult to justify. As discussed above, genetic counseling for psychiatric conditions involves discussing both the genetic and environmental contributions to these conditions in a holistic manner; it does not involve advising people against having children. In fact, promoting and supporting patient autonomy is central to the ethos of the genetic counseling practice (Veach et al. 2007).

To address this issue, I have considered alternative names for the intervention over time. All are inadequate for a variety of reasons. "Nido-genetic counseling"—in Italian, *nido* refers to the nest, the environmental element of the counseling—would be meaningless to most people. "Attributional therapy" or "etiological counseling" are accurately descriptive, but again unclear. Critically, it is important to remember that regardless of name, the content of the intervention is founded on a genetic counseling practice model. Moving away from the genetic counseling label brings the risk of the intervention being perceived as atheoretical or lacking foundation.

Finally, stigma is relevant as a barrier to broader implementation of psychiatric genetic counseling because research shows that physicians primarily consider referring to this service only after patients ask about it explicitly (Leach et al. 2016). Unfortunately, many patients who could benefit most from psychiatric genetic counseling are the same people who are least likely to inquire about it. People often fear being told by an expert that they are somehow responsible for their illness, that there is nothing they can do about it, that they now have to accept being in a state of poor mental health for the rest of their lives, or that any children they might have will certainly develop the same condition. These ideas are antithetical to the content and values of genetic counseling practice in the context of psychiatric conditions.

Psychiatric Genetic Counseling May Be a Cost Saver, Not a Revenue Generator

In nonpublic healthcare settings, services are prioritized, at least in part, according to the potential for revenue generation. Genetic testing is a revenue generator: When a genetic condition has been identified in one individual, interventions can sometimes be offered to that individual (e.g., prophylactic mastectomies in the context of BRCA testing). Testing can also be offered to relatives, which enhances revenue generation. Psychiatric genetic counseling does not demonstrate such obvious routes for revenue generation, though it is possible that a genetic counselor providing this service could be considered a "physician extender," allowing the physician to bill for more patients by providing oversight to the genetic counselor.

If psychiatric genetic counseling does indeed have an influence on mental health outcomes, the expectation would be that it would involve cost savings for the healthcare system because people would be better equipped to self-manage their own risk for psychiatric illness. This is an appealing concept from a public health perspective and would potentially be attractive to publicly funded healthcare systems, but it potentially fits less easily within the context of private healthcare systems.

Literature Silos

Many researchers are interested in and publishing papers on various aspects of the potential applications of genetic testing in the context of psychiatric conditions. Though genetic counseling is not yet firmly established as an academic discipline, a large body of data is emerging from this community about the process and outcomes of genetic counseling in the context of various kinds of conditions and in relation to different kinds of genetic testing. To date, however, there is little cross referencing of the genetic counseling literature in the psychology, psychiatry, or psychiatric genetics literature. This perpetuates the misconceptions about genetic counseling (Gershon and Alliey-Rodriguez 2013; Moreno-De-Luca et al. 2018) and could ultimately act as a barrier to its implementation. As a potentially related issue, the genetic counseling community is female dominated, and accordingly, papers published in this community tend to be by female authors. Data shows that female-authored papers are less cited than male authored papers (Dworkin et al. 2020).

Summary

Genetic counseling for psychiatric conditions is of interest to families and is associated with meaningful positive outcomes for patients even in the absence of any genetic testing being provided. Despite these advantages and ongoing efforts to provide training, it remains limited in its availability to patients worldwide. With this article, I hope to further discussion about the barriers to implementation of psychiatric genetic counseling and how they might be overcome. This work is growing increasingly urgent, given the increasing interest in the application of various forms of genetic testing in psychiatry. This urgency is further underscored by the many ethical issues around implementation of genetic testing, and the fact that many of these ethical issues can be readily addressed in the context of evidence-based genetic counseling.

16

Concluding Summary

Joshua A. Gordon and Elisabeth B. Binder

Introduction

As discussed throughout this volume, our understanding of the genetic basis of psychiatric disorders has advanced tremendously. This understanding now needs to be translated into actionable biology to help patients. The chapters in this volume represent an earnest attempt to clarify just how much our understanding has progressed, and what might be necessary to complete the translation process. As we noted in Chapter 1, during the course of the Forum, four distinct groups captured the progress to date and discussed pathways forward for next steps, tackling a set of questions the groups posed of themselves and then set about to answer. Here we will recap the progress made toward answering these questions in the four groups, summarizing the principal conclusions. We will then close by considering some cross-cutting themes that link ideas across multiple groups.

Delineating Additional Risk Factors

Discussion in the first group focused on whether and how to explore additional genetic risk factors. The progress and conclusions reached by Ronald et al. are detailed in Chapter 2. Despite the undeniable success in identifying hundreds of loci predisposing to multiple psychiatric disorders, Ronald et al. rapidly recognized that there remained considerable work to be done. First, they note that there remain relatively few known genetic risk factors for some less-studied disorders. Second, they recognized the evidence, reviewed by Robinson et al. (Chapter 3), that even for the well-studied disorders, there are likely more risk factors that can be identified in regions of the allelic spectrum that remain underexplored. There was a fair degree of consensus that the most important reason to continue the search for additional genetic risk factors was the lack of diversity in current genetic samples. Indeed, in considering next steps, Ronald et al. place the highest priority on ensuring that future data collection focus exclusively, or nearly exclusively, on incorporating individuals from genetically ancestral populations, to ensure both scientific progress and equity.

They also emphasize the need to consider the phenotypes being explored to maximize the return on investments in future gene discovery efforts. Phenotypes discussed included quantitative phenotypes related to brain and behavior; developmental and other longitudinally assessed phenotypes, including co-occurring disorders; and environmental exposures. Ronald et al. note that these and other nondisease, nonbinary phenotypes are more challenging (and expensive) to obtain at scale. They point to several seminal examples of the potential power of exploiting these phenotypes to reveal additional biological and environmental influences on psychiatric disorders. In the final section of Chapter 2, Ronald et al. identify several potential strategies to efficiently gather this phenotypic data. They also addressed the methodology to be used to characterize genetic variation. Here, consensus was more challenging to reach. Some argued that whole-genome sequencing was the appropriate level to interrogate genetic variation, maximizing the information to be gained from each individual and permitting a wide range of analyses to be conducted. Others noted that the trade-off in cost compared to whole-exome sequencing or chip-based genotyping and argued that it was more important to prioritize larger sample sizes and/or deeper phenotyping given potential budgetary constraints. Ronald et al. settled in on the notion that these trade-offs be considered when designing gene discovery projects and that the project should utilize the highest feasible level of genotyping depth possible.

Rare Variation

A second group was tasked with discussing pathways for translating knowledge about rare variants into neurobiological understanding and/or novel therapies. The deliberations and recommendations reached by Bearden et al. are included in Chapter 5. Recognizing the progress made in gene therapy for other monogenic disorders of the central nervous system, they note that much of this progress followed an understanding of the neurobiological consequences of these rare variants. Thus, they consider the pursuits of neurobiology and therapeutics to be intertwined.

Given the large number of rare variants that have now been shown to be causal for disorders such as autism (and to a lesser extent, schizophrenia), Bearden et al. discussed the need to prioritize among these variants for further follow-up. In Chapter 5, they detail a number of important factors to be considered in such a prioritization. These factors include those relevant to the clinical condition—including the strength of the association, the natural history of the illness, etc. —as well as biological variables—including the nature of the variant, its functional implications, and the dependence on gene dosage. Some of these factors are more relevant for studies aimed at understanding the neurobiology of the variants, while others are more relevant for therapeutic development.

Bearden et al. also considered the importance of identifying mechanistic convergence, both between different rare variant causes of a disorder as well as between rare and common variants. They note that in autism, in particular, there is already considerable evidence for convergence, both in terms of biological pathways and in terms of the tissues and developmental time periods during which risk genes are most likely to be expressed. Further, they delineate a number of model systems that might be utilized to identify these functional consequences.

Finally, Bearden et al. note that therapeutic development for rare variants is conceivable in the not-too-distant future, given advances in gene therapy and targeting methodologies. Accordingly, they considered the preparatory studies that are necessary to lay the groundwork for future clinical trials aimed at testing such therapies. Given the importance of understanding when and where such interventions should be targeted, Bearden et al. prioritize studies of the natural history of rare variant-associated illness as well as the development of biomarkers that could be used to identify individuals who might benefit from a particular treatment or to measure therapeutic effects during the course of treatment.

Common Variation

In terms of understanding the neurobiological and clinical consequences of common risk variants, the third group acknowledge the considerable, additional challenges that exist at present, as described in Chapter 8 by Won et al. The small effect size of each variant leads to questions of how this risk is summed mechanistically. Moreover, most of these variants are found in intergenic regions rather than within sequences that code for genes, leading to uncertainty as to which biological pathways are altered by the variants. As a result, Won et al. hold that unlike the case for common variation, where clinical and neurobiological implications can be explored simultaneously, further understanding of the biological consequences are the primary priority for rare variation. To help facilitate this understanding, Won et al. considered both experimental approaches and resources.

Experimentally, Won et al. note the importance of both human genetic and model system approaches. They articulate the need to establish a pathway leading from causal risk variant to gene that begins with increased sample sizes and increased diversity in existing genome-wide association studies (GWASs). Next, they note the necessity for refining approaches to statistical fine mapping to utilize these GWAS-derived data to identify the specific single nucleotide polymorphisms most likely responsible for the risk signal. Further, they describe a range of different approaches, including experimental in model systems, to validate these fine-mapping results and link them to altered gene and/or protein regulation. This pathway is crucial to understand the impact of common risk variants on cellular functions.

Refining this pathway of approaches is not in and of itself sufficient, in part due to the sheer magnitude of the task at hand. With hundreds and perhaps thousands of risk variants playing a role in psychiatric disorders, Won et al. recognize that a coordinated, resource-based approach will be key to elucidating a biological understanding. Accordingly, they suggest prioritizing the development of large-scale resources such as molecular atlases, validated gene ontologies specific to the brain, and stem cell banks and other biological material repositories linked to deeply clinically phenotyped individuals. These resources will assist at various points along the experimental pathway to speed progress and ensure a comprehensive treatment of the biological consequences of common risk variation.

Clinical Opportunities

The fourth group was tasked with discussing how to maximize the near-term potential for clinical opportunities stemming from progress in understanding of genetic risk. While acknowledging that the principal outcome of clinical benefit—novel therapies—is a long-term objective, Davis et al. recognize that there is a potential for more immediate impact, particularly regarding the explanatory power and predictive capacity of genetic testing. In Chapter 12, they consider the current and potential near-term future clinical use of various types of genetic information, the ethical and clinical implications of such use, as well as the barriers to effective use of genetic information in current clinical practice.

On several issues, Davis et al. achieved a principled consensus. Regarding rare variation, they note that in many countries, routine clinical care for autism and neurodevelopmental disorders already involves genetic testing for rare variants. The consensus was that this return of results was an informative and useful clinical endeavor. Regarding common variation, Davis et al. evaluated the clinical evidence for the utility of polygenic scores (PGSs) and found it lacking. They reached conclusions, including that current iterations of PGSs are not sufficiently predictive of psychiatric risk to be of utility in the general population; that the utility of PGS use in high-risk populations requires further study; and that equity in the application of PGSs in the future will require significant diversification of the samples used to conduct GWAS.

Cross-Cutting Themes

Several cross-cutting themes emerged that played significant roles in the discussions that took place across multiple groups at the Forum. First and perhaps foremost, each of the four groups independently recognized the importance of enriching diversity and considering community-driven goals as we progress along the path from genetics to biological knowledge and novel treatments. Diverse samples, especially those that include ancestral populations, serve multiple goals. Diverse samples may facilitate the discovery of additional genetic and environmental risk factors. Moreover, the inclusion of ancestral populations, with greater haplotype heterogeneity, can facilitate more precise fine mapping of known risk factors. Application of genetic information to clinical use requires diverse samples if the clinical utility is to be capable of being applied broadly across the globe. Finally, genetic studies that utilize diverse communities across the globe need to ensure that they are working in the service of those communities. The importance of engaging deeply with these communities to understand their needs and design genetic studies accordingly was emphasized in several chapters in this volume.

Another cross-cutting theme centered on the importance of moving beyond consideration of binary diagnostics and capturing deeper phenotypes. From ensuring that we fully capture meaningful genetic risk factors, to enabling a greater understanding of developmental events and capturing gene–environment interactions, deeper phenotyping has the potential to enhance dramatically our understanding of the biological implications of genetic risk. Moreover, increasing the breadth and depth of phenotyping has implications for clinical approaches. Characterization of genetic associations with neurodevelopmental phenotypes raises the possibility of novel preventative interventions, while physiological or behavioral phenotypes might lead to novel biomarkers. Meanwhile, translation of these genetically characterized phenotypes into model systems, such as human cell preparations or animal models, could enable progress in both clinical and biological spheres.

Developmental and translatable phenotypes are aspects of two additional themes that cut across the groups. All developmental events, phases of illness, and sequencing of co-occuring disorders are important for gene discovery, biological understanding, and clinical translation. Translatable phenotypes have the potential to confirm gene-phenotype associations, which will be especially useful for priorizing common variants. Moreover, translation of these phenotypes into model systems will facilitate exploration of biological pathways influenced by genetic risk, as well as testing of potential therapeutic targets.

A final cross-cutting theme that influenced much of the conclusions drawn by each of the groups is the importance of searching for convergence. With hundreds of risk variants, both common and rare, identifying convergent effects of these variants on biological mechanisms will allow neurobiologists to focus their efforts. Convergence between rare and common alleles will be particularly telling for clinical relevance; for most psychiatric disorders, rare alleles will likely only contribute to a minority of cases. The degree of convergence between the mechanisms implicated by rare and common variation will predict the degree to which knowledge and treatments that emerge from rare variants (which are much easier to study in model systems) will be relevant for clinical translation to the larger majority of individuals who have "idiopathic" illness that is not explained by a large effect size, rare variant.

Conclusion: Strategic Coordination to Speed Progess

These and other priorities articulated throughout this volume represent a potential strategic framework for advancing biological discovery and clinical translation in the wake of the many advances made in psychiatric genetics over the past decade. A noteable commonality worth underscoring here is the notion, articulated again across all the groups, that strategic coordination will be the key to accelerating furture progress. Both for large-scale efforts (e.g., developmental resources, multi-omics on single cells) and for smaller-scale efforts (deep phenotyping of individual variants, convergence from multiple common variants), vigorous coordination can ensure complete coverage of the variance space, reduce duplication, and ensure harmonization for rigor, reproducibility, and future meta- and mega-analyses. The enthusiasm for a coordinated approach was uniformly expressed and can be seen in the myriad recommendations detailed here and in the individual chapters. Such coordination, applied to the challenges and opportunities noted throughout the volume, holds the promise to transform the understanding, prevention, and treatment of mental illnesses over the coming decades.

Disclaimer The views expressed in this chapter/introduction do not necessarily represent the views of the NIH, HHS, or the United States Government.

Bibliography

Note: Numbers in square brackets denote the chapter in which an entry is cited.

Abell, N. S., M. K. DeGorter, M. J. Gloudemans, et al. 2022. Multiple Causal Variants Underlie Genetic Associations in Humans. *Science* **375**:1247–1254. [8]

Abud, E. M., R. N. Ramirez, E. S. Martinez, et al. 2017. iPSC-Derived Human Microglia-Like Cells to Study Neurological Diseases. *Neuron* **94**:278–293. [7]

Adams, M. J., W. D. Hill, D. M. Howard, et al. 2020. Factors Associated with Sharing E-Mail Information and Mental Health Survey Participation in Large Population Cohorts. *Int. J. Epidemiol.* **49**:410–421. [2]

Ahn, K., N. Gotay, T. M. Andersen, et al. 2014. High Rate of Disease-Related Copy Number Variations in Childhood Onset Schizophrenia. *Mol. Psychiatry* **19**:568–572. [3]

Aibar, S., C. B. González-Blas, T. Moerman, et al. 2017. Scenic: Single-Cell Regulatory Network Inference and Clustering. *Nat. Methods* **14**:1083–1086. [11]

Aittokallio, J., A. Kauko, F. Vaura, et al. 2022. Polygenic Risk Scores for Predicting Adverse Outcomes after Coronary Revascularization. *Am. J. Cardiol.* **167**:9–14. [13]

Alareeki, A., B. Lashewicz, and L. Shipton. 2019. "Get Your Child in Order": Illustrations of Courtesy Stigma from Fathers Raising Both Autistic and Non-Autistic Children. *Disabil. Stud. Q.* **39**: [14]

Alasoo, K., J. Rodrigues, S. Mukhopadhyay, et al. 2018. Shared Genetic Effects on Chromatin and Gene Expression Indicate a Role for Enhancer Priming in Immune Response. *Nat. Genet.* **50**:424–431. [10]

Alkelai, A., L. Greenbaum, A. R. Docherty, et al. 2022. The Benefit of Diagnostic Whole Genome Sequencing in Schizophrenia and Other Psychotic Disorders. *Mol. Psychiatry* **27**:1435–1447. [13]

Alver, M., V. Mancini, K. Lall, et al. 2022. Contribution of Schizophrenia Polygenic Burden to Longitudinal Phenotypic Variance in 22q11.2 Deletion Syndrome. *Mol. Psychiatry* **27**:4191–4200. [13]

Amar, M., A. B. Pramod, N. K. Yu, et al. 2021. Autism-Linked Cullin3 Germline Haploinsufficiency Impacts Cytoskeletal Dynamics and Cortical Neurogenesis through RhoA Signaling. *Mol. Psychiatry* **26**:3586–3613. [5]

Amiri, A., G. Coppola, S. Scuderi, et al. 2018. Transcriptome and Epigenome Landscape of Human Cortical Development Modeled in Organoids. *Science* **362**:eaat6720. [5]

Anderson, K., and J. C. Austin. 2012. Effects of a Documentary Film on Public Stigma Related to Mental Illness Among Genetic Counselors. *J. Genet. Counsel.* **21**:573–581. [15]

Anderson, N. C., P. F. Chen, K. Meganathan, et al. 2021. Balancing Serendipity and Reproducibility: Pluripotent Stem Cells as Experimental Systems for Intellectual and Developmental Disorders. *Stem Cell Rep.* **16**:1446–1457. [5, 6]

Andlauer, T. F. M., J. Link, D. Martin, et al. 2020. Treatment- and Population-Specific Genetic Risk Factors for Anti-Drug Antibodies against Interferon-Beta: A GWAS. *BMC Med.* **18**:298. [2]

Anzalone, A. V., P. B. Randolph, J. R. Davis, et al. 2019. Search-and-Replace Genome Editing without Double-Strand Breaks or Donor DNA. *Nature* **576**:149–157. [7]

Appelbaum, P. S., and S. Benston. 2017. Anticipating the Ethical Challenges of Psychiatric Genetic Testing. *Curr. Psychiatry Rep.* **19**:39. [14]

Aragam, K. G., A. Dobbyn, R. Judy, et al. 2020. Limitations of Contemporary Guidelines for Managing Patients at High Genetic Risk of Coronary Artery Disease. *J. Am. Coll. Cardiol.* **75**:2769–2780. [13]

Araki, Y., I. Hong, T. R. Gamache, et al. 2020. SynGAP Isoforms Differentially Regulate Synaptic Plasticity and Dendritic Development. *eLife* **9**:e56273. [5]

Arango, C., C. M. Diaz-Caneja, P. D. McGorry, et al. 2018. Preventive Strategies for Mental Health. *Lancet Psychiatry* **5**:591–604. [13]

Araújo, D. S., and H. E. Wheeler. 2022. Genetic and Environmental Variation Impact Transferability of Polygenic Risk Scores. *Cell Rep. Med.* **3**:100687. [12]

Arnberg, F. K., R. Gudmundsdóttir, A. Butwicka, et al. 2015. Psychiatric Disorders and Suicide Attempts in Swedish Survivors of the 2004 Southeast Asia Tsunami: A 5 Year Matched Cohort Study. *Lancet Psychiatry* **2**:817–824. [4]

Arnett, D. K., R. S. Blumenthal, M. A. Albert, et al. 2019. 2019 ACC/AHA Guideline on the Primary Prevention of Cardiovascular Disease: Executive Summary: A Report of the American College of Cardiology/American Heart Association Task Force on Clinical Practice Guidelines. *J. Am. Coll. Cardiol.* **74**:1376–1414. [13]

Aschard, H., V. Guillemot, B. Vilhjalmsson, et al. 2017. Covariate Selection for Association Screening in Multiphenotype Genetic Studies. *Nat. Genet.* **49**:1789–1795. [2]

Ashburn, T. T., and K. B. Thor. 2004. Drug Repositioning: Identifying and Developing New Uses for Existing Drugs. *Nat. Rev. Drug Discov.* **3**:673–683. [6]

Attardo, A., J. E. Fitzgerald, and M. J. Schnitzer. 2015. Impermanence of Dendritic Spines in Live Adult CA1 Hippocampus. *Nature* **523** 592–596. [5]

Austin, J. C. 2015. The Effect of Genetic Test-Based Risk Information on Behavioral Outcomes: A Critical Examination of Failed Trials and a Call to Action. *Am. J. Med. Genet. A* **167**:2913–2915. [15]

———. 2019. Evidence-Based Genetic Counseling for Psychiatric Disorders: A Road Map. *Cold Spring Harb. Perspect. Med.* **10**:a036608. [15]

Austin, J. C., and W. G. Honer. 2004. The Potential Impact of Genetic Counseling for Mental Illness. *Clin. Genet.* **67**:134–142. [15]

———. 2008. Psychiatric Genetic Counselling for Parents of Individuals Affected with Psychotic Disorders: A Pilot Study. *Early. Interv. Psychiatry* **2**:80–89. [15]

Austin, J. C., C. G. S. Palmer, B. Rosen-Sheidley, et al. 2008. Psychiatric Disorders in Clinical Genetics II: Individualizing Recurrence Risks. *J. Genet. Counsel.* **17**:18–29. [15]

Austin, J. C., A. Semaka, and G. Hadjipavlou. 2014. Conceptualizing Genetic Counseling as Psychotherapy in the Era of Genomic Medicine. *J. Genet. Counsel.* **23**:903–909. [15]

Austin, J. C., G. N. Smith, and W. G. Honer. 2006. The Genomic Era and Perceptions of Psychotic Disorders: Genetic Risk Estimation, Associations with Reproductive Decisions and Views About Predictive Testing. *Am. J. Med. Genet. B Neuropsychiatr. Genet.* **141B**:926–928. [15]

Auton, A., G. R. Abecasis, D. M. Altshuler, et al. 2015. A Global Reference for Human Genetic Variation. *Nature* **526**:68–74. [2]

Auwerx, C., M. Lepamets, M. C. Sadler, et al. 2022. The Individual and Global Impact of Copy-Number Variants on Complex Human Traits. *Am. J. Hum. Genet.* **109**:647–668. [12]

Badini, I., J. R. I. Coleman, S. P. Hagenaars, et al. 2022. Depression with Atypical Neurovegetative Symptoms Shares Genetic Predisposition with Immuno-Metabolic Traits and Alcohol Consumption. *Psychol. Med.* **52**:726–736. [2]

Baglioni, C., G. Battagliese, B. Feige, et al. 2011. Insomnia as a Predictor of Depression: A Meta-Analytic Evaluation of Longitudinal Epidemiological Studies. *J. Affect. Disord.* **135**:10–19. [15]

Ballouz, S., and J. Gillis. 2017. Strength of Functional Signature Correlates with Effect Size in Autism. *Genome Med.* **9**:64. [7]

Baselmans, B. M. L., L. Yengo, W. van Rheenen, and N. R. Wray. 2021. Risk in Relatives, Heritability, Snp-Based Heritability, and Genetic Correlations in Psychiatric Disorders: A Review. *Biol. Psychiatry* **89**:11–19. [9]

Bashford, A., and P. Levine. 2010. The Oxford Handbook of the History of Eugenics. New York: Oxford Univ. Press. [14]

Bauer, M. S., and J. Kirchner. 2020. Implementation Science: What Is It and Why Should I Care? *Psychiatry Res.* **283**:112376. [13]

Bear, M. F., K. M. Huber, and S. T. Warren. 2004. The mGluR Theory of Fragile X Mental Retardation. *Trends Neurosci.* **27**:370–377. [5]

Beauchamp, M. R., R. E. Rhodes, C. Kreutzer, and J. L. Rupert. 2011. Experiential versus Genetic Accounts of Inactivity: Implications for Inactive Individuals' Self-Efficacy Beliefs and Intentions to Exercise. *Behav. Med.* **37**:8–14. [14]

Bélanger, S. A., and J. Caron. 2018. Evaluation of the Child with Global Developmental Delay and Intellectual Disability. *Paediatr. Child Health* **23**:403–419. [12]

Ben-David, E., and S. Shifman. 2013. Combined Analysis of Exome Sequencing Points toward a Major Role for Transcription Regulation during Brain Development in Autism. *Mol. Psychiatry* **18**:1054–1056. [11]

Bennett, C. F., B. F. Baker, N. Pham, E. Swayze, and R. S. Geary. 2017. Pharmacology of Antisense Drugs. *Annu. Rev. Pharmacol. Toxicol.* **57**:81–105. [6]

Ben-Shalom, R., C. M. Keeshen, K. N. Berrios, et al. 2017. Opposing Effects on Nav1.2 Function Underlie Differences between SCN2A Variants Observed in Individuals with Autism Spectrum Disorder or Infantile Seizures. *Biol. Psychiatry* **82**:224–232. [7]

Bentley, A. R., S. L. Callier, and C. N. Rotimi. 2020. Evaluating the Promise of Inclusion of African Ancestry Populations in Genomics. *NPJ Genom. Med.* **5**:5. [2]

Berendzen, K. M., R. Sharma, M. A. Mandujano, et al. 2023. Oxytocin Receptor Is Not Required for Social Attachment in Prairie Voles. *Neuron*, in press. [5]

Bergen, S. E., A. Ploner, D. Howrigan, et al. 2019. Joint Contributions of Rare Copy Number Variants and Common SNPs to Risk for Schizophrenia. *Am. J. Psychiatry* **176**:29–35. [13]

Berry-Kravis, E., V. Des Portes, R. Hagerman, et al. 2016. Mavoglurant in Fragile X Syndrome: Results of Two Randomized, Double-Blind, Placebo-Controlled Trials. *Sci. Transl. Med.* **8**:321. [5, 6]

Bershteyn, M., T. J. Nowakowski, A. A. Pollen, et al. 2017. Human iPSC-Derived Cerebral Organoids Model Cellular Features of Lissencephaly and Reveal Prolonged Mitosis of Outer Radial Glia. *Cell Stem Cell* **20**:435–449. [5]

Bhaduri, A., M. G. Andrews, W. Mancia Leon, et al. 2020. Cell Stress in Cortical Organoids Impairs Molecular Subtype Specification. *Nature* **578**:142–148. [5]

Bhakar, A. L., G. Dolen, and M. F. Bear. 2012. The Pathophysiology of Fragile X (and What It Teaches Us About Synapses). *Annu. Rev. Neurosci.* **35**:417–443. [6]

Biesecker, B. B. 2001. Goals of Genetic Counseling. *Clin. Genet.* **60**:323–330. [15]

Bigdeli, T. B., S. Ripke, R. E. Peterson, et al. 2017. Genetic Effects Influencing Risk for Major Depressive Disorder in China and Europe. *Transl. Psychiatry* **7**:e1074. [2]

Birey, F., J. Andersen, C. D. Makinson, et al. 2017. Assembly of Functionally Integrated Human Forebrain Spheroids. *Nature* **545**:54–59. [5, 7]

Birey, F., M. Y. Li, A. Gordon, et al. 2022. Dissecting the Molecular Basis of Human Interneuron Migration in Forebrain Assembloids from Timothy Syndrome. *Cell Stem Cell* **29**:248–264. [7]

Biroli, P., T. J. Galama, S. von Hinke, et al. 2022. The Economics and Econometrics of Gene–Environment Interplay. *arXiv* 00729. [4]

Bishop, S. L., A. Thurm, E. Robinson, and S. J. Sanders. 2021. *Preprint*: Prevalence of Returnable Genetic Results Based on Recognizable Phenotypes among Children with Autism Spectrum Disorder. *medRxiv* 2021.2005.2028.21257736. [3]

Bloss, C. S., N. J. Schork, and E. J. Topol. 2011. Effect of Direct-to-Consumer Genomewide Profiling to Assess Disease Risk. *N. Engl. J. Med.* **364**:524–534. [15]

Blout Zawatsky, C. L., N. Shah, K. Machini, et al. 2021. Returning Actionable Genomic Results in a Research Biobank: Analytic Validity, Clinical Implementation, and Resource Utilization. *Am. J. Hum. Genet.* **108**:2224–2237. [13]

Bodnar, L. M., and K. L. Wisner. 2005. Nutrition and Depression: Implications for Improving Mental Health Among Childbearing-Aged Women. *Biol. Psychiatry* **1**:679–685. [15]

Boeschoten, R. E., A. M. J. Braamse, A. T. F. Beekman, et al. 2017. Prevalence of Depression and Anxiety in Multiple Sclerosis: A Systematic Review and Meta-Analysis. *J. Neurologic. Sci.* **372**:331–341. [2]

Bonanno, S., R. Giossi, R. Zanin, et al. 2022. Amifampridine Safety and Efficacy in Spinal Muscular Atrophy Ambulatory Patients: A Randomized, Placebo-Controlled, Crossover Phase 2 Trial. *J. Neurol.* **269**:5858–5867. [5]

Booke, S., J. Austin, L. Calderwood, and M. Campion. 2020. Genetic Counselors' Attitudes toward and Practice Related to Psychiatric Genetic Counseling. *J. Genet. Counsel.* **29**:25–34. [15]

Borle, K., E. Morris, A. Inglis, and J. Austin. 2018. Risk Communication in Genetic Counseling: Exploring Uptake and Perception of Recurrence Numbers, and Their Impact on Patient Outcomes. *Clin. Genet.* **94**:239–245. [15]

Botkin, J. R., J. W. Belmont, J. S. Berg, et al. 2015. Points to Consider: Ethical, Legal, and Psychosocial Implications of Genetic Testing in Children and Adolescents. *Am. J. Hum. Genet.* **97**:6–21. [15]

Boyd Ritsher, J., and J. C. Phelan. 2005. Internalized Stigma Predicts Erosion of Morale among Psychiatric Outpatients. *Psychiatry Res.* **129**:257–265. [15]

Boyle, E. A., Y. I. Li, and J. K. Pritchard. 2017. An Expanded View of Complex Traits: From Polygenic to Omnigenic. *Cell* **169**:1177–1186. [9]

BRAIN Initiative Cell Census Network. 2021. A Multimodal Cell Census and Atlas of the Mammalian Primary Motor Cortex. *Nature* **598**:86–102. [8]

BrainSeq Consortium. 2015. Neurogenomics to Drive Novel Target Discovery for Neuropsychiatric Disorders. *Neuron* **88**:1078–1083. [10]

Brainstorm Consortium, V. Anttila, B. Bulik-Sullivan, et al. 2018. Analysis of Shared Heritability in Common Disorders of the Brain. *Science* **360**:eaap8757. [1, 2]

Breen, M. S., T. Rusielewicz, H. N. Bader, et al. 2021. Modeling Gene X Environment Interactions in PTSD Using Glucocorticoid-Induced Transcriptomics in Human Neurons. *bioRxiv* 433391. [7]

Brennand, K., J. N. Savas, Y. Kim, et al. 2015. Phenotypic Differences in hiPSC NPCs Derived from Patients with Schizophrenia. *Mol. Psychiatry* **20**:361–368. [7]

Brennand, K. J., A. Simone, J. Jou, et al. 2011. Modelling Schizophrenia Using Human Induced Pluripotent Stem Cells. *Nature* **473**:221–225. [7]

Bristow, G. C., D. M. Thomson, R. L. Openshaw, et al. 2020. 16p11 Duplication Disrupts Hippocampal-Orbitofrontal-Amygdala Connectivity, Revealing a Neural Circuit Endophenotype for Schizophrenia. *Cell Rep.* **31**:107536. [7]

Brown, R. C., E. C. Berenz, S. H. Aggen, et al. 2014. Trauma Exposure and Axis I Psychopathology: A Cotwin Control Analysis in Norwegian Young Adults. *Psychol. Trauma* **6**:652–660. [4]

Brownstein, C. A., E. Douard, J. Mollon, et al. 2022. Similar Rates of Deleterious Copy Number Variants in Early-Onset Psychosis and Autism Spectrum Disorder. *Am. J. Psychiatry* **179**:853–861. [12]

Brunner, C., M. Grillet, A. Sans-Dublanc, et al. 2020. A Platform for Brain-Wide Volumetric Functional Ultrasound Imaging and Analysis of Circuit Dynamics in Awake Mice. *Neuron* **108**:861–875. [8]

Brunner, C., M. Grillet, A. Urban, et al. 2021. Whole-Brain Functional Ultrasound Imaging in Awake Head-Fixed Mice. *Nat. Protoc.* **16**:3547–3571. [8]

Brunner, D., P. Kabitzke, D. He, et al. 2015. Comprehensive Analysis of the 16p11.2 Deletion and Null Cntnap2 Mouse Models of Autism Spectrum Disorder. *PLOS ONE* **10**:e0134572. [7]

Bryois, J., D. Calini, W. Macnair, et al. 2022. Cell-Type-Specific *cis*-eQTLs in Eight Human Brain Cell Types Identify Novel Risk Genes for Psychiatric and Neurological Disorders. *Nat. Neurosci.* **25**:1104–1112. [10, 11]

Bryois, J., M. E. Garrett, L. Song, et al. 2018. Evaluation of Chromatin Accessibility in Prefrontal Cortex of Individuals with Schizophrenia. *Nat. Commun.* **9**:3121. [10]

Butcher, L. M., and R. Plomin. 2008. The Nature of Nurture: A Genomewide Association Scan for Family Chaos. *Behav. Genet.* **38**:361–371. [2]

Butler, M. G., D. Moreno-De-Luca, and A. M. Persico. 2022. Actionable Genomics in Clinical Practice: Paradigmatic Case Reports of Clinical and Therapeutic Strategies Based Upon Genetic Testing. *Genes* **13**:323. [12]

Buxbaum, J. D., D. J. Cutler, M. J. Daly, et al. 2020. Not All Autism Genes Are Created Equal: A Response to Myers et al. *Am. J. Hum. Genet.* **107**:1000–1003. [6]

Byrne, L., and A. E. Toland. 2021. Polygenic Risk Scores in Prostate Cancer Risk Assessment and Screening. *Urol. Clin. North Am.* **48**:387–399. [13]

Bzdok, D., G. Varoquaux, and E. W. Steyerberg. 2021. Prediction, Not Association, Paves the Road to Precision Medicine. *JAMA Psychiatry* **78**:127–128. [13]

Cadwell, C. R., A. Palasantza, X. Jiang, et al. 2016. Electrophysiological, Transcriptomic and Morphologic Profiling of Single Neurons Using Patch-Seq. *Nat. Biotechnol.* **34**:199–203. [11]

Cai, N., K. W. Choi, and E. I. Fried. 2020a. Reviewing the Genetics of Heterogeneity in Depression: Operationalizations, Manifestations and Etiologies. *Hum. Mol. Genet.* **29**:R10–R18. [2]

Cai, N., J. A. Revez, M. J. Adams, et al. 2020b. Minimal Phenotyping Yields Genome-Wide Association Signals of Low Specificity for Major Depression. *Nat. Genet.* **52**:437–447. [2]

Cai, Z., S. Li, D. Matuskey, N. Nabulsi, and Y. Huang. 2019. PET Imaging of Synaptic Density: A New Tool for Investigation of Neuropsychiatric Diseases. *Neurosci. Lett.* **691**:44–50. [8]

Cakir, B., Y. Xiang, Y. Tanaka, et al. 2019. Engineering of Human Brain Organoids with a Functional Vascular-Like System. *Nat. Methods* **16**:1169–1175. [7]

Calderon, D., A. Bhaskar, D. A. Knowles, et al. 2017. Inferring Relevant Cell Types for Complex Traits by Using Single-Cell Gene Expression. *Am. J. Hum. Genet.* **101**:686–699. [11]

Califf, R. M. 2018. Biomarker Definitions and Their Applications. *Exp. Biol. Med.* **243**:213–221. [5]

Camp, J. G., F. Badsha, M. Florio, et al. 2015. Human Cerebral Organoids Recapitulate Gene Expression Programs of Fetal Neocortex Development. *PNAS* **112**:15672–15677. [5]

Campos, A. I., A. Mulcahy, J. G. Thorp, et al. 2021. Understanding Genetic Risk Factors for Common Side Effects of Antidepressant Medications. *Commun. Med.* **1**:45. [14]

Cantor-Graae, E., C. B. Pedersen, T. F. McNeil, and P. B. Mortensen. 2003. Migration as a Risk Factor for Schizophrenia: A Danish Population-Based Cohort Study. *Br. J. Psychiatry* **182**:117–122. [4]

Cantor-Graae, E., and J.-P. Selten. 2005. Schizophrenia and Migration: A Meta-Analysis and Review. *Am. J. Psychiatry* **162**:12–24. [4]

Cao, Z., H. Yang, Y. Ye, et al. 2021. Polygenic Risk Score, Healthy Lifestyles, and Risk of Incident Depression. *Transl. Psychiatry* **11**:189. [13]

Carlyle, B. C., R. R. Kitchen, J. E. Kanyo, et al. 2017. A Multiregional Proteomic Survey of the Postnatal Human Brain. *Nat. Neurosci.* **20**:1787–1795. [11]

Carrion, P., A. Semaka, R. Batallones, et al. 2022. Reflections of Parents of Children with 22q11.2 Deletion Syndrome on the Experience of Receiving Psychiatric Genetic Counseling: Awareness to Act. *J. Genet. Couns.* **31**:140–152. [12]

Carver, T., S. Hartley, A. Lee, et al. 2021. Canrisk Tool-a Web Interface for the Prediction of Breast and Ovarian Cancer Risk and the Likelihood of Carrying Genetic Pathogenic Variants. *Cancer Epidemiol. Biomarkers Prev.* **30**:469–473. [13]

Casale, F. P., D. Horta, B. Rakitsch, and O. Stegle. 2017. Joint Genetic Analysis Using Variant Sets Reveals Polygenic Gene-Context Interactions. *PLoS genetics* **13**:e1006693. [2]

Caspi, A., R. M. Houts, D. W. Belsky, et al. 2014. The P Factor: One General Psychopathology Factor in the Structure of Psychiatric Disorders? *Clin. Psychol. Sci.* **2**:119–137. [2]

Caswell-Jin, J. L., T. Gupta, E. Hall, et al. 2018. Racial/Ethnic Differences in Multiple-Gene Sequencing Results for Hereditary Cancer Risk. *Genet. Med.* **20**:234–239. [3]

Cearns, M., A. T. Amare, K. O. Schubert, et al. 2022. Using Polygenic Scores and Clinical Data for Bipolar Disorder Patient Stratification and Lithium Response Prediction: Machine Learning Approach. *Br. J. Psychiatry* **Feb. 28**:1–10. [13]

Cederquist, G. Y., J. Tchieu, S. J. Callahan, et al. 2020. A Multiplex Human Pluripotent Stem Cell Platform Defines Molecular and Functional Subclasses of Autism-Related Genes. *Cell Stem Cell* **27**:35–49. [7]

Centers for Disease Control and Prevention. 2022. Facts About Suicide. https://www.cdc.gov/suicide/facts/index.html. [14]

Chailangkarn, T., C. Noree, and A. R. Muotri. 2018. The Contribution of GTF2I Haploinsufficiency to Williams Syndrome. *Mol. Cell Probes* **40**:45–51. [5]

Chang, J., S. R. Gilman, A. H. Chiang, S. J. Sanders, and D. Vitkup. 2015. Genotype to Phenotype Relationships in Autism Spectrum Disorders. *Nat. Neurosci.* **18**:191–198. [5]

Chang, X., L. A. Lima, Y. Liu, et al. 2018. Common and Rare Genetic Risk Factors Converge in Protein Interaction Networks Underlying Schizophrenia. *Front. Genet.* **9**:434. [7]

Chanouha, N., D. L. Cragun, V. Y. Pan, J. C. Austin, and C. Hoell. 2022. Healthcare Decision Makers' Perspectives on the Creation of New Genetic Counselor Positions in North America: Exploring the Case for Psychiatric Genetic Counseling. *J. Genet. Counsel.* **31**:1– 12. [12, 15]

Charney, A. W., E. A. Stahl, E. K. Green, et al. 2018. Contribution of Rare Copy Number Variants to Bipolar Disorder Risk Is Limited to Schizoaffective Cases. *Biol. Psychiatry* **86**:110–119. [3]

Charvet, C. J. 2020. Closing the Gap from Transcription to the Structural Connectome Enhances the Study of Connections in the Human Brain. *Dev. Dynamics* **249**:1047–1061. [8]

Charvet, C. J., and B. L. Finlay. 2018. Comparing Adult Hippocampal Neurogenesis across Species: Translating Time to Predict the Tempo in Humans. *Front. Neurosci.* **12**:706. [8]

Charvet, C. J., K. Ofori, C. Baucum, et al. 2022. Tracing Modification to Cortical Circuits in Human and Nonhuman Primates from High-Resolution Tractography, Transcription, and Temporal Dimensions. *The Journal of Neuroscience* **42**:3749–3767. [8]

Chau, K. K., P. Zhang, J. Urresti, et al. 2021. Full-Length Isoform Transcriptome of the Developing Human Brain Provides Further Insights into Autism. *Cell Rep.* **36**:109631. [5]

Chawner, S., J. L. Doherty, R. J. L. Anney, et al. 2021. A Genetics-First Approach to Dissecting the Heterogeneity of Autism: Phenotypic Comparison of Autism Risk Copy Number Variants. *Am. J. Psychiatry* **178**:77–86. [1]

Chen, P. J., J. A. Hussmann, J. Yan, et al. 2021. Enhanced Prime Editing Systems by Manipulating Cellular Determinants of Editing Outcomes. *Cell* **184**:5635–5652. [6]

Chen, S., R. Fragoza, L. Klei, et al. 2018. An Interactome Perturbation Framework Prioritizes Damaging Missense Mutations for Developmental Disorders. *Nat. Genet.* **50**:1032–1040. [11]

Chen, X., S. Ravindra Kumar, C. D. Adams, et al. 2022. Engineered Aavs for Non-Invasive Gene Delivery to Rodent and Non-Human Primate Nervous Systems. *Neuron* **110**:2242–2257. [6]

Cheung, R., K. D. Insigne, D. Yao, et al. 2019. A Multiplexed Assay for Exon Recognition Reveals That an Unappreciated Fraction of Rare Genetic Variants Cause Large-Effect Splicing Disruptions. *Mol. Cell* **73**:183–194. [8]

Choi, K. W., C. Y. Chen, R. J. Ursano, et al. 2019. Prospective Study of Polygenic Risk, Protective Factors, and Incident Depression Following Combat Deployment in US Army Soldiers. *Psychol. Med.* **50**:737–745. [13]

Choi, K. W., M. B. Stein, K. M. Nishimi, et al. 2020a. An Exposure-Wide and Mendelian Randomization Approach to Identifying Modifiable Factors for the Prevention of Depression. *Am. J. Psychiatry* **177**:944–954. [13]

Choi, K. W., A. B. Zheutlin, R. A. Karlson, et al. 2020b. Physical Activity Offsets Genetic Risk for Incident Depression Assessed via Electronic Health Records in a Biobank Cohort Study. *Depress. Anxiety* **37**:106–114. [13]

Choi, S. W., T. S. Mak, and P. F. O'Reilly. 2020c. Tutorial: A Guide to Performing Polygenic Risk Score Analyses. *Nat. Protoc.* **15**:2759–2772. [13]

Clarke, M. C., A. Tanskanen, M. O. Huttunen, and M. Cannon. 2013. Sudden Death of Father or Sibling in Early Childhood Increases Risk for Psychotic Disorder. *Schizophr. Res.* **143**:363–366. [4]

Cleynen, I., W. Engchuan, M. S. Hestand, et al. 2021. Genetic Contributors to Risk of Schizophrenia in the Presence of a 22q11.2 Deletion. *Mol. Psychiatry* **26**:4496–4510. [13]

Clifton, N. E., E. Rees, P. A. Holmans, et al. 2020. Genetic Association of FMRP Targets with Psychiatric Disorders. *Mol. Psychiatry* **26**:2977–2990. [11]

Coffee and Caffeine Genetics Consortium, M. C. Cornelis, E. M. Byrne, et al. 2015. Genome-Wide Meta-Analysis Identifies Six Novel Loci Associated with Habitual Coffee Consumptions. *Mol. Psychiatry* **20**:647–656. [4]

Colasante, G., G. Lignani, S. Brusco, et al. 2020. dCas9-Based Scn1a Gene Activation Restores Inhibitory Interneuron Excitability and Attenuates Seizures in Dravet Syndrome Mice. *Mol. Ther.* **28**:235–253. [5]

Coleman, J. R. I., W. J. Peyrot, K. L. Purves, et al. 2020. Genome-Wide Gene–Environment Analyses of Major Depressive Disorder and Reported Lifetime Traumatic Experiences in UK Biobank. *Mol. Psychiatry* **25**:1430–1446. [4]

Collado-Torres, L., E. E. Burke, A. Peterson, et al. 2019. Regional Heterogeneity in Gene Expression, Regulation, and Coherence in the Frontal Cortex and Hippocampus across Development and Schizophrenia. *Neuron* **103**:203–216. [11]

Collins, R. E., A. J. Wright, and T. M. Marteau. 2010. Impact of Communicating Personalized Genetic Risk Information on Perceived Control over the Risk: A Systematic Review. *Genet. Med.* **13**:273–277. [15]

Colloca, L., and A. J. Barsky. 2020. Placebo and Nocebo Effects. *N. Engl. J. Med.* **382**:554–561. [14]

Converge Consortium. 2015. Sparse Whole-Genome Sequencing Identifies Two Loci for Major Depressive Disorder. *Nature* **523**:588–591. [2, 7]

Conway, C. C., M. K. Forbes, S. C. South, and HiTOP Consortium. 2022. A Hierarchical Taxonomy of Psychopathology (HiTOP) Primer for Mental Health Researchers. *Clin. Psychol. Sci.* **10**:236–258. [2]

Cook, N. R. 2018. Quantifying the Added Value of New Biomarkers: How and How Not. *Diagn. Progn. Res.* **2**:14. [13]

Corominas, R., X. Yang, G. N. Lin, et al. 2014. Protein Interaction Network of Alternatively Spliced Isoforms from Brain Links Genetic Risk Factors for Autism. *Nat. Commun.* **5**:3650. [11]

Corrigan, P. W., and A. C. Watson. 2002. The Paradox of Self-Stigma and Mental Illness. *Clin. Psychol.* **9**:35–53. [15]

Corvin, A., and P. F. Sullivan. 2016. What Next in Schizophrenia Genetics for the Psychiatric Genomics Consortium? *Schizophr. Bull.* **42**:538–541. [5]

Costain, G., M. J. Esplen, B. Toner, K. A. Hodgkinson, and A. S. Bassett. 2012. Evaluating Genetic Counseling for Family Members of Individuals with Schizophrenia in the Molecular Age. *Schizophr. Bull.* **40**:88–99. [15]

Costain, G., M. J. Esplen, B. Toner, et al. 2014. Evaluating Genetic Counseling for Individuals with Schizophrenia in the Molecular Age. *Schizophr. Bull.* **40**:78–87. [15]

Costello, E. J., A. Erkanli, W. Copeland, and A. Angold. 2010. Association of Family Income Supplements in Adolescence with Development of Psychiatric and Substance Use Disorders in Adulthood among an American Indian Population. *JAMA* **303**:1954–1960. [4]

Cox, N. J. 2017. Comments on Pritchard Paper. *J. Psychiatry Brain Sci.* **2**:S5. [9]

Cross-Disorder Group of the Psychiatric Genomics Consortium. 2019. Genomic Relationships, Novel Loci, and Pleiotropic Mechanisms across Eight Psychiatric Disorders. *Cell* **179**:1469–1482. [1, 7, 11]

Cross-Disorder Group of the Psychiatric Genomics Consortium, C. Lee, S. Ripke, et al. 2013. Genetic Relationship between Five Psychiatric Disorders Estimated from Genome-Wide SNPs. *Nat. Genet.* **45**:984–994. [9]

Cruceanu, C., L. Dony, A. C. Krontira, et al. 2021. Cell-Type-Specific Impact of Glucocorticoid Receptor Activation on the Developing Brain: A Cerebral Organoid Study. *Am. J. Psychiatry* **179**:21010095. [7]

Cuomo, A. S. E., D. D. Seaton, D. J. McCarthy, et al. 2020. Single-Cell RNA-Sequencing of Differentiating iPS Cells Reveals Dynamic Genetic Effects on Gene Expression. *Nat. Commun.* **11**:810. [7]

Curran, G. M., M. Bauer, B. Mittman, J. M. Pyne, and C. Stetler. 2012. Effectiveness-Implementation Hybrid Designs: Combining Elements of Clinical Effectiveness and Implementation Research to Enhance Public Health Impact. *Med. Care* **50**:217–226. [13]

Curtis, D. 2018. Polygenic Risk Score for Schizophrenia Is More Strongly Associated with Ancestry Than with Schizophrenia. *Psychiatr. Genet.* **28**:85–89. [2]

Dagani, J., G. Signorini, O. Nielssen, et al. 2017. Meta-Analysis of the Interval between the Onset and Management of Bipolar Disorder. *Can. J. Psychiatry* **62**:247–258. [13]

Daghlas, I., J. M. Lane, R. Saxena, and C. Vetter. 2021. Genetically Proxied Diurnal Preference, Sleep Timing, and Risk of Major Depressive Disorder. *JAMA Psychiatry* **78**:903–910. [4]

D'Agostino, R. S., R. Vasan, M. Pencina, et al. 2008. General Cardiovascular Risk Profile for Use in Primary Care: The Framingham Heart Study. *Circulation* **117**:743–753. [13]

Dahl, A., V. Guillemot, J. Mefford, H. Aschard, and N. Zaitlen. 2019. Adjusting for Principal Components of Molecular Phenotypes Induces Replicating False Positives. *Genetics* **211**:1179–1189. [2]

Dahl, A., K. Nguyen, N. Cai, et al. 2020. A Robust Method Uncovers Significant Context-Specific Heritability in Diverse Complex Traits. *Am. J. Hum. Genet.* **106**:71–91. [2]

Dai, J., J. Aoto, and T. C. Südhof. 2019. Alternative Splicing of Presynaptic Neurexins Differentially Controls Postsynaptic NMDA and AMPA Receptor Responses. *Neuron* **102**:993–1008. [5]

Daily, J. L., K. Nash, U. Jinwal, et al. 2011. Adeno-Associated Virus-Mediated Rescue of the Cognitive Defects in a Mouse Model for Angelman Syndrome. *PLOS ONE* **6**:e27221. [6]

Damask, A., P. G. Steg, G. G. Schwartz, et al. 2020. Patients with High Genome-Wide Polygenic Risk Scores for Coronary Artery Disease May Receive Greater Clinical Benefit from Alirocumab Treatment in the Odyssey Outcomes Trial. *Circulation* **141**:624–636. [13]

Dana, K., J. Finik, S. Koenig, et al. 2019. Prenatal Exposure to Famine and Risk for Development of Psychopathology in Adulthood: A Meta-Analysis. *J. Psychiatry Psychiatr. Disord.* **3**:227–240. [4]

D'Angelo, D., S. Lebon, Q. Chen, et al. 2016. Defining the Effect of the 16p11.2 Duplication on Cognition, Behavior, and Medical Comorbidities. *JAMA Psychiatry* **73**:20–30. [5]

Darnell, R. B. 2013. RNA Protein Interaction in Neurons. *Annu. Rev. Neurosci.* **36**:243–270. [11]

Dar-Nimrod, I., B. Y. Cheung, M. B. Ruby, and S. J. Heine. 2014. Can Merely Learning About Obesity Genes Affect Eating Behavior? *Appetite* **81**:269–276. [14]

Dar-Nimrod, I., M. Zuckerman, and P. R. Duberstein. 2012. The Effects of Learning About One's Own Genetic Susceptibility to Alcoholism: A Randomized Experiment. *Genet. Med.* **15**:132–138. [15]

Daskalakis, N. P., H. Cohen, G. Cai, J. D. Buxbaum, and R. Yehuda. 2014. Expression Profiling Associates Blood and Brain Glucocorticoid Receptor Signaling with Trauma-Related Individual Differences in Both Sexes. *PNAS* **111**:13529–13534. [7]

Davey Smith, G., and G. Hemani. 2014. Mendelian Randomization: Genetic Anchors for Causal Inference in Epidemiological Studies. *Hum. Mol. Genet.* **23**:R89–98. [2]

Daviaud, N., R. H. Friedel, and H. Zou. 2018. Vascularization and Engraftment of Transplanted Human Cerebral Organoids in Mouse Cortex. *eNeuro* **5**:0219–182018. [5]

Davidson, B. L., G. Gao, E. Berry-Kravis, et al. 2022. Gene-Based Therapeutics for Rare Genetic Neurodevelopmental Psychiatric Disorders. *Mol. Ther.* **30**:2416–2428. [6]

Davidsson, M., G. Wang, P. Aldrin-Kirk, et al. 2019. A Systematic Capsid Evolution Approach Performed *in Vivo* for the Design of AAV Vectors with Tailored Properties and Tropism. *PNAS* **116**:27053–27062. [6]

Davies, N. M., D. Gunnell, K. H. Thomas, et al. 2013. Physicians' Prescribing Preferences Were a Potential Instrument for Patients' Actual Prescriptions of Antidepressants. *J. Clin. Epidemiol.* **66**:1386–1396. [4]

Davies, R. W., A. M. Fiksinski, E. J. Breetvelt, et al. 2020. Using Common Genetic Variation to Examine Phenotypic Expression and Risk Prediction in 22q11.2 Deletion Syndrome. *Nat. Med.* **26**:1912–1918. [5, 12, 13]

Defelipe, J. 2011. The Evolution of the Brain, the Human Nature of Cortical Circuits, and Intellectual Creativity. *Front. Neuroanat.* **5**:29. [7]

de Klein, N., E. A. Tsai, M. Vochteloo, et al. 2023. Brain Expression Quantitative Trait Locus and Network Analyses Reveal Downstream Effects and Putative Drivers for Brain-Related Diseases. *Nat. Genet.* **55**:377–388. [10]

de la Torre-Ubieta, L., J. L. Stein, H. Won, et al. 2018. The Dynamic Landscape of Open Chromatin during Human Cortical Neurogenesis. *Cell* **172**:289–304. [10]

de la Torre-Ubieta, L., H. Won, J. L. Stein, and D. H. Geschwind. 2016. Advancing the Understanding of Autism Disease Mechanisms through Genetics. *Nat. Med.* **22**:345–361. [7]

de Leeuw, C., N. Y. A. Sey, D. Posthuma, and H. Won. 2020. *Preprint*: A Response to Yurko et al.: H-MAGMA, Inheriting a Shaky Statistical Foundation, Yields Excess False Positives. *bioRxiv* 310722 [10]

DeLisi, L. E., and H. Bertisch. 2006. A Preliminary Comparison of the Hopes of Researchers, Clinicians, and Families for the Future Ethical Use of Genetic Findings on Schizophrenia. *Am. J. Med. Genet. B Neuropsychiatr. Genet.* **141B**:110–115. [15]

Demange, P. A., M. Malanchini, T. T. Mallard, et al. 2021. Investigating the Genetic Architecture of Noncognitive Skills Using GWAS-by-Subtraction. *Nat. Genet.* **53**:35–44. [2]

Demontis, D., R. K. Walters, J. Martin, et al. 2019. Discovery of the First Genome-Wide Significant Risk Loci for Attention Deficit/Hyperactivity Disorder. *Nat. Genet.* **51**:63–75. [2, 3]

Demro, C., B. A. Mueller, J. S. Kent, et al. 2021. The Psychosis Human Connectome Project: An Overview. *Neuroimage* **241**:118439. [8]

Deng, C., S. Whalen, M. Steyert, et al. 2023. *Preprint*: Massively Parallel Characterization of Psychiatric Disorder-Associated and Cell-Type-Specific Regulatory Elements in the Developing Human Cortex. *bioRxiv* 2023.2002.2015.528663. [10]

De Rubeis, S., X. He, A. P. Goldberg, et al. 2014. Synaptic, Transcriptional and Chromatin Genes Disrupted in Autism. *Nature* **515**:209–215. [3, 5, 7, 11]

Deverman, B. E., P. L. Pravdo, B. P. Simpson, et al. 2016. Cre-Dependent Selection Yields AAV Variants for Widespread Gene Transfer to the Adult Brain. *Nat. Biotechnol.* **34**:204–209. [6]

Devlin, B., N. Melhem, and K. Roeder. 2011. Do Common Variants Play a Role in Risk for Autism? Evidence and Theoretical Musings. *Brain Res.* **1380**:78–84. [3]

Dezonne, R. S., R. C. Sartore, J. M. Nascimento, et al. 2017. Derivation of Functional Human Astrocytes from Cerebral Organoids. *Sci. Rep.* **7**:45091. [7]

Diefenbach, M. A., and H. Leventhal. 2010. The Common-Sense Model of Illness Representation: Theoretical and Practical Considerations. *J. Soc. Distress Homeless* **5**:11–38. [15]

Dillon, A., J. Austin, K. McGhee, and M. Watson. 2022. The Impact of a "Psychiatric Genetics for Genetic Counselors" Workshop on Genetic Counselor Attendees: An Exploratory Study. *Am. J. Med. Genet. B Neuropsychiatr. Genet.* **189**:108–115. [12, 15]

Ding, Y., K. Hou, K. S. Burch, et al. 2022. Large Uncertainty in Individual Polygenic Risk Score Estimation Impacts PRS-Based Risk Stratification. *Nat. Genet.* **54**:30–39. [13]

Dixit, A., O. Parnas, B. Li, et al. 2016. Perturb-Seq: Dissecting Molecular Circuits with Scalable Single-Cell RNA Profiling of Pooled Genetic Screens. *Cell* **167**:1853–1866. [7]

Doan, R. N., E. T. Lim, S. De Rubeis, et al. 2019. Recessive Gene Disruptions in Autism Spectrum Disorder. *Nat. Genet.* **51**:1092–1098. [3]

Dobrindt, K., H. Zhang, D. Das, et al. 2021. Publicly Available hiPSC Lines with Extreme Polygenic Risk Scores for Modeling Schizophrenia. *Complex Psychiatry* **6**:68–82. [8, 9]

Dölen, G., E. Osterweil, B. S. Rao, et al. 2007. Correction of Fragile X Syndrome in Mice. *Neuron* **56**:955–962. [5]

Domingue, B. W., L. Duncan, A. Harrati, and D. W. Belsky. 2021a. Short-Term Mental Health Sequelae of Bereavement Predict Long-Term Physical Health Decline in Older Adults: U.S. Health and Retirement Study Analysis. *J. Gerontol. B Psychol. Sci. Soc. Sci.* **76**:1231–1240. [4]

Domingue, B. W., K. Kanopka, S. Trejo, M. Rhemtulla, and E. M. Tucker-Drob. 2021b. *Preprint*: Ubiquitous Bias & False Discovery Due to Model Misspecification in Analysis of Statistical Interactions: The Role of the Outcome's Distribution and Metric Properties. *PsyArXiv* 1–21. [4]

Dominguez, A. A., W. A. Lim, and L. S. Qi. 2016. Beyond Editing: Repurposing CRISPR-Cas9 for Precision Genome Regulation and Interrogation. *Nat. Rev. Mol. Cell Biol.* **17**:5–15. [5]

Donsante, A., D. G. Miller, Y. Li, et al. 2007. AAV Vector Integration Sites in Mouse Hepatocellular Carcinoma. *Science* **317**:477. [6]

Douard, E., A. Zeribi, C. Schramm, et al. 2021. Effect Sizes of Deletions and Duplications on Autism Risk across the Genome. *Am. J. Psychiatry* **178**:87–98. [1]

Doyle Jr., J. J. 2008. Child Protection and Adult Crime: Using Investigator Assignment to Estimate Causal Effects of Foster Care. *J. Polit. Econ.* **116**:746–770. [4]

Dworkin, J. D., K. A. Linn, E. G. Teich, et al. 2020. The Extent and Drivers of Gender Imbalance in Neuroscience Reference Lists. *Nat. Neurosci.* **23**:918–926. [15]

Eichler, F., C. Duncan, P. L. Musolino, et al. 2017. Hematopoietic Stem-Cell Gene Therapy for Cerebral Adrenoleukodystrophy. *N. Engl. J. Med.* **377**:1630–1638. [6]

Eichmüller, O. L., N. S. Corsini, Á. Vértesy, et al. 2022. Amplification of Human Interneuron Progenitors Promotes Brain Tumors and Neurological Defects. *Science* **375**:eabf5546. [5]

Eisman, A. B., A. M. Kilbourne, A. R. Dopp, L. Saldana, and D. Eisenberg. 2020. Economic Evaluation in Implementation Science: Making the Business Case for Implementation Strategies. *Psychiatry Res.* **283**:112433. [13]

Ellenbroek, B., and J. Youn. 2016. Rodent Models in Neuroscience Research: Is It a Rat Race? *Dis. Model Mech.* **9**:1079–1087. [5]

Elliott, J., B. Bodinier, T. A. Bond, et al. 2020. Predictive Accuracy of a Polygenic Risk Score-Enhanced Prediction Model vs a Clinical Risk Score for Coronary Artery Disease. *JAMA* **323**:636–645. [13]

Ellison, S. M., A. Liao, S. Wood, et al. 2019. Pre-Clinical Safety and Efficacy of Lentiviral Vector-Mediated *ex Vivo* Stem Cell Gene Therapy for the Treatment of Mucopolysaccharidosis IIIA. *Mol. Ther. Methods Clin. Dev.* **13**:399–413. [6]

Engle, S. J., L. Blaha, and R. J. Kleiman. 2018. Best Practices for Translational Disease Modeling Using Human iPSC-Derived Neurons. *Neuron* **100**:783–797. [6]

Erickson, J. A., L. Kuzmich, K. E. Ormond, et al. 2014. Genetic Testing of Children for Predisposition to Mood Disorders: Anticipating the Clinical Issues. *J. Genet. Counsel.* **23**:566–577. [15]

Escamilla, C. O., I. Filonova, A. K. Walker, et al. 2017. *Kctd13* Deletion Reduces Synaptic Transmission via Increased RhoA. *Nature* **551**:227–231. [5]

Etherton, M. R., C. A. Blaiss, C. M. Powell, and T. C. Sudhof. 2009. Mouse Neurexin-1α Deletion Causes Correlated Electrophysiological and Behavioral Changes Consistent with Cognitive Impairments. *PNAS* **106**:17998–18003. [7]

Faden, J., and L. Citrome. 2020. Intravenous Brexanolone for Postpartum Depression: What It Is, How Well Does It Work, and Will It Be Used? *Ther. Adv. Psychopharmacol.* **10**:2045125320968658. [5]

Fagiolini, A., and D. J. Kupfer. 2003. Is Treatment-Resistant Depression a Unique Subtype of Depression? *Biol. Psychiatry* **53**:640–648. [2]

Fahed, A. C., A. A. Philippakis, and A. V. Khera. 2022. The Potential of Polygenic Scores to Improve Cost and Efficiency of Clinical Trials. *Nat. Commun.* **13**:2922. [13]

Fahed, A. C., M. Wang, J. R. Homburger, et al. 2020. Polygenic Background Modifies Penetrance of Monogenic Variants for Tier 1 Genomic Conditions. *Nat. Commun.* **11**:3635. [9, 13]

Falconer, D. S. 1965. The Inheritance of Liability to Certain Diseases, Estimated from the Incidence among Relatives. *Ann. Hum. Health* **29**:51–76. [9]

Fallesen, P., N. Emanuel, and C. Wildeman. 2014. Cumulative Risks of Foster Care Placement for Danish Children. *PLOS ONE* **9**:e109207. [4]

Fanelli, G., K. Domschke, A. Minelli, et al. 2022. A Meta-Analysis of Polygenic Risk Scores for Mood Disorders, Neuroticism, and Schizophrenia in Antidepressant Response. *Eur. Neuropsychopharmacol.* **55**:86–95. [13]

Farrell, M. S., T. Werge, P. Sklar, et al. 2015. Evaluating Historical Candidate Genes for Schizophrenia. *Mol. Psychiatry* **20**:555–562. [7]

Fatumo, S., T. Chikowore, M. Ayub, A. R. Martin, and K. Kuchenbaecker. 2022. A Roadmap to Increase Diversity in Genomic Studies. *Nat. Med.* **28**:243–250. [3]

Feinberg, I. 1982. Schizophrenia: Caused by a Fault in Programmed Synaptic Elimination during Adolescence? *J. Psychiatr. Res.* **17**:319–334. [11]

Fergusson, D., S. Doucette, K. C. Glass, et al. 2005. Association between Suicide Attempts and Selective Serotonin Reuptake Inhibitors: Systematic Review of Randomised Controlled Trials. *BMJ* **330**:396. [4]

Fernandes, G., P. K. Mishra, M. S. Nawaz, et al. 2021. Correction of Amygdalar Dysfunction in a Rat Model of Fragile X Syndrome. *Cell Rep.* **37**:109805. [5]

Ferrat, L. A., K. Vehik, S. A. Sharp, et al. 2020. A Combined Risk Score Enhances Prediction of Type 1 Diabetes among Susceptible Children. *Nat. Med.* **26**:1247–1255. [13]

Finkel, R. S., E. Mercuri, B. T. Darras, et al. 2017. Nusinersen versus Sham Control in Infantile-Onset Spinal Muscular Atrophy. *N. Engl. J. Med.* **377**:1723–1732. [5, 6]

Finn, C. T., and J. W. Smoller. 2006. Genetic Counseling in Psychiatry. *Harv. Rev. Psychiatry* **14**:109–121. [15]

Finn, C. T., M. A. Wilcox, B. R. Korf, et al. 2005. Psychiatric Genetics: A Survey of Psychiatrists' Knowledge, Opinions, and Practice Patterns. *J. Clin. Psychiatry* **66**:821–830. [15]

Finucane, B. M., D. H. Ledbetter, and J. A. Vorstman. 2021. Diagnostic Genetic Testing for Neurodevelopmental Psychiatric Disorders: Closing the Gap between Recommendation and Clinical Implementation. *Curr. Opin. Genet. Dev.* **68**:1–8. [12]

Finucane, B. M., S. M. Myers, C. L. Martin, and D. H. Ledbetter. 2020. Long Overdue: Including Adults with Brain Disorders in Precision Health Initiatives. *Curr. Opin. Genet. Dev.* **65**:47–52. [1, 12]

Finucane, B. M., M. T. Oetjens, A. Johns, et al. 2022. Medical Manifestations and Health Care Utilization among Adult Mycode Participants with Neurodevelopmental Psychiatric Copy Number Variants. *Genet. Med.* **24**:703–711. [12]

Finucane, H. K., B. Bulik-Sullivan, A. Gusev, et al. 2015. Partitioning Heritability by Functional Annotation Using Genome-Wide Association Summary Statistics. *Nat. Genet.* **47**:1228–1235. [11]

Finucane, H. K., Y. A. Reshef, V. Anttila, et al. 2018. Heritability Enrichment of Specifically Expressed Genes Identifies Disease-Relevant Tissues and Cell Types. *Nat. Genet.* **50**:621–629. [11]

Fitzjohn, S. M., M. J. Palmer, J. E. May, et al. 2001. A Characterisation of Long-Term Depression Induced by Metabotropic Glutamate Receptor Activation in the Rat Hippocampus *in vitro*. *J. Physiol.* **537**:421–430. [5]

Flaherty, E., S. Zhu, N. Barretto, et al. 2019. Neuronal Impact of Patient-Specific Aberrant NRXN1α Splicing. *Nat. Genet.* **51**:1679–1690. [7, 11]

Flint, J., and K. S. Kendler. 2014. The Genetics of Major Depression. *Neuron* **81**:484–503. [7]

Folkersen, L., O. Pain, A. Ingason, et al. 2020. Impute.Me: An Open-Source, Non-Profit Tool for Using Data from Direct-to-Consumer Genetic Testing to Calculate and Interpret Polygenic Risk Scores. *Front. Genet.* **11**:578. [13, 15]

Forrest, M. P., H. Zhang, W. Moy, et al. 2017. Open Chromatin Profiling in hiPSC-Derived Neurons Prioritizes Functional Noncoding Psychiatric Risk Variants and Highlights Neurodevelopmental Loci. *Cell Stem Cell* **21**:305–318. [7]

Foust, K. D., E. Nurre, C. L. Montgomery, et al. 2009. Intravascular AAV9 Preferentially Targets Neonatal Neurons and Adult Astrocytes. *Nat. Biotechnol.* **27**:59–65. [6]

Frances, A. J. 2013. Last Plea to DSM 5: Save Grief from the Drug Companies: Let Us Respect the Dignity of Love and Loss. *Psychology Today* Jan. 3, 2013. [4]

Franklin, J. C., J. D. Ribeiro, K. R. Fox, et al. 2017. Risk Factors for Suicidal Thoughts and Behaviors: A Meta-Analysis of 50 Years of Research. *Psychol. Bull.* **143**:187–232. [14]

Franz, D. N., J. Leonard, C. Tudor, et al. 2006. Rapamycin Causes Regression of Astrocytomas in Tuberous Sclerosis Complex. *Ann. Neurol.* **59**:490–498. [6]

French, J. A., J. A. Lawson, Z. Yapici, et al. 2016. Adjunctive Everolimus Therapy for Treatment-Resistant Focal-Onset Seizures Associated with Tuberous Sclerosis (Exist-3): A Phase 3, Randomised, Double-Blind, Placebo-Controlled Study. *Lancet* **388**:2153–2163. [6]

Fried, E. I. 2015. Problematic Assumptions Have Slowed Down Depression Research: Why Symptoms, Not Syndromes Are the Way Forward. *Front. Psychol.* **6**:309. [2]

Fried, E. I. 2017. The 52 Symptoms of Major Depression: Lack of Content Overlap among Seven Common Depression Scales. *J. Affect. Disord.* **208**:191–197. [2]

Frisell, T. 2021. Invited Commentary: Sibling-Comparison Designs, Are They Worth the Effort? *Am. J. Epidemiol.* **190**:738–741. [4]

Fromer, M., A. J. Pocklington, D. H. Kavanagh, et al. 2014. *De Novo* Mutations in Schizophrenia Implicate Synaptic Networks. *Nature* **506**:179–184. [7, 11]

Fromer, M., P. Roussos, S. K. Sieberts, et al. 2016. Gene Expression Elucidates Functional Impact of Polygenic Risk for Schizophrenia. *Nat. Neurosci.* **19**:1442–1453. [3, 8, 11]

Fry, A., T. J. Littlejohns, C. Sudlow, et al. 2017. Comparison of Sociodemographic and Health-Related Characteristics of UK Biobank Participants with Those of the General Population. *Am. J. Epidemiol.* **186**:1026–1034. [2]

Fu, J. M., F. K. Satterstrom, M. Peng, et al. 2022. Rare Coding Variation Provides Insight into the Genetic Architecture and Phenotypic Context of Autism. *Nat. Genet.* **54**:1320–1331. [3, 5, 6]

Fulco, C. P., J. Nasser, T. R. Jones, et al. 2019. Activity-by-Contact Model of Enhancer-Promoter Regulation from Thousands of CRISPR Perturbations. *Nat. Genet.* **51**:1664–1669. [7, 8, 10]

Fumagalli, F., V. Calbi, M. G. Natali Sora, et al. 2022. Lentiviral Haematopoietic Stem-Cell Gene Therapy for Early-Onset Metachromatic Leukodystrophy: Long-Term Results from a Non-Randomised, Open-Label, Phase 1/2 Trial and Expanded Access. *Lancet* **399**:372–383. [6]

Fusar-Poli, P., S. Borgwardt, A. Bechdolf, et al. 2013. The Psychosis High-Risk State: A Comprehensive State-of-the-Art Review. *JAMA Psychiatry* **70**:107–120. [13]

Gadalla, K. K., M. E. Bailey, R. C. Spike, et al. 2013. Improved Survival and Reduced Phenotypic Severity Following AAV9/MECP2 Gene Transfer to Neonatal and Juvenile Male Mecp2 Knockout Mice. *Mol. Ther.* **21**:18–30. [6]

Gallois, A., J. Mefford, A. Ko, et al. 2019. A Comprehensive Study of Metabolite Genetics Reveals Strong Pleiotropy and Heterogeneity across Time and Context. *Nat. Commun.* **10**:4788. [2]

Gandal, M. J., J. R. Haney, N. N. Parikshak, et al. 2018a. Shared Molecular Neuropathology across Major Psychiatric Disorders Parallels Polygenic Overlap. *Science* **359**:693–697. [2, 11]

Gandal, M. J., V. Leppa, H. Won, N. N. Parikshak, and D. H. Geschwind. 2016. The Road to Precision Psychiatry: Translating Genetics into Disease Mechanisms. *Nat. Neurosci.* **19**:1397–1407. [11]

Gandal, M. J., P. Zhang, E. Hadjimichael, et al. 2018b. Transcriptome-Wide Isoform-Level Dysregulation in ASD, Schizophrenia, and Bipolar Disorder. *Science* **362**:eaat8127. [10, 11]

Ganesalingam, J., and R. Bowser. 2010. The Application of Biomarkers in Clinical Trials for Motor Neuron Disease. *Biomark. Med.* **4**:281–297. [5]

Gariepy, G., H. Honkaniemi, and A. Quesnel-Vallee. 2016. Social Support and Protection from Depression: Systematic Review of Current Findings in Western Countries. *Br. J. Psychiatry* **209**:284–293. [13]

Garrido, M. M., H. G. Prigerson, S. Neupane, et al. 2017. Mental Illness and Mental Healthcare Receipt among Hospitalized Veterans with Serious Physical Illnesses. *J. Palliat. Med.* **20**:247–252. [2]

Garrido-Martín, D., B. Borsari, M. Calvo, F. Reverter, and R. Guigó. 2021. Identification and Analysis of Splicing Quantitative Trait Loci across Multiple Tissues in the Human Genome. *Nat. Commun.* **12**:727. [11]

Gasperini, M., A. J. Hill, J. L. McFaline-Figueroa, et al. 2019. A Genome-Wide Framework for Mapping Gene Regulation via Cellular Genetic Screens. *Cell* **176**:1516. [7, 8]

Gaugler, T., L. Klei, S. J. Sanders, et al. 2014. Most Genetic Risk for Autism Resides with Common Variation. *Nat. Genet.* **46**:881–885. [6]

Gaynes, B. N., D. Warden, M. H. Trivedi, et al. 2009. What Did Star*D Teach Us? Results from a Large-Scale, Practical, Clinical Trial for Patients with Depression. *Psychiatr. Serv.* **60**:1439–1445. [13]

GBD 2016 Disease and Injury Incidence and Prevalence Collaborators. 2017. Global, Regional, and National Incidence, Prevalence, and Years Lived with Disability for 328 Diseases and Injuries for 195 Countries, 1990–2016: A Systematic Analysis for the Global Burden of Disease Study 2016. *Lancet* **390**:1211–1259. [7]

Ge, T., A. Patki, V. Srinivasasainagendra, et al. 2021. Development and Validation of a Trans-Ancestry Polygenic Risk Score for Type 2 Diabetes in Diverse Populations. *Genome Med.* **14**:70. [13]

Geller, E., J. Gockley, D. Emera, et al. 2019. *Preprint*: Massively Parallel Disruption of Enhancers Active during Human Corticogenesis. *bioRxiv* 852673. [7, 8]

Gentner, B., F. Tucci, S. Galimberti, et al. 2021. Hematopoietic Stem- and Progenitor-Cell Gene Therapy for Hurler Syndrome. *N. Engl. J. Med.* **385**:1929–1940. [6]

Germain, P. L., and G. Testa. 2017. Taming Human Genetic Variability: Transcriptomic Meta-Analysis Guides the Experimental Design and Interpretation of iPSC-Based Disease Modeling. *Stem Cell Rep.* **8**:1784–1796. [6]

Gerrard, S., A. Inglis, E. Morris, and J. Austin. 2020. Relationships between Patient- and Session-Related Variables and Outcomes of Psychiatric Genetic Counseling. *Eur. J. Hum. Genet.* **28**:907–914. [12, 15]

Gershon, E. S., and N. Alliey-Rodriguez. 2013. New Ethical Issues for Genetic Counseling in Common Mental Disorders. *Am. J. Psychiatry* **170**:968–976. [15]

Giannakopoulou, O., K. Lin, X. Meng, et al. 2021. The Genetic Architecture of Depression in Individuals of East Asian Ancestry: A Genome-Wide Association Study. *JAMA Psychiatry* **78**:1258–1269. [2, 3]

Gidaro, T., and L. Servais. 2019. Nusinersen Treatment of Spinal Muscular Atrophy: Current Knowledge and Existing Gaps. *Dev. Med. Child Neurol.* **61**:19–24. [5]

Gilman, S. R., J. Chang, B. Xu, et al. 2012. Diverse Types of Genetic Variation Converge on Functional Gene Networks Involved in Schizophrenia. *Nat. Neurosci.* **15**:1723–1728. [11]

Girdhar, K., G. E. Hoffman, Y. Jiang, et al. 2018. Cell-Specific Histone Modification Maps in the Human Frontal Lobe Link Schizophrenia Risk to the Neuronal Epigenome. *Nat. Neurosci.* **21**:1126–1136. [11]

Glessner, J. T., K. Wang, G. Cai, et al. 2009. Autism Genome-Wide Copy Number Variation Reveals Ubiquitin and Neuronal Genes. *Nature* **459**:569–573. [11]

Golan, D., E. S. Lander, and S. Rosset. 2014. Measuring Missing Heritability: Inferring the Contribution of Common Variants. *PNAS* **111**:E5272–E5281. [4]

Golzio, C., J. Willer, M. E. Talkowski, et al. 2012. *KCTD13* Is a Major Driver of Mirrored Neuroanatomical Phenotypes of the 16p11.2 Copy Number Variant. *Nature* **485**:363–367. [5]

Gong, S., M. Doughty, C. R. Harbaugh, et al. 2007. Targeting Cre Recombinase to Specific Neuron Populations with Bacterial Artificial Chromosome Constructs. *J. Neurosci.* **27**:9817–9823. [7]

Goodman, R. 1997. The Strengths and Difficulties Questionnaire: A Research Note. *J. Child Psychol. Psychiatry* **38**:581–586. [2]

Goorden, S. M., G. M. van Woerden, L. van der Weerd, J. P. Cheadle, and Y. Elgersma. 2007. Cognitive Deficits in $Tsc1^{+/-}$ Mice in the Absence of Cerebral Lesions and Seizures. *Ann. Neurol.* **62**:648–655. [7]

Gorzynski, J. E., S. D. Goenka, K. Shafin, et al. 2022. Ultrarapid Nanopore Genome Sequencing in a Critical Care Setting. *N. Engl. J. Med.* **386**:700–702. [1]

Govek, E. E., M. E. Hatten, and L. Van Aelst. 2011. The Role of Rho GTPase Proteins in CNS Neuronal Migration. *Dev. Neurobiol.* **71**:528–553. [5]

Grabb, M. C., and W. Z. Potter. 2022. Central Nervous System Trial Failures: Using the Fragile X Syndrome-mGluR5 Drug Target to Highlight the Complexities of Translating Preclinical Discoveries into Human Trials. *J. Clin. Psychopharmacol.* **42**:234–237. [5]

Graham, D. B., and R. J. Xavier. 2020. Pathway Paradigms Revealed from the Genetics of Inflammatory Bowel Disease. *Nature* **578**:527–539. [9]

Grasby, K. L., N. Jahanshad, J. N. Painter, et al. 2020. The Genetic Architecture of the Human Cerebral Cortex. *Science* **367**:eaay6690. [8]

Gray, S. J., V. Matagne, L. Bachaboina, et al. 2011. Preclinical Differences of Intravascular AAV9 Delivery to Neurons and Glia: A Comparative Study of Adult Mice and Nonhuman Primates. *Mol. Ther.* **19**:1058–1069. [6]

Green, R. C., J. S. Roberts, L. A. Cupples, et al. 2009. Disclosure of APOE Genotype for Risk of Alzheimer's Disease. *N. Engl. J. Med.* **361**:245–254. [14, 15]

Gregory, G., K. Das Gupta, B. Meiser, et al. 2022. Polygenic Risk in Familial Breast Cancer: Changing the Dynamics of Communicating Genetic Risk. *J. Genet. Couns.* **31**:120–129. [13]

Griesemer, D., J. R. Xue, S. K. Reilly, et al. 2021. Genome-Wide Functional Screen of 3'UTR Variants Uncovers Causal Variants for Human Disease and Evolution. *Cell* **184**:5247–5260. [8]

Grob, R. 2019. Qualitative Research on Expanded Prenatal and Newborn Screening: Robust but Marginalized. *Hastings Cent. Rep.* **49**:S72–S81. [14]

Groenendyk, J. W., P. Greenland, and S. S. Khan. 2022. Incremental Value of Polygenic Risk Scores in Primary Prevention of Coronary Heart Disease: A Review. *JAMA Intern. Med.* **182**:1082–1088. [13]

Grotzinger, A. D., T. T. Mallard, W. A. Akingbuwa, et al. 2022. Genetic Architecture of 11 Major Psychiatric Disorders at Biobehavioral, Functional Genomic and Molecular Genetic Levels of Analysis. *Nat. Genet.* **54**:548–559. [2]

Grotzinger, A. D., M. Rhemtulla, R. de Vlaming, et al. 2019. Genomic Structural Equation Modelling Provides Insights into the Multivariate Genetic Architecture of Complex Traits. *Nat. Hum. Behav.* **3**:513–525. [2]

Grove, J., S. Ripke, T. D. Als, et al. 2019. Identification of Common Genetic Risk Variants for Autism Spectrum Disorder. *Nat. Genet.* **51**:431–444. [3, 7, 11]

GTEx Consortium. 2017. Genetic Effects on Gene Expression across Human Tissues. *Nature* **550**:204–213. [3]

———. 2020. The GTEx Consortium Atlas of Genetic Regulatory Effects across Human Tissues. *Science* **369**:1318–1330. [3, 8, 10, 11]

Gudmundsson, S., M. Singer-Berk, N. A. Watts, et al. 2022. Variant Interpretation Using Population Databases: Lessons from Gnomad. *Hum. Mutat.* **43**:1012–1030. [3]

Gulinello, M., H. A. Mitchell, Q. Chang, et al. 2019. Rigor and Reproducibility in Rodent Behavioral Research. *Neurobiol. Learn. Mem.* **165**:106780. [5]

Gulsuner, S., T. Walsh, A. C. Watts, et al. 2013. Spatial and Temporal Mapping of *de Novo* Mutations in Schizophrenia to a Fetal Prefrontal Cortical Network. *Cell* **154**:518–529. [7, 11]

Gunnell, D., J. Saperia, and D. Ashby. 2005. Selective Serotonin Reuptake Inhibitors (SSRIs) and Suicide in Adults: Meta-Analysis of Drug Company Data from Placebo Controlled, Randomised Controlled Trials Submitted to the MHRA's Safety Review. *BMJ* **330**:385. [4]

Gupta, A., G. de Bruyn, S. Tousseyn, et al. 2020. Epilepsy and Neurodevelopmental Comorbidities in Tuberous Sclerosis Complex: A Natural History Study. *Pediatr. Neurol.* **106**:10–16. [5]

Guy, J., J. Gan, J. Selfridge, S. Cobb, and A. Bird. 2007. Reversal of Neurological Defects in a Mouse Model of Rett Syndrome. *Science* **315**:1143–1147. [5]

Haaker, J., S. Maren, M. Andreatta, et al. 2019. Making Translation Work: Harmonizing Cross-Species Methodology in the Behavioural Neuroscience of Pavlovian Fear Conditioning. *Neurosci. Biobehav. Rev.* **107**:329–345. [2]

Hamilton, J. G., and M. E. Robson. 2019. Psychosocial Effects of Multigene Panel Testing in the Context of Cancer Genomics. *Hastings Cent. Rep.* **49**:S44–S52. [14]

Han, S. K., D. Kim, H. Lee, I. Kim, and S. Kim. 2018. Divergence of Noncoding Regulatory Elements Explains Gene-Phenotype Differences between Human and Mouse Orthologous Genes. *Mol. Biol. Evol.* **35**:1653–1667. [8]

Haney, J. R., B. Wamsley, G. T. Chen, et al. 2020. *Preprint*: Broad Transcriptomic Dysregulation across the Cerebral Cortex in ASD. *bioRxiv* 423129. [11]

Hannon, E., H. Spiers, J. Viana, et al. 2016. Methylation QTLs in the Developing Brain and Their Enrichment in Schizophrenia Risk Loci. *Nat. Neurosci.* **19**:48–54. [11]

Hansen, B. T., K. M. Sønderskov, I. Hageman, P. T. Dinesen, and S. D. Østergaard. 2017. Daylight Savings Time Transitions and the Incidence Rate of Unipolar Depressive Episodes. *Epidemiology* **28**:346–353. [4]

Hansen, D. V., J. H. Lui, P. R. Parker, and A. R. Kriegstein. 2010. Neurogenic Radial Glia in the Outer Subventricular Zone of Human Neocortex. *Nature* **464**:554–561. [7]

Harrington, R., M. Rutter, and E. Fombonne. 1996. Developmental Pathways in Depression: Multiple Meanings, Antecedents, and Endpoints. *Dev. Psychopathol.* **8**:601–616. [2]

Hartl, C. L., G. Ramaswami, W. G. Pembroke, et al. 2021. Coexpression Network Architecture Reveals the Brain-Wide and Multiregional Basis of Disease Susceptibility. *Nat. Neurosci.* **24**:1313–1323. [11]

Harvey, S. B., S. Øverland, S. L. Hatch, et al. 2018. Exercise and the Prevention of Depression: Results of the Hunt Cohort Study. *Am. J. Psychiatry* **175**:28–36. [15]

Hawrylycz, M. J., E. S. Lein, A. L. Guillozet-Bongaarts, et al. 2012. An Anatomically Comprehensive Atlas of the Adult Human Brain Transcriptome. *Nature* **489**:391–399. [5, 11]

He, X., S. J. Sanders, L. Liu, et al. 2013. Integrated Model of *de Novo* and Inherited Genetic Variants Yields Greater Power to Identify Risk Genes. *PLOS Genet.* **9**:e1003671. [5]

Hebebrand, J., A. Scherag, B. G. Schimmelmann, and A. Hinney. 2010. Child and Adolescent Psychiatric Genetics. *Eur. Child Adolesc. Psychiatry* **19**:259–279. [6]

Herculano-Houzel, S., B. Mota, and R. Lent. 2006. Cellular Scaling Rules for Rodent Brains. *PNAS* **103**:12138–12143. [7]

Hernandez, L. M., M. Kim, G. D. Hoftman, et al. 2021. Transcriptomic Insight into the Polygenic Mechanisms Underlying Psychiatric Disorders. *Biol. Psychiatry* **89**:54–64. [11]

Herzeg, A., G. Almeida-Porada, R. A. Charo, et al. 2022. Prenatal Somatic Cell Gene Therapies: Charting a Path toward Clinical Applications (Proc. of the Cersi-FDA Meeting). *J. Clin. Pharmacol.* **62(Suppl 1)**:S36–S52. [5]

Hess, J. L., D. S. Tylee, M. Mattheisen, et al. 2021. A Polygenic Resilience Score Moderates the Genetic Risk for Schizophrenia. *Mol. Psychiatry* **26**:800–815. [7]

Hikishima, K., M. M. Quallo, Y. Komaki, et al. 2011. Population-Averaged Standard Template Brain Atlas for the Common Marmoset (*Callithrix jacchus*). *Neuroimage* **54**:2741–2749. [5]

Hill, R. S., and C. A. Walsh. 2005. Molecular Insights into Human Brain Evolution. *Nature* **437**:64–67. [7]

Hill, S. F., and M. H. Meisler. 2021. Antisense Oligonucleotide Therapy for Neurodevelopmental Disorders. *Dev. Neurosci.* **43**:247–252. [5]

Hill, W. D., S. P. Hagenaars, R. E. Marioni, et al. 2016. Molecular Genetic Contributions to Social Deprivation and Household Income in UK Biobank. *Curr. Biol.* **26**:3083–3089. [2]

Hilton, I. B., A. M. D'Ippolito, C. M. Vockley, et al. 2015. Epigenome Editing by a CRISPR-Cas9-Based Acetyltransferase Activates Genes from Promoters and Enhancers. *Nat. Biotechnol.* **33**:510–517. [7]

Hinderer, C., N. Katz, E. L. Buza, et al. 2018. Severe Toxicity in Nonhuman Primates and Piglets Following High-Dose Intravenous Administration of an Adeno-Associated Virus Vector Expressing Human Smn. *Hum. Gene Ther.* **29**:285–298. [6]

Hindy, G., K. G. Aragam, K. Ng, et al. 2020. Genome-Wide Polygenic Score, Clinical Risk Factors, and Long-Term Trajectories of Coronary Artery Disease. *Arterioscler. Thromb. Vasc. Biol.* **40**:2738–2746. [13]

Hinshaw, S. P., and A. Stier. 2008. Stigma as Related to Mental Disorders. *Clin. Psychol.* **4**:367. [15]

Hippman, C., A. Ringrose, A. Inglis, et al. 2016. A Pilot Randomized Clinical Trial Evaluating the Impact of Genetic Counseling for Serious Mental Illnesses. *J. Clin. Psychiatry* **77**:e190–e198. [15]

Hirschfeld, R. M. 2000. History and Evolution of the Monoamine Hypothesis of Depression. *J. Clin. Psychiatry* **61 Suppl 6**:4–6. [7]

Ho, S. M., B. J. Hartley, E. Flaherty, et al. 2017. Evaluating Synthetic Activation and Repression of Neuropsychiatric-Related Genes in hiPSC-Derived NPCs, Neurons, and Astrocytes. *Stem Cell Rep.* **9**:615–628. [7]

Hodge, R. D., T. E. Bakken, J. A. Miller, et al. 2019. Conserved Cell Types with Divergent Features in Human versus Mouse Cortex. *Nature* **573**:61–68. [7]

Hodgkinson, K. A., J. Murphy, S. O'Neill, L. Brzustowicz, and A. S. Bassett. 2001. Genetic Counselling for Schizophrenia in the Era of Molecular Genetics. *Can. J. Psychiatry* **46**:123–130. [15]

Hoek, H. W., A. S. Brown, and E. Susser. 1998. The Dutch Famine and Schizophrenia Spectrum Disorders. *Soc. Psychiatry Psychiatr. Epidemiol.* **33**:373–379. [4]

Hoffman, G. E., B. J. Hartley, E. Flaherty, et al. 2017. Transcriptional Signatures of Schizophrenia in hiPSC-Derived NPCs and Neurons Are Concordant with Post-Mortem Adult Brains. *Nat. Commun.* **8**:2225. [7]

Hoffman, G. E., N. Schrode, E. Flaherty, and K. J. Brennand. 2019. New Considerations for hiPSC-Based Models of Neuropsychiatric Disorders. *Mol. Psychiatry* **24**:49–66. [5]

Hoge, S. K., and P. S. Appelbaum. 2012. Ethics and Neuropsychiatric Genetics: A Review of Major Issues. *Int. J. Neuropsychopharmacol.* **15**:1547–1557. [14]

Holloway, A., and H. E. Watson. 2002. Role of Self-Efficacy and Behaviour Change. *Int. J. Nurs. Pract.* **8**:106–115. [15]

Holm, I. A., P. B. Agrawal, O. Ceyhan-Birsoy, et al. 2018. The BabySeq Project: Implementing Genomic Sequencing in Newborns. *BMC Pediatr.* **18**:225. [14]

Hook, V., K. J. Brennand, Y. Kim, et al. 2014. Human iPSC Neurons Display Activity-Dependent Neurotransmitter Secretion: Aberrant Catecholamine Levels in Schizophrenia Neurons. *Stem Cell Rep.* **3**:531–538. [7]

Hoop, J. G., L. W. Roberts, K. A. G. Hammond, and N. J. Cox. 2008. Psychiatrists' Attitudes, Knowledge, and Experience Regarding Genetics: A Preliminary Study. *Genet. Med.* **10**:439. [15]

Hoop, J. G., and G. Salva. 2010. The Current State of Genetics Training in Psychiatric Residency: Views of 235 US Educators and Trainees. *Acad. Psychiatry* **34**:109–114. [15]

Hordeaux, J., C. Hinderer, T. Goode, et al. 2018. Toxicology Study of Intra-Cisterna Magna Adeno-Associated Virus 9 Expressing Human Alpha-L-Iduronidase in Rhesus Macaques. *Mol. Ther. Methods Clin. Dev.* **10**:79–88. [6]

Horev, G., J. Ellegood, J. P. Lerch, et al. 2011. Dosage-Dependent Phenotypes in Models of 16p11.2 Lesions Found in Autism. *PNAS* **108**:17076–17081. [7]

Horváth, S., and K. Mirnics. 2015. Schizophrenia as a Disorder of Molecular Pathways. *Biol. Psychiatry* **77**:22–28. [11]

Hoskovec, J. M., R. L. Bennett, M. E. Carey, et al. 2018. Projecting the Supply and Demand for Certified Genetic Counselors: A Workforce Study. *J. Genet. Counsel.* **27**:16–20. [15]

Hou, L., M. D. Antion, D. Hu, et al. 2006. Dynamic Translational and Proteasomal Regulation of Fragile X Mental Retardation Protein Controls mGluR-Dependent Long-Term Depression. *Neuron* **51**:441–454. [5]

Hou, L., U. Heilbronner, F. Degenhardt, et al. 2016. Genetic Variants Associated with Response to Lithium Treatment in Bipolar Disorder: A Genome-Wide Association Study. *Lancet* **387**:1085–1093. [7]

Howard, D. M., M. J. Adams, T. K. Clarke, et al. 2019. Genome-Wide Meta-Analysis of Depression Identifies 102 Independent Variants and Highlights the Importance of the Prefrontal Brain Regions. *Nat. Neurosci.* **22**:343–352. [3, 7]

Howard, D. M., L. Folkersen, J. R. I. Coleman, et al. 2020. Genetic Stratification of Depression in UK Biobank. *Transl. Psychiatry* **10**:163. [2]

Howe, J. R., M. F. Bear, P. Golshani, et al. 2018. The Mouse as a Model for Neuropsychiatric Drug Development. *Curr. Biol.* **28**:R909–R914. [5, 6]

Hsu, P. D., E. S. Lander, and F. Zhang. 2014. Development and Applications of CRISPR-Cas9 for Genome Engineering. *Cell* **157**:1262–1278. [7]

Hu, B., H. Won, W. Mah, et al. 2021. Neuronal and Glial 3D Chromatin Architecture Informs the Cellular Etiology of Brain Disorders. *Nat. Commun.* **12**:3968. [10]

Hua, Y., K. Sahashi, G. Hung, et al. 2010. Antisense Correction of SMN2 Splicing in the CNS Rescues Necrosis in a Type III SMA Mouse Model. *Genes Dev.* **24**:1634–1644. [5]

Hua, Y., T. A. Vickers, B. F. Baker, C. F. Bennett, and A. R. Krainer. 2007. Enhancement of SMN2 Exon 7 Inclusion by Antisense Oligonucleotides Targeting the Exon. *PLOS Biol.* **5**:e73. [5]

Huan, T., J. Rong, C. Liu, et al. 2015. Genome-Wide Identification of microRNA Expression Quantitative Trait Loci. *Nat. Commun.* **6**:6601. [8]

Huang, S., K. Chaudhary, and L. X. Garmire. 2017. More Is Better: Recent Progress in Multi-Omics Data Integration Methods. *Front. Genet.* **8**:84. [11]

Huber, K. M., S. M. Gallagher, S. T. Warren, and M. F. Bear. 2002. Altered Synaptic Plasticity in a Mouse Model of Fragile X Mental Retardation. *PNAS* **99**:7746–7750. [5]

Hurson, A. N., P. Pal Choudhury, C. Gao, et al. 2022. Prospective Evaluation of a Breast-Cancer Risk Model Integrating Classical Risk Factors and Polygenic Risk in 15 Cohorts from Six Countries. *Int. J. Epidemiol.* **50**:1897–1911. [13]

Hyde, C. L., M. W. Nagle, C. Tian, et al. 2016. Identification of 15 Genetic Loci Associated with Risk of Major Depression in Individuals of European Descent. *Nat. Genet.* **48**:1031–1036. [2, 7]

Hyman, S. E. 2012. Revolution Stalled. *Sci. Transl. Med.* **4**:155cm111. [7]

Iakoucheva, L. M., A. R. Muotri, and J. Sebat. 2019. Getting to the Cores of Autism. *Cell* **178**:1287–1298. [1]

Iglewicz, A., K. Seay, S. D. Zetumer, and S. Zisook. 2013. The Removal of the Bereavement Exclusion in the DSM-5: Exploring the Evidence. *Curr. Psychiatry Rep.* **15**:413. [4]

Inglis, A., D. Koehn, B. McGillivray, S. E. Stewart, and J. Austin. 2015. Evaluating a Unique, Specialist Psychiatric Genetic Counseling Clinic: Uptake and Impact. *Clin. Genet.* **87**:218–224. [15]

Inoue, F., A. Kreimer, T. Ashuach, N. Ahituv, and N. Yosef. 2019. Identification and Massively Parallel Characterization of Regulatory Elements Driving Neural Induction. *Cell Stem Cell* **25**:713–727. [7]

International Common Disease Alliance. 2020. Recommendations and White Paper. https://drive.google.com/file/d/16SVJ5lbneN9hB9E03PZMhpescAN527HO/view. (accessed Jan. 18, 2023). [8]

International Consortium on Lithium Genetics, A. T. Amare, K. O. Schubert, et al. 2018. Association of Polygenic Score for Schizophrenia and HLA Antigen and Inflammation Genes with Response to Lithium in Bipolar Affective Disorder: A Genome-Wide Association Study. *JAMA Psychiatry* **75**:65–74. [13]

International Schizophrenia Consortium, S. M. Purcell, N. R. Wray, et al. 2009. Common Polygenic Variation Contributes to Risk of Schizophrenia and Bipolar Disorder. *Nature* **460**:748–752. [7]

Iossifov, I., B. J. O'Roak, S. J. Sanders, et al. 2014. The Contribution of *de Novo* Coding Mutations to Autism Spectrum Disorder. *Nature* **515**:216–221. [11]

Iossifov, I., M. Ronemus, D. Levy, et al. 2012. *De Novo* Gene Disruptions in Children on the Autistic Spectrum. *Neuron* **74**:285–299. [7, 11]

Iwanami, A., J. Yamane, H. Katoh, et al. 2005. Establishment of Graded Spinal Cord Injury Model in a Nonhuman Primate: The Common Marmoset. *J. Neurosci. Res.* **80**:172–181. [5]

Jacquemont, S., G. Huguet, M. Klein, et al. 2022. Genes to Mental Health (G2MH): A Framework to Map the Combined Effects of Rare and Common Variants on Dimensions of Cognition and Psychopathology. *Am. J. Psychiatry* **179**:189–203. [5]

Jaffe, A. E., Y. Gao, A. Deep-Soboslay, et al. 2016. Mapping DNA Methylation across Development, Genotype and Schizophrenia in the Human Frontal Cortex. *Nat. Neurosci.* **19**:40–47. [11]

Jaffe, A. E., D. J. Hoeppner, T. Saito, et al. 2020. Profiling Gene Expression in the Human Dentate Gyrus Granule Cell Layer Reveals Insights into Schizophrenia and Its Genetic Risk. *Nat. Neurosci.* **23**:510–519. [11]

Jaffe, A. E., R. E. Straub, J. H. Shin, et al. 2018. Developmental and Genetic Regulation of the Human Cortex Transcriptome Illuminate Schizophrenia Pathogenesis. *Nat. Neurosci.* **21**:1117–1125. [11]

Janssens, A. C. J. W. 2019. Proprietary Algorithms for Polygenic Risk: Protecting Scientific Innovation or Hiding the Lack of It? *Genes* **10**:448–447. [15]

Javierre, B. M., O. S. Burren, S. P. Wilder, et al. 2016. Lineage-Specific Genome Architecture Links Enhancers and Non-Coding Disease Variants to Target Gene Promoters. *Cell* **167**:1369–1384. [10]

Jehuda, R. B., Y. Shemer, and B. Ofer. 2018. Genome Editing in Induced Pluripotent Stem Cells Using CRISPR/Cas9. *Stem Cell Rev. Rep.* **14**:323–336. [5]

Jerber, J., D. D. Seaton, A. S. E. Cuomo, et al. 2021. Population-Scale Single-Cell RNA-Seq Profiling across Dopaminergic Neuron Differentiation. *Nat. Genet.* **53**:304–312. [7, 8]

Jermy, B. S., S. P. Hagenaars, K. P. Glanville, et al. 2022. Using Major Depression Polygenic Risk Scores to Explore the Depressive Symptom Continuum. *Psychol. Med.* **52**:149–158. [2]

Jia, P., X. Chen, A. H. Fanous, and Z. Zhao. 2018. Convergent Roles of *de Novo* Mutations and Common Variants in Schizophrenia in Tissue-Specific and Spatiotemporal Co-Expression Network. *Transl. Psychiatry* **8**:105. [7]

Jin, X., S. K. Simmons, A. Guo, et al. 2020. *In Vivo* Perturb-Seq Reveals Neuronal and Glial Abnormalities Associated with Autism Risk Genes. *Science* **370**:eaaz6063. [7, 10]

Johnston, J., and L. J. Matthews. 2022. Polygenic Embryo Testing: Understated Ethics, Unclear Utility. *Nat. Med.* **28**:446–448. [14]

Jonas, K. G., T. Lencz, K. Li, et al. 2019. Schizophrenia Polygenic Risk Score and 20-Year Course of Illness in Psychotic Disorders. *Transl. Psychiatry* **9**:300. [13]

Jørgensen, K. T., M. Bøg, M. Kabra, et al. 2021. Predicting Time to Relapse in Patients with Schizophrenia According to Patients' Relapse History: A Historical Cohort Study Using Real-World Data in Sweden. *BMC Psychiatry* **21**:634. [4]

Juanatey, A., L. Blanco-Garcia, and N. Tellez. 2018. Ocrelizumab: Its Efficacy and Safety in Multiple Sclerosis. *Rev. Neurol.* **66**:423–433. [5]

Judson, M. C., C. Shyng, J. M. Simon, et al. 2021. Dual-Isoform hUBE3A Gene Transfer Improves Behavioral and Seizure Outcomes in Angelman Syndrome Model Mice. *JCI Insight* **6**:e144712. [5]

Kadoshima, T., H. Sakaguchi, T. Nakano, et al. 2013. Self-Organization of Axial Polarity, inside-out Layer Pattern, and Species-Specific Progenitor Dynamics in Human Es Cell-Derived Neocortex. *PNAS* **110**:20284–20289. [7]

Kahn-Greene, E. T., D. B. Killgore, G. H. Kamimori, T. J. Balkin, and W. D. S. Killgore. 2007. The Effects of Sleep Deprivation on Symptoms of Psychopathology in Healthy Adults. *Sleep Med.* **8**:215–221. [4]

Kalb, F. M., V. Vincent, T. Herzog, and J. Austin. 2017. Genetic Counseling for Alcohol Addiction: Assessing Perceptions and Potential Utility in Individuals with Lived Experience and Their Family Members. *J. Genet. Counsel.* **26**:963–970. [15]

Kalman, J. L., L. M. Olde Loohuis, A. Vreeker, et al. 2021. Characterisation of Age and Polarity at Onset in Bipolar Disorder. *Br. J. Psychiatry* **219**:659–669. [2]

Kang, H. J., Y. I. Kawasawa, F. Cheng, et al. 2011a. Spatio-Temporal Transcriptome of the Human Brain. *Nature* **478**:483–489. [8, 10, 11]

Kaplanis, J., K. E. Samocha, L. Wiel, et al. 2020. Evidence for 28 Genetic Disorders Discovered by Combining Healthcare and Research Data. *Nature* **586**:757–762. [3]

Karamihalev, S., C. Flachskamm, N. Eren, M. Kimura, and A. Chen. 2019. Social Context and Dominance Status Contribute to Sleep Patterns and Quality in Groups of Freely-Moving Mice. *Sci. Rep.* **9**:15190. [8]

Karayiorgou, M., M. A. Morris, B. Morrow, et al. 1995. Schizophrenia Susceptibility Associated with Interstitial Deletions of Chromosome 22q11. *PNAS* **92**:7612–7616. [7]

Karczewski, K. J., L. C. Francioli, G. Tiao, et al. 2020. The Mutational Constraint Spectrum Quantified from Variation in 141,456 Humans. *Nature* **581**:434–443. [3, 5]

Katayama, Y., M. Nishiyama, H. Shoji, et al. 2016. CHD8 Haploinsufficiency Results in Autistic-Like Phenotypes in Mice. *Nature* **537**:675–679. [7]

Ke, S., J. Lai, T. Sun, et al. 2015. Healthy Young Minds: The Effects of a 1-Hour Classroom Workshop on Mental Illness Stigma in High School Students. *Comm. Ment. Health J.* **51**:329–337. [12]

Keinath, M. C., D. E. Prior, and T. W. Prior. 2021. Spinal Muscular Atrophy: Mutations, Testing, and Clinical Relevance. *Appl. Clin. Genet.* **14**:11–25. [5]

Keller, M. C. 2014. Gene × Environment Interaction Studies Have Not Properly Controlled for Potential Confounders: The Problem and the (Simple) Solution. *Biol. Psychiatry* **75**:18–24. [4]

Kelley, K. W., H. Nakao-Inoue, A. V. Molofsky, and M. C. Oldham. 2018. Variation among Intact Tissue Samples Reveals the Core Transcriptional Features of Human CNS Cell Classes. *Nat. Neurosci.* **21**:1171–1184. [11]

Kelley, K. W., and S. P. Paşca. 2022. Human Brain Organogenesis: Toward a Cellular Understanding of Development and Disease. *Cell* **185**:42–61. [5]

Kendall, K. M., E. Rees, M. Bracher-Smith, et al. 2019. Association of Rare Copy Number Variants with Risk of Depression. *JAMA Psychiatry* **76**:818–825. [3]

Kendler, K. S. 2021. The Prehistory of Psychiatric Genetics: 1780-1910. *Am. J. Psychiatry* **178**:490–508. [1]

Kendler, K. S., C. M. Bulik, J. Silberg, et al. 2000. Childhood Sexual Abuse and Adult Psychiatric and Substance Use Disorders in Women: An Epidemiological and Cotwin Control Analysis. *Arch. Gen. Psychiatry* **57**:953. [4]

Kendler, K. S., L. M. Karkowski, and C. A. Prescott. 1999. Causal Relationship between Stressful Life Events and the Onset of Major Depression. *Am. J. Psychiatry* **156**:837–841. [4]

Kendler, K. S., J. Myers, and S. Zisook. 2008. Does Bereavement-Related Major Depression Differ from Major Depression Associated with Other Stressful Life Events? *Am. J. Psychiatry* **165**:1449–1455. [4]

Kendler, K. S., H. Ohlsson, J. Sundquist, and K. Sundquist. 2021. The Rearing Environment and the Risk for Alcohol Use Disorder: A Swedish National High-Risk Home-Reared V. Adopted Co-Sibling Control Study. *Psychol. Med.* **51**:2370–2377. [4]

Kendler, K. S., and K. F. Schaffner. 2011. The Dopamine Hypothesis of Schizophrenia: An Historical and Philosophical Analysis. *Philos. Psychiatr. Psychol.* **18**:41–63 [7]

Kerin, M., and J. Marchini. 2020. Inferring Gene-by-Environment Interactions with a Bayesian Whole-Genome Regression Model. *Am. J. Hum. Genet.* **107**:698–713. [2]

Kessler, R. C., W. T. Chiu, O. Demler, K. R. Merikangas, and E. E. Walters. 2005. Prevalence, Severity, and Comorbidity of 12-Month DSM-IV Disorders in the National Comorbidity Survey Replication. *Arch. Gen. Psychiatry* **62**:617–627. [2]

Khan, A., M. C. Turchin, A. Patki, et al. 2022. Genome-Wide Polygenic Score to Predict Chronic Kidney Disease across Ancestries. *Nat. Med.* **28**:1412–1420. [13]

Khan, T. A., O. Revah, A. Gordon, et al. 2020. Neuronal Defects in a Human Cellular Model of 22q11.2 Deletion Syndrome. *Nat. Med.* **26**:1888–1898. [3, 7]

Khera, A. V., M. Chaffin, K. G. Aragam, et al. 2018. Genome-Wide Polygenic Scores for Common Diseases Identify Individuals with Risk Equivalent to Monogenic Mutations. *Nat. Genet.* **50**:1219–1224. [13]

Khera, A. V., C. A. Emdin, and S. Kathiresan. 2017. Genetic Risk, Lifestyle, and Coronary Artery Disease. *N. Engl. J. Med.* **376**:1194–1195. [13]

Kiiskinen, T., N. J. Mars, T. Palviainen, et al. 2020. Genomic Prediction of Alcohol-Related Morbidity and Mortality. *Transl. Psychiatry* **10**:23. [13]

Kilpinen, H., A. Goncalves, A. Leha, et al. 2017. Common Genetic Variation Drives Molecular Heterogeneity in Human iPSCs. *Nature* **546**:370–375. [8]

Kim, J., C. Hu, C. Moufawad El Achkar, et al. 2019. Patient-Customized Oligonucleotide Therapy for a Rare Genetic Disease. *N. Engl. J. Med.* **381**:1644–1652. [5, 6]

Kim, M., J. R. Haney, P. Zhang, et al. 2021a. Brain Gene Co-Expression Networks Link Complement Signaling with Convergent Synaptic Pathology in Schizophrenia. *Nat. Neurosci.* **24**:799–809. [11]

Kim, S. S., K. Jagadeesh, K. K. Dey, et al. 2021b. *Preprint*: Leveraging Single-Cell ATAC-Seq to Identify Disease-Critical Fetal and Adult Brain Cell Types. *bioRxiv* 445067. [11]

Kim-Hellmuth, S., F. Aguet, M. Oliva, et al. 2020. Cell Type-Specific Genetic Regulation of Gene Expression across Human Tissues. *Science* **369**:eaaz8528. [10]

Kinge, J. M., S. Øverland, M. Flatø, et al. 2021. Parental Income and Mental Disorders in Children and Adolescents: Prospective Register-Based Study. *Int. J. Epidemiol.* **50**:1615–1627. [4]

Kious, B. M., A. R. Docherty, J. R. Botkin, et al. 2021. Ethical and Public Health Implications of Genetic Testing for Suicide Risk: Family and Survivor Perspectives. *Genet. Med.* **23**:289–297. [14]

Kishi, N., K. Sato, E. Sasaki, and H. Okano. 2014. Common Marmoset as a New Model Animal for Neuroscience Research and Genome Editing Technology. *Dev. Growth Differ.* **56**:53–62. [5]

Kita, Y., H. Nishibe, Y. Wang, et al. 2021. Cellular-Resolution Gene Expression Profiling in the Neonatal Marmoset Brain Reveals Dynamic Species- and Region-Specific Differences. *PNAS* **118**:e2020125118. [5]

Kleiman, R. J., and M. D. Ehlers. 2016. Data Gaps Limit the Translational Potential of Preclinical Research. *Sci. Transl. Med.* **8**:320. [6]

Knevel, R., S. le Cessie, C. C. Terao, et al. 2020. Using Genetics to Prioritize Diagnoses for Rheumatology Outpatients with Inflammatory Arthritis. *Sci. Transl. Med.* **12**:eaay1548. [13]

Koblan, L. W., M. R. Erdos, L. B. Gordon, et al. 2021. Base Editor Treats Progeria in Mice. *Nature* **589**:608–614. [6]

Koene, L. M., E. Niggl, I. Wallaard, et al. 2021. Identifying the Temporal Electrophysiological and Molecular Changes That Contribute to TSC-Associated Epileptogenesis. *JCI Insight* **6**:e150120. [5]

Kolberg, L., N. Kerimov, H. Peterson, and K. Alasoo. 2020. Co-Expression Analysis Reveals Interpretable Gene Modules Controlled by Trans-Acting Genetic Variants. *eLife* **9**:e58705. [11]

Konermann, S., P. Lotfy, N. J. Brideau, et al. 2018. Transcriptome Engineering with RNA-Targeting Type VI-D CRISPR Effectors. *Cell* **173**:665–676. [7]

Kong, A., G. Thorleifsson, M. L. Frigge, et al. 2018. The Nature of Nurture: Effects of Parental Genotypes. *Science* **359**:424–428. [2]

Konjarski, M., G. Murray, V. V. Lee, and M. L. Jackson. 2018. Reciprocal Relationships between Daily Sleep and Mood: A Systematic Review of Naturalistic Prospective Studies. *Sleep Med. Rev.* **42**:47–58. [4]

Koopmans, F., P. van Nierop, M. Andres-Alonso, et al. 2019. SynGO: An Evidence-Based, Expert-Curated Knowledge Base for the Synapse. *Neuron* **103**:217–234. [8, 11]

Krebs, M. D., G. E. Themudo, M. E. Benros, et al. 2021. Associations between Patterns in Comorbid Diagnostic Trajectories of Individuals with Schizophrenia and Etiological Factors. *Nat. Commun.* **12**:6617. [2]

Krey, J. F., S. P. Paşca, A. Shcheglovitov, et al. 2013. Timothy Syndrome Is Associated with Activity-Dependent Dendritic Retraction in Rodent and Human Neurons. *Nat. Neurosci.* **16**:201–209. [5]

Krieg, A. M. 2006. Therapeutic Potential of Toll-Like Receptor 9 Activation. *Nat. Rev. Drug Discov.* **5**:471–484. [6]

Krishnan, A., R. Zhang, V. Yao, et al. 2016. Genome-Wide Prediction and Functional Characterization of the Genetic Basis of Autism Spectrum Disorder. *Nat. Neurosci.* **19**:1454–1462. [11]

Krueger, D. A., M. M. Care, K. Holland, et al. 2010. Everolimus for Subependymal Giant-Cell Astrocytomas in Tuberous Sclerosis. *N. Engl. J. Med.* **363**:1801–1811. [6]

Krueger, D. A., A. Sadhwani, A. W. Byars, et al. 2017. Everolimus for Treatment of Tuberous Sclerosis Complex-Assocaited Neuropsychiatric Disorders. *Ann. Clin. Transl. Neurol.* **4**:877–887. [6]

Ksinan, A. J., R. L. Smith, P. B. Barr, and A. T. Vazsonyi. 2022. The Associations of Polygenic Scores for Risky Behaviors and Parenting Behaviors with Adolescent Externalizing Problems. *Behav. Genet.* **52**:26–37. [13]

Kuchenbaecker, K. B., L. McGuffog, D. Barrowdale, et al. 2017. Evaluation of Polygenic Risk Scores for Breast and Ovarian Cancer Risk Prediction in BRCA1 and BRCA2 Mutation Carriers. *J. Natl. Cancer Inst.* **109**: [12]

Kuleshov, M. V., M. R. Jones, A. D. Rouillard, et al. 2016. Enrichr: A Comprehensive Gene Set Enrichment Analysis Web Server 2016 Update. *Nucleic Acids Res.* **44**:W90–W97. [11]

Kullo, I. J., H. Jouni, E. E. Austin, et al. 2016. Incorporating a Genetic Risk Score into Coronary Heart Disease Risk Estimates: Effect on Low-Density Lipoprotein Cholesterol Levels (the MI-Genes Clinical Trial). *Circulation* **133**:1181–1188. [13]

Kumar, M., L. Atwoli, R. A. Burgess, et al. 2022. What Should Equity in Global Health Research Look Like? *Lancet* **400**:145–147. [2]

Kumar, P. 1968. Genetic Counselling in Family Planning. *Antiseptic* **65**:831–834. [15]

Kuzmin, D. A., M. V. Shutova, N. R. Johnston, et al. 2021. The Clinical Landscape for AAV Gene Therapies. *Nat. Rev. Drug Discov.* **20**:173–174. [5]

Laegsgaard, M. M., A. S. Kristensen, and O. Mors. 2009. Potential Consumers' Attitudes toward Psychiatric Genetic Research and Testing and Factors Influencing Their Intentions to Test. *Genet. Test. Mol. Biomarkers* **13**:57–65. [14]

Lake, B. B., S. Chen, B. C. Sos, et al. 2018. Integrative Single-Cell Analysis of Transcriptional and Epigenetic States in the Human Adult Brain. *Nat. Biotechnol.* **36**:70–80. [11]

Lakhan, S. E., and K. F. Vieira. 2008. Nutritional Therapies for Mental Disorders. *Nutr. J.* 7:2. [15]

Lam, M., C. Y. Chen, Z. Li, et al. 2019. Comparative Genetic Architectures of Schizophrenia in East Asian and European Populations. *Nat. Genet.* **51**:1670–1678. [2, 3]

Lamb, J., E. D. Crawford, D. Peck, et al. 2006. The Connectivity Map: Using Gene-Expression Signatures to Connect Small Molecules, Genes, and Disease. *Science* **313**:1929–1935. [8]

Lancaster, M. A., M. Renner, C. A. Martin, et al. 2013. Cerebral Organoids Model Human Brain Development and Microcephaly. *Nature* **501**:373–379. [5]

Landes, S. J., S. A. McBain, and G. M. Curran. 2019. An Introduction to Effectiveness-Implementation Hybrid Designs. *Psychiatry Res.* **280**:112513. [13]

Landi, I., D. A. Kaji, L. Cotter, et al. 2021. Prognostic Value of Polygenic Risk Scores for Adults with Psychosis. *Nat. Med.* **27**:1576–1581. [13]

Langfelder, P., and S. Horvath. 2008. WGCNA: An R Package for Weighted Correlation Network Analysis. *BMC Bioinformat.* **9**:559. [11]

Lázaro-Muñoz, G., S. Pereira, S. Carmi, and T. Lencz. 2021. Screening Embryos for Polygenic Conditions and Traits: Ethical Considerations for an Emerging Technology. *Genet. Med.* **23**:432–434. [13]

Leach, E., E. Morris, H. J. White, et al. 2016. How Do Physicians Decide to Refer Their Patients for Psychiatric Genetic Counseling? A Qualitative Study of Physicians' Practice. *J. Genet. Counsel.* **25**:1235–1242. [15]

Leader, L. D., M. O'Connell, and A. VandenBerg. 2019. Brexanolone for Postpartum Depression: Clinical Evidence and Practical Considerations. *Pharmacotherapy* **39**:1105–1112. [5]

Lebowitz, M. S., and W.-K. Ahn. 2017. Testing Positive for a Genetic Predisposition to Depression Magnifies Retrospective Memory for Depressive Symptoms. *J. Consult. Clin. Psychol.* **85**:1052–1063. [15]

Lebowitz, M. S., and W.-K. Ahn. 2018. Blue Genes? Understanding and Mitigating Negative Consequences of Personalized Information About Genetic Risk for Depression. *J. Genet. Couns.* **27**:204–216. [14]

Lebowitz, M. S., W.-K. Ahn, and S. Nolen-Hoeksema. 2013. Fixable or Fate? Perceptions of the Biology of Depression. *J. Consult. Clin. Psychol.* **81**:518–527. [14]

Lebowitz, M. S., and P. S. Appelbaum. 2019. Biomedical Explanations of Psychopathology and Their Implications for Attitudes and Beliefs About Mental Disorders. *Annu. Rev. Clin. Psychol.* **15**:555–577. [14]

Lebowitz, M. S., P. S. Appelbaum, L. B. Dixon, R. R. Girgis, and M. M. Wall. 2021. Experimentally Exploring the Potential Behavioral Effects of Personalized Genetic Information About Marijuana and Schizophrenia Risk. *J. Psychiatr. Res.* **140**:316–322. [14]

Lee, A., N. Mavaddat, A. N. Wilcox, et al. 2019a. BOADICEA: A Comprehensive Breast Cancer Risk Prediction Model Incorporating Genetic and Nongenetic Risk Factors. *Genet. Med.* **21**:1708–1718. [13]

Lee, J.-M., K. Correia, J. Loupe, et al. 2019b. CAG Repeat Not Polyglutamine Length Determines Timing of Huntington's Disease Onset. *Cell* **178**:887–900. [9]

Lee, P. H., V. Anttila, H. Won, et al. 2019c. Genomic Relationships, Novel Loci, and Pleiotropic Mechanisms across Eight Psychiatric Disorders. *Cell* **179**:1469–1482. [2]

Lee, P. H., V. Anttila, H. Won, et al. 2019d. *Preprint*: Genome Wide Meta-Analysis Identifies Genomic Relationships, Novel Loci, and Pleiotropic Mechanisms across Eight Psychiatric Disorders. *bioRxiv* 528117. [7]

Lee, P. H., Y. A. Feng, and J. W. Smoller. 2021. Pleiotropy and Cross-Disorder Genetics Among Psychiatric Disorders. *Biol. Psychiatry* **89**:20–31. [1, 13]

Lee, Y. H., T. Thaweethai, Y.-C. A. Feng, et al. 2022. *Preprint*: Impact of Selection Bias on Polygenic Risk Score Estimates in Healthcare Settings. *medRxiv* 22277710. [2]

Leiserson, M. D. M., J. V. Eldridge, S. Ramachandran, and B. J. Raphael. 2013. Network Analysis of GWAS Data. *Curr. Opin. Genet. Dev.* **23**:602–610. [11]

Lek, M., K. J. Karczewski, E. V. Minikel, et al. 2016. Analysis of Protein-Coding Genetic Variation in 60,706 Humans. *Nature* **536**:285–291. [3]

Lencz, T., D. Backenroth, E. Granot-Hershkovitz, et al. 2021. Utility of Polygenic Embryo Screening for Disease Depends on the Selection Strategy. *eLife* **10**:e64716. [13]

Leonard, H., S. Cobb, and J. Downs. 2017. Clinical and Biological Progress over 50 Years in Rett Syndrome. *Nat. Rev. Neurol.* **13**:37–51. [6]

Levey, D. F., J. Gerlernter, R. Polimanti, et al. 2020. Reproducible Genetic Risk Loci for Anxiety: Results from ~200,000 Participants in the Million Veteran Program. *Am. J. Psychiatry* **177**:223–232. [3]

Levey, D. F., M. B. Stein, F. R. Wendt, et al. 2021. Bi-Ancestral Depression GWAS in the Million Veteran Program and Meta-Analysis in >1.2 Million Individuals Highlight New Therapeutic Directions. *Nat. Neurosci.* **24**:954–963. [7]

Lewis, A. C. F., R. C. Green, and J. L. Vassy. 2021. Polygenic Risk Scores in the Clinic: Translating Risk into Action. *HGG Adv.* **2**:100047. [13]

Lewis, A. C. F., E. F. Perez, A. E. R. Prince, et al. 2022. Patient and Provider Perspectives on Polygenic Risk Scores: Implications for Clinical Reporting and Utilization. *Genome Med.* **14**:114. [12]

Lewis, C. M., and E. Vassos. 2022. Polygenic Scores in Psychiatry: On the Road from Discovery to Implementation. *Am. J. Psychiatry* **179**:800–806. [12]

Li, J., Z. Ma, M. Shi, et al. 2015. Identification of Human Neuronal Protein Complexes Reveals Biochemical Activities and Convergent Mechanisms of Action in Autism Spectrum Disorders. *Cell Syst.* **1**:361–374. [11]

Li, J. H., C. A. Mazur, T. Berisa, and J. K. Pickrell. 2021a. Low-Pass Sequencing Increases the Power of GWAS and Decreases Measurement Error of Polygenic Risk Scores Compared to Genotyping Arrays. *Genome Res.* **31**:529–537. [2]

Li, L., K.-L. Huang, Y. Gao, et al. 2021b. An Atlas of Alternative Polyadenylation Quantitative Trait Loci Contributing to Complex Trait and Disease Heritability. *Nat. Genet.* **53**:994–1005. [8]

Li, M., N. Jancovski, P. Jafar-Nejad, et al. 2021c. Antisense Oligonucleotide Therapy Reduces Seizures and Extends Life Span in an SCN2A Gain-of-Function Epilepsy Model. *J. Clin. Invest.* **131**:e152079. [5]

Li, M., G. Santpere, Y. Imamura Kawasawa, et al. 2018. Integrative Functional Genomic Analysis of Human Brain Development and Neuropsychiatric Risks. *Science* **362**:eaat7615. [5, 10, 11]

Li, Q. S., C. Tian, D. Hinds, and 23andMe Research Team. 2020. Genome-Wide Association Studies of Antidepressant Class Response and Treatment-Resistant Depression. *Transl. Psychiatry* **10**:360. [13]

Li, S. X., R. L. Milne, T. Nguyen-Dumont, et al. 2021d. Prospective Evaluation of the Addition of Polygenic Risk Scores to Breast Cancer Risk Models. *JNCI Cancer Spectr.* **5**:pkab021. [13]

Li, Y. I., B. van de Geijn, A. Raj, et al. 2016. RNA Splicing Is a Primary Link between Genetic Variation and Disease. *Science* **352**:600–604. [10, 11]

Liang, H., J. Olsen, W. Yuan, et al. 2016. Early Life Bereavement and Schizophrenia: A Nationwide Cohort Study in Denmark and Sweden. *Medicine* **95**:e2434. [4]

Liang, L., S. Fazel Darbandi, S. Pochareddy, et al. 2021. Developmental Dynamics of Voltage-Gated Sodium Channel Isoform Expression in the Human and Mouse Brain. *Genome Med.* **13**:135. [5]

Liang, X. H., H. Sun, W. Shen, et al. 2017. Antisense Oligonucleotides Targeting Translation Inhibitory Elements in 5' UTRs Can Selectively Increase Protein Levels. *Nucleic Acids Res.* **45**:9528–9546. [5]

Lichtenstein, P., B. H. Yip, C. Björk, et al. 2009. Common Genetic Determinants of Schizophrenia and Bipolar Disorder in Swedish Families: A Population-Based Study. *Lancet Psychiatry* **373**:234–239. [4]

Liebers, D. T., M. Pirooznia, A. Ganna, S. Bipolar Genome, and F. S. Goes. 2021. Discriminating Bipolar Depression from Major Depressive Disorder with Polygenic Risk Scores. *Psychol. Med.* **51**:1451–1458. [13]

Lim, E. T., S. Raychaudhuri, S. J. Sanders, et al. 2013. Rare Complete Knockouts in Humans: Population Distribution and Significant Role in Autism Spectrum Disorders. *Neuron* **77**:235–242. [3]

Lin, G. N., R. Corominas, I. Lemmens, et al. 2015. Spatiotemporal 16p11.2 Protein Network Implicates Cortical Late Mid-Fetal Brain Development and KCTD13-Cul3-RhoA Pathway in Psychiatric Diseases. *Neuron* **85**:742–754. [5]

Lin, K., X. Zhong, L. Li, et al. 2020. AAV9-Retro Mediates Efficient Transduction with Axon Terminal Absorption and Blood-Brain Barrier Transportation. *Mol. Brain* **13**:138. [6]

Lineweaver, T. T., M. W. Bondi, D. Galasko, and D. P. Salmon. 2014. Effect of Knowledge of APOE Genotype on Subjective and Objective Memory Performance in Healthy Older Adults. *Am. J. Psychiatry* **171**:201–208. [14, 15]

Liu, L., J. Lei, S. J. Sanders, et al. 2014. Dawn: A Framework to Identify Autism Genes and Subnetworks Using Gene Expression and Genetics. *Mol. Autism* **5**:22. [11]

Liu, P., M. Chen, Y. Liu, L. S. Qi, and S. Ding. 2018a. CRISPR-Based Chromatin Remodeling of the Endogenous Oct4 or Sox2 Locus Enables Reprogramming to Pluripotency. *Cell Stem Cell* **22**:252–261. [7]

Liu, X. S., H. Wu, M. Krzisch, et al. 2018b. Rescue of Fragile X Syndrome Neurons by DNA Methylation Editing of the Fmr1 Gene. *Cell* **172**:979–992. [7]

Liu, Y., C. Yu, T. P. Daley, et al. 2018c. CRISPR Activation Screens Systematically Identify Factors That Drive Neuronal Fate and Reprogramming. *Cell Stem Cell* **23**:758–771. [7]

Livingston, J. D., and J. E. Boyd. 2010. Correlates and Consequences of Internalized Stigma for People Living with Mental Illness: A Systematic Review and Meta-Analysis. *Soc. Sci. Med.* **71**:2150–2161. [15]

Loh, K. H., P. S. Stawski, A. S. Draycott, et al. 2016. Proteomic Analysis of Unbounded Cellular Compartments: Synaptic Clefts. *Cell* **166**:1295–1307. [11]

Loh, P. R., G. Bhatia, A. Gusev, et al. 2015. Contrasting Genetic Architectures of Schizophrenia and Other Complex Diseases Using Fast Variance-Components Analysis. *Nat. Genet.* **47**:1385–1392. [3]

Loohuis, L. M., J. A. Vorstman, A. P. Ori, et al. 2015. Genome-Wide Burden of Deleterious Coding Variants Increased in Schizophrenia. *Nat. Commun.* **6**:7501. [7]

Lourida, I., E. Hannon, T. J. Littlejohns, et al. 2019. Association of Lifestyle and Genetic Risk with Incidence of Dementia. *JAMA* **322**:430–437. [13]

Lowther, C., G. Costain, D. A. Baribeau, and A. S. Bassett. 2017. Genomic Disorders in Psychiatry: What Does the Clinician Need to Know? *Curr. Psychiatry Rep.* **19**:82. [13]

Lu, C., X. Shi, A. Allen, et al. 2019. Overexpression of $NEUROG_2$ and $NEUROG_1$ in Human Embryonic Stem Cells Produces a Network of Excitatory and Inhibitory Neurons. *FASEB J.* **33**:5287–5299. [7]

Lukashchuk, V., K. E. Lewis, I. Coldicott, A. J. Grierson, and M. Azzouz. 2016. AAV9-Mediated Central Nervous System-Targeted Gene Delivery via Cisterna magna Route in Mice. *Mol. Ther. Methods Clin. Dev.* **3**:15055. [6]

Lund, C., M. De Silva, S. Plagerson, et al. 2011. Poverty and Mental Disorders: Breaking the Cycle in Low-Income and Middle-Income Countries. *Lancet Psychiatry* **378**:1502–1514. [4]

Luningham, J. M., A. M. Hendriks, E. Krapohl, et al. 2020. Harmonizing Behavioral Outcomes across Studies, Raters, and Countries: Application to the Genetic Analysis of Aggression in the Action Consortium. *J. Child Psychol. Psychiatry* **61**:807–817. [2]

Luningham, J. M., D. B. McArtor, A. M. Hendriks, et al. 2019. Data Integration Methods for Phenotype Harmonization in Multi-Cohort Genome-Wide Association Studies with Behavioral Outcomes. *Front. Genet.* **10**:1227. [2]

Luo, C., M. A. Lancaster, R. Castanon, et al. 2016. Cerebral Organoids Recapitulate Epigenomic Signatures of the Human Fetal Brain. *Cell Rep.* **17**:3369–3384. [5]

Luo, C., H. Liu, F. Xie, et al. 2022. Single Nucleus Multi-Omics Identifies Human Cortical Cell Regulatory Genome Diversity. *Cell Genom.* **2**: [11]

Luo, Y., K. M. de Lange, L. Jostins, et al. 2017. Exploring the Genetic Architecture of Inflammatory Bowel Disease by Whole-Genome Sequencing Identifies Association at ADCY7. *Nat. Genet.* **49**:186–192. [2]

Luoni, M., S. Giannelli, M. T. Indrigo, et al. 2020. Whole Brain Delivery of an Instability-Prone *Mecp2* Transgene Improves Behavioral and Molecular Pathological Defects in Mouse Models of Rett Syndrome. *eLife* **9**:e52629. [5]

Lyus, V. L. 2007. The Importance of Genetic Counseling for Individuals with Schizophrenia and Their Relatives: Potential Clients' Opinions and Experiences. *Am. J. Med. Genet. B Neuropsychiatr. Genet.* **144B**:1014–1021. [15]

Ma, S., M. Skarica, Q. Li, et al. 2022. Molecular and Cellular Evolution of the Primate Dorsolateral Prefrontal Cortex. *Science* **377**:eabo7257. [5]

Ma, S., B. Zhang, L. M. LaFave, et al. 2020. Chromatin Potential Identified by Shared Single-Cell Profiling of RNA and Chromatin. *Cell* **183**:1103–1116. [10]

MacDonald, M. L., M. Garver, J. Newman, et al. 2020. Synaptic Proteome Alterations in the Primary Auditory Cortex of Individuals with Schizophrenia. *JAMA Psychiatry* **77**:86–95. [11]

Madisen, L., T. Mao, H. Koch, et al. 2012. A Toolbox of Cre-Dependent Optogenetic Transgenic Mice for Light-Induced Activation and Silencing. *Nat. Neurosci.* **15**:793–802. [7]

Magnus, P., C. Birke, K. Vejrup, et al. 2016. Cohort Profile Update: The Norwegian Mother and Child Cohort Study (MoBa). *Int. J. Epidemiol.* **45**:382–388. [2]

Mah, W., and H. Won. 2020. The Three-Dimensional Landscape of the Genome in Human Brain Tissue Unveils Regulatory Mechanisms Leading to Schizophrenia Risk. *Schizophr. Res.* **217**:17–25. [8, 10]

Mahjani, B., S. De Rubeis, C. Gustavsson Mahjani, et al. 2021. Prevalence and Phenotypic Impact of Rare Potentially Damaging Variants in Autism Spectrum Disorder. *Mol. Autism* **12**:65. [6]

Maier, R., G. Moser, G. B. Chen, et al. 2015. Joint Analysis of Psychiatric Disorders Increases Accuracy of Risk Prediction for Schizophrenia, Bipolar Disorder, and Major Depressive Disorder. *Am. J. Hum. Genet.* **96**:283–294. [2]

Major Depressive Disorder Working Group of the Psychiatric GWAS Consortium. 2013. A Mega-Analysis of Genome-Wide Association Studies for Major Depressive Disorder. *Mol. Psychiatry* **18**:497–511. [7]

Maltzberg, B. 1936. Migration and Mental Disease among Negroes in New York State. *Am. J. Biol. Anthropol.* **21**:107–113. [4]

Maltzberg, B. 1962. NIVARD

Mancini, M., A. Karakuzu, J. Cohen-Adad, et al. 2020. An Interactive Meta-Analysis of MRI Biomarkers of Myelin. *eLife* **9**:e61523. [5]

Manickam, K., M. R. McClain, L. A. Demmer, et al. 2021. Exome and Genome Sequencing for Pediatric Patients with Congenital Anomalies or Intellectual Disability: an Evidence-Based Clinical Guideline of the American College of Medical Genetics and Genomics. *Genet. Med.* **23**:2029–2037. [6, 12]

Mansfield, K. 2003. Marmoset Models Commonly Used in Biomedical Research. *Comp. Med.* **53**:383–392. [5]

Mansour, A. A., J. T. Gonçalves, C. W. Bloyd, et al. 2018. An *in Vivo* Model of Functional and Vascularized Human Brain Organoids. *Nat. Biotechnol.* **36**:432–441. [5, 7]

Marbach, D., D. Lamparter, G. Quon, et al. 2016. Tissue-Specific Regulatory Circuits Reveal Variable Modular Perturbations across Complex Diseases. *Nat. Methods* **13**:366–370. [11]

Marchetto, M. C., C. Carromeu, A. Acab, et al. 2010. A Model for Neural Development and Treatment of Rett Syndrome Using Human Induced Pluripotent Stem Cells. *Cell* **143**:527–539. [7]

Marek, S., B. Tervo-Clemmens, F. J. Calabro, et al. 2022. Reproducible Brain-Wide Association Studies Require Thousands of Individuals. *Nature* **603**:654–660. [8]

Mariani, J., G. Coppola, P. Zhang, et al. 2015. FOXG1-Dependent Dysregulation of GABA/Glutamate Neuron Differentiation in Autism Spectrum Disorders. *Cell* **162**:375–390. [5, 7]

Mariani, J., M. V. Simonini, D. Palejev, et al. 2012. Modeling Human Cortical Development *in vitro* Using Induced Pluripotent Stem Cells. *PNAS* **109**:12770–12775. [7]

Marouli, E., M. Graff, C. Medina-Gomez, et al. 2017. Rare and Low-Frequency Coding Variants Alter Human Adult Height. *Nature* **542**:186–190. [2]

Marro, S. G., S. Chanda, N. Yang, et al. 2019. Neuroligin-4 Regulates Excitatory Synaptic Transmission in Human Neurons. *Neuron* **103**:617–626. [7]

Mars, N., S. Kerminen, Y. A. Feng, et al. 2022. Genome-Wide Risk Prediction of Common Diseases across Ancestries in One Million People. *Cell Genom.* **2**:None. [13]

Mars, N., J. T. Koskela, P. Ripatti, et al. 2020. Polygenic and Clinical Risk Scores and Their Impact on Age at Onset and Prediction of Cardiometabolic Diseases and Common Cancers. *Nat. Med.* **26**:549–557. [13]

Marshall, C. R., D. P. Howrigan, D. Merico, et al. 2017. Contribution of Copy Number Variants to Schizophrenia from a Genome-Wide Study of 41,321 Subjects. *Nat. Genet.* **49**:27–35. [3, 7, 11]

Marshall, C. R., A. Noor, J. B. Vincent, et al. 2008. Structural Variation of Chromosomes in Autism Spectrum Disorder. *Am. J. Hum. Genet.* **82**:477–488. [5]

Marshall, J. J., and J. O. Mason. 2019. Mouse vs Man: Organoid Models of Brain Development & Disease. *Brain Res.* **1724**:146427. [5]

Marteau, T., D. French, and S. Griffin. 2010. Effects of Communicating DNA-Based Disease Risk Estimates on Risk-Reducing Behaviours. *Cochrane Database Syst. Rev.* **Oct 6**:CD007275. [15]

Martin, A. R., E. G. Atkinson, S. B. Chapman, et al. 2021. Low-Coverage Sequencing Cost-Effectively Detects Known and Novel Variation in Underrepresented Populations. *Am. J. Hum. Genet.* **108**:656–668. [2]

Martin, A. R., M. J. Daly, E. B. Robinson, S. E. Hyman, and B. M. Neale. 2019a. Predicting Polygenic Risk of Psychiatric Disorders. *Biol. Psychiatry* **86**:97–109. [13, 14]

Martin, A. R., C. R. Gignoux, R. K. Walters, et al. 2017. Human Demographic History Impacts Genetic Risk Prediction across Diverse Populations. *Am. J. Hum. Genet.* **100**:635–649. [2]

Martin, A. R., M. Kanai, Y. Kamatani, et al. 2019b. Clinical Use of Current Polygenic Risk Scores May Exacerbate Health Disparities. *Nat. Genet.* **51**:584–591. [2, 3, 8, 13]

Martin, A. R., R. E. Stroud 2nd, T. Abebe, et al. 2022. Increasing Diversity in Genomics Requires Investment in Equitable Partnerships and Capacity Building. *Nat. Genet.* **54**:740–745. [2]

Martin, J., K. Tilling, L. Hubbard, et al. 2016. Association of Genetic Risk for Schizophrenia with Nonparticipation over Time in a Population-Based Cohort Study. *Am. J. Epidemiol.* **183**:1149–1158. [2]

Martin-Brevet, S., B. Rodríguez-Herreros, J. A. Nielsen, et al. 2018. Quantifying the Effects of 16p11.2 Copy Number Variants on Brain Structure: A Multisite Genetic-First Study. *Biol. Psychiatry* **84**:253–264. [5]

Marton, R. M., Y. Miura, S. A. Sloan, et al. 2019. Differentiation and Maturation of Oligodendrocytes in Human Three-Dimensional Neural Cultures. *Nat. Neurosci.* **22**:484–491. [7]

Mashiko, H., A. C. Yoshida, S. S. Kikuchi, et al. 2012. Comparative Anatomy of Marmoset and Mouse Cortex from Genomic Expression. *J. Neurosci.* **32**:5039–5053. [5]

Matharu, N., S. Rattanasopha, S. Tamura, et al. 2019. CRISPR-Mediated Activation of a Promoter or Enhancer Rescues Obesity Caused by Haploinsufficiency. *Science* **363**:eaau0629. [6]

Matoba, N., D. Liang, H. Sun, et al. 2020. Common Genetic Risk Variants Identified in the Spark Cohort Support Ddhd2 as a Candidate Risk Gene for Autism. *Transl. Psychiatry* **10**:265. [8]

Matzner, U., E. Herbst, K. K. Hedayati, et al. 2005. Enzyme Replacement Improves Nervous System Pathology and Function in a Mouse Model for Metachromatic Leukodystrophy. *Hum. Mol. Genet.* **14**:1139–1152. [6]

McAfee, J. C., J. L. Bell, O. Krupa, et al. 2022a. Focus on Your Locus with a Massively Parallel Reporter Assay. *J. Neurodev. Disord.* **14**:50. [10]

McAfee, J. C., S. Lee, J. Lee, et al. 2022b. *Preprint*: Systematic Investigation of Allelic Regulatory Activity of Schizophrenia-Associated Common Variants. *medRxiv* 22279954. [8, 10]

McAllister, M., G. Dunn, and C. Todd. 2010. Empowerment: Qualitative Underpinning of a New Clinical Genetics-Specific Patient-Reported Outcome. *Eur. J. Hum. Genet.* **19**:125–130. [15]

McCarthy, M. I. 2017. Painting a New Picture of Personalised Medicine for Diabetes. *Diabetologia* **60**:793–799. [9]

McCarthy, S. E., V. Makarov, G. Kirov, et al. 2009. Microduplications of 16p11.2 Are Associated with Schizophrenia. *Nat. Genet.* **41**:1223–1227. [5]

McGillivray, P., D. Clarke, W. Meyerson, et al. 2018. Network Analysis as a Grand Unifier in Biomedical Data Science. *Annu. Rev. Biomed. Data Sci.* **1**:153–180. [11]

McGinty, E. E., and M. D. Eisenberg. 2022. Mental Health Treatment Gap: The Implementation Problem as a Research Problem. *JAMA Psychiatry* **79**:746–747. [13]

McIntyre, R. S., M. Berk, E. Brietzke, et al. 2020. Bipolar Disorders. *Lancet* **396**:1841–1856. [13]

McPhie, D. L., R. Nehme, C. Ravichandran, et al. 2018. Oligodendrocyte Differentiation of Induced Pluripotent Stem Cells Derived from Subjects with Schizophrenias Implicate Abnormalities in Development. *Transl. Psychiatry* **8**:230. [7]

Meehan, A. J., S. J. Lewis, S. Fazel, et al. 2022. Clinical Prediction Models in Psychiatry: A Systematic Review of Two Decades of Progress and Challenges. *Mol. Psychiatry* **27**:2700–2708. [13]

Meerman, J. J., S. E. Ter Hark, J. G. E. Janzing, and M. J. H. Coenen. 2022. The Potential of Polygenic Risk Scores to Predict Antidepressant Treatment Response in Major Depression: A Systematic Review. *J. Affect. Disord.* **304**:1–11. [13]

Mega, J. L., N. O. Stitziel, J. G. Smith, et al. 2015. Genetic Risk, Coronary Heart Disease Events, and the Clinical Benefit of Statin Therapy: an Analysis of Primary and Secondary Prevention Trials. *Lancet* **385**:2264–2271. [13]

Meikle, L., K. Pollizzi, A. Egnor, et al. 2008. Response of a Neuronal Model of Tuberous Sclerosis to Mammalian Target of Rapamycin (mTOR) Inhibitors: Effects on mTORC1 and Akt Signaling Lead to Improved Survival and Function. *J. Neurosci.* **28**:5422–5432. [6]

Meiser, B., N. A. Kasparian, P. B. Mitchell, et al. 2008. Attitudes to Genetic Testing in Families with Multiple Cases of Bipolar Disorder. *Genet. Test.* **12**:233–243. [15]

Meiser, B., P. B. Mitchell, N. A. Kasparian, et al. 2007. Attitudes Towards Childbearing, Causal Attributions for Bipolar Disorder and Psychological Distress: A Study of Families with Multiple Cases of Bipolar Disorder. *Psychol. Med.* **37**:1601–1611. [14]

Meiser, B., P. B. Mitchell, H. McGirr, M. Van Herten, and P. R. Schofield. 2005. Implications of Genetic Risk Information in Families with a High Density of Bipolar Disorder: an Exploratory Study. *Soc. Sci. Med.* **60**:109–118. [15]

Melby, M. K., L. C. Loh, J. Evert, et al. 2016. Beyond Medical "Missions" to Impact-Driven Short-Term Experiences in Global Health (STEGHs): Ethical Principles to Optimize Community Benefit and Learner Experience. *Acad. Med.* **91**:633–638. [2]

Meng, L., A. J. Ward, S. Chun, et al. 2015. Towards a Therapy for Angelman Syndrome by Targeting a Long Non-Coding RNA. *Nature* **518**:409–412. [6]

Merikangas, K. R., W. Wicki, and J. Angst. 1994. Heterogeneity of Depression. Classification of Depressive Subtypes by Longitudinal Course. *Br. J. Psychiatry* **164**:342–348. [2]

Mertens, J., Q. W. Wang, Y. Kim, et al. 2015. Differential Responses to Lithium in Hyperexcitable Neurons from Patients with Bipolar Disorder. *Nature* **527**:95–99. [7]

Meseck, E. K., G. Guibinga, S. Wang, et al. 2022. Intrathecal sc-AAV9-CB-GFP: Systemic Distribution Predominates Following Single-Dose Administration in Cynomolgus Macaques. *Toxicol. Pathol.* **50**:415–431. [6]

Messina, S., and M. Sframeli. 2020. New Treatments in Spinal Muscular Atrophy: Positive Results and New Challenges. *J. Clin. Med.* **9**:2222. [5]

Meyer, J. E. 1988. The Fate of the Mentally Ill in Germany during the Third Reich. *Psychol. Med.* **18**:575–581. [14]

Micali, N., E. Simonoff, and J. Treasure. 2007. Risk of Major Adverse Perinatal Outcomes in Women with Eating Disorders. *BMC Psychiatry* **190**:255–259. [4]

Michael, J. E., C. M. Bulik, S. J. Hart, L. Doyle, and J. Austin. 2020. Perceptions of Genetic Risk, Testing, and Counseling among Individuals with Eating Disorders. *Int. J. Eat. Disord.* **53**:1496–1505. [15]

Mikl, M., D. Eletto, M. Nijim, et al. 2022. A Massively Parallel Reporter Assay Reveals Focused and Broadly Encoded RNA Localization Signals in Neurons. *Nucleic Acids Res.* **50**:10643–10664. [8]

Milaneschi, Y., F. Lamers, M. Berk, and B. Penninx. 2020. Depression Heterogeneity and Its Biological Underpinnings: Toward Immunometabolic Depression. *Biol. Psychiatry* **88**:369–380. [2]

Milaneschi, Y., F. Lamers, W. J. Peyrot, et al. 2016. Polygenic Dissection of Major Depression Clinical Heterogeneity. *Mol. Psychiatry* **21**:516–522. [2]

Milaneschi, Y., F. Lamers, W. J. Peyrot, et al. 2017. Genetic Association of Major Depression with Atypical Features and Obesity-Related Immunometabolic Dysregulations. *JAMA Psychiatry* **74**:1214–1225. [2]

Milazzo, C., E. J. Mientjes, I. Wallaard, et al. 2021. Antisense Oligonucleotide Treatment Rescues *UBE3A* Expression and Multiple Phenotypes of an Angelman Syndrome Mouse Model. *JCI Insight* **6**:e145991. [5, 7]

Miller, D. T., M. P. Adam, S. Aradhya, et al. 2010. Consensus Statement: Chromosomal Microarray Is a First-Tier Clinical Diagnostic Test for Individuals with Developmental Disabilities or Congenital Anomalies. *Am. J. Hum. Genet.* **86**:749–764. [12]

Miller, J. A., S.-L. Ding, S. M. Sunkin, et al. 2014. Transcriptional Landscape of the Prenatal Human Brain. *Nature* **508**:199–206. [11]

Milosavljevic, F., N. Bukvic, Z. Pavlovic, et al. 2021. Association of CYP2C19 and CYP2D6 Poor and Intermediate Metabolizer Status with Antidepressant and Antipsychotic Exposure: A Systematic Review and Meta-Analysis. *JAMA Psychiatry* **78**:270–280. [13]

Mimitou, E. P., A. Cheng, A. Montalbano, et al. 2019. Multiplexed Detection of Proteins, Transcriptomes, Clonotypes and CRISPR Perturbations in Single Cells. *Nat. Methods* **16**:409–412. [7]

Mitchell, J. M., J. Nemesh, S. Ghosh, et al. 2020. *Preprint*: Mapping Genetic Effects on Cellular Phenotypes with "Cell Villages" *BioRxiv* 174383 [7, 8]

Modi, M. E., and M. Sahin. 2017. Translational Use of Event-Related Potentials to Assess Circuit Integrity in ASD. *Nat. Rev. Neurol.* **13**:160–170. [5]

Moldovan, R., K. McGhee, D. A. Coviello, et al. 2019. Psychiatric Genetic Counseling: A Mapping Exercise. *Am. J. Med. Genet. B Neuropsychiatr. Genet.* **180**:523–532. [15]

Moldovan, R., S. Pintea, and J. Austin. 2017. The Efficacy of Genetic Counseling for Psychiatric Disorders: A Meta-Analysis. *J. Genet. Counsel.* **26**:1341–1347. [15]

Monteys, A. M., A. A. Hundley, P. T. Ranum, et al. 2021. Regulated Control of Gene Therapies by Drug-Induced Splicing. *Nature* **596**:291–295. [6]

Moore, R., F. P. Casale, M. J. Bonder, et al. 2019. A Linear Mixed-Model Approach to Study Multivariate Gene–Environment Interactions. *Nat. Genet.* **51**:180–186. [2]

Moreno-De-Luca, D., M. E. Ross, and D. A. Ross. 2018. Leveraging the Power of Genetics to Bring Precision Medicine to Psychiatry: Too Little of a Good Thing? *Biol. Psychiatry* **83**:e45–e46. [15]

Morris, E., R. Batallones, J. Ryan, et al. 2021. Psychiatric Genetic Counseling for Serious Mental Illness: Impact on Psychopathology and Psychotropic Medication Adherence. *Psychiatry Res.* **296**:113663. [12, 15]

Morris, E., M. O'Donovan, A. Virani, and J. Austin. 2022. An Ethical Analysis of Divergent Clinical Approaches to the Application of Genetic Testing for Autism and Schizophrenia. *Hum. Genet.* **141**:1069–1084. [12, 15]

Mosley, J. D., D. K. Gupta, J. Tan, et al. 2020. Predictive Accuracy of a Polygenic Risk Score Compared with a Clinical Risk Score for Incident Coronary Heart Disease. *JAMA* **323**:627–635. [13]

Mostafavi, H., A. Harpak, I. Agarwal, et al. 2020. Variable Prediction Accuracy of Polygenic Scores within an Ancestry Group. *eLife* **9**:e48376. [13]

Mostafavi, H., J. P. Spence, S. Naqvi, and J. K. Pritchard. 2022. *Preprint*: Limited Overlap of eQTLs and GWAS Hits Due to Systematic Differences in Discovery. *bioRxiv* 491045. [10]

Mueller, C., J. D. Berry, D. M. McKenna-Yasek, et al. 2020. SOD1 Suppression with Adeno-Associated Virus and MicroRNA in Familial Als. *N. Engl. J. Med.* **383**:151–158. [6]

Mukai, J., E. Cannavo, G. W. Crabtree, et al. 2019. Recapitulation and Reversal of Schizophrenia-Related Phenotypes in Setd1a-Deficient Mice. *Neuron* **104**:471–487. [7]

Mullins, N., A. J. Forstner, K. S. O'Connell, et al. 2021. Genome-Wide Association Study of over 40,000 Bipolar Disorder Cases Provides New Insights into the Underlying Biology. *Nat. Genet.* **53**:817–829. [3]

Mullins, N., J. Kang, A. I. Campos, et al. 2022. Dissecting the Shared Genetic Architecture of Suicide Attempt, Psychiatric Disorders, and Known Risk Factors. *Biol. Psychiatry* **91**:313–327. [14]

Mulvey, B., and J. D. Dougherty. 2021. Transcriptional-Regulatory Convergence across Functional Mdd Risk Variants Identified by Massively Parallel Reporter Assays. *Transl. Psychiatry* **11**:403. [7]

Mumbach, M. R., A. T. Satpathy, E. A. Boyle, et al. 2017. Enhancer Connectome in Primary Human Cells Identifies Target Genes of Disease-Associated DNA Elements. *Nat. Genet.* **49**:1602–1612. [10]

Muñoz-Castañeda, R., B. Zingg, K. S. Matho, et al. 2021. Cellular Anatomy of the Mouse Primary Motor Cortex. *Nature* **598**:159–166. [11]

Muntoni, F., and M. J. Wood. 2011. Targeting RNA to Treat Neuromuscular Disease. *Nat. Rev. Drug Discov.* **10**:621–637. [5]

Murphy, L. E., T. M. Fonseka, C. A. Bousman, and D. J. Muller. 2022. Gene-Drug Pairings for Antidepressants and Antipsychotics: Level of Evidence and Clinical Application. *Mol. Psychiatry* **27**:593–605. [13]

Murray, G. K., T. Lin, J. Austin, et al. 2021. Could Polygenic Risk Scores Be Useful in Psychiatry? A Review. *JAMA Psychiatry* **78**:210–219. [13, 14]

Musliner, K. L., E. Agerbo, B. J. Vilhjálmsson, et al. 2021. Polygenic Liability and Recurrence of Depression in Patients with First-Onset Depression Treated in Hospital-Based Settings. *JAMA Psychiatry* **78**:792–795. [13]

Musliner, K. L., M. D. Krebs, C. Albiñana, et al. 2020. Polygenic Risk and Progression to Bipolar or Psychotic Disorders Among Individuals Diagnosed with Unipolar Depression in Early Life. *Am. J. Psychiatry* **177**:936–943. [13]

Myers, S. M., T. D. Challman, R. Bernier, et al. 2020a. Insufficient Evidence for "Autism-Specific" Genes. *Am. J. Hum. Genet.* **106**:587–595. [6]

Myers, S. M., T. D. Challman, C. L. Martin, and D. H. Ledbetter. 2020b. Response to Buxbaum et Al. *Am. J. Hum. Genet.* **107**:1004. [6]

Myint, L., R. Wang, L. Boukas, et al. 2020. A Screen of 1,049 Schizophrenia and 30 Alzheimer's-Associated Variants for Regulatory Potential. *Am. J. Med. Genet. B Neuropsychiatr. Genet.* **183**:61–73. [7, 8]

Nagahama, K., K. Sakoori, T. Watanabe, et al. 2020. Setd1a Insufficiency in Mice Attenuates Excitatory Synaptic Function and Recapitulates Schizophrenia-Related Behavioral Abnormalities. *Cell Rep.* **32**:108126. [7]

Nakamoto, M., V. Nalavadi, M. P. Epstein, et al. 2007. Fragile X Mental Retardation Protein Deficiency Leads to Excessive mGluR5-Dependent Internalization of AMPA Receptors. *PNAS* **104**:15537–15542. [5]

Namjou, B., M. Lape, E. Malolepsza, et al. 2022. Multiancestral Polygenic Risk Score for Pediatric Asthma. *J. Allergy Clin. Immunol.* **150**:1086–1109. [13]

Narcisa, V., M. Discenza, E. Vaccari, et al. 2013. Parental Interest in a Genetic Risk Assessment Test for Autism Spectrum Disorders. *Clin. Pediatr.* **52**:139–146. [14]

Natarajan, P., R. Young, N. O. Stitziel, et al. 2017. Polygenic Risk Score Identifies Subgroup with Higher Burden of Atherosclerosis and Greater Relative Benefit from Statin Therapy in the Primary Prevention Setting. *Circulation* **135**:2091–2101. [13]

Neale, B. M., Y. Kou, L. Liu, et al. 2012. Patterns and Rates of Exonic *de Novo* Mutations in Autism Spectrum Disorders. *Nature* **485**:242–245. [7]

Neavin, D., Q. Nguyen, M. S. Daniszewski, et al. 2021a. Single Cell eQTL Analysis Identifies Cell Type-Specific Genetic Control of Gene Expression in Fibroblasts and Reprogrammed Induced Pluripotent Stem Cells. *Genome Biol.* **22**:76. [7]

Neavin, D. R., A. M. Steinmann, H. S. Chiu, et al. 2021b. *Preprint*: Village in a Dish: A Model System for Population-Scale hiPSC Studies. *BioRxiv* 457030. [8]

Nehme, R., O. Pietiläine, M. Artomov, et al. 2021. *Preprint*: The 22q11.2 Region Regulates Presynaptic Gene-Products Linked to Schizophrenia. *bioRxiv* 461360. [7]

Nelson, A. D., A. M. Catalfio, J. M. Gupta, et al. 2022. *Preprint*: Physical and Functional Convergence of the Autism Risk Genes *Scn2a* and *Ank2* in Neocortical Pyramidal Cell Dendrites. *bioRxiv*2022.2005.2031.494205. [5]

Nelson, C. A., Z. A. Bhutta, N. B. Harris, A. Danese, and M. Samara. 2020. Adversity in Childhood Is Linked to Mental and Physical Health Throughout Life. *BMJ* **371**:m3048. [2]

Nelson, E. C., A. C. Heath, P. A. F. Madden, et al. 2002. Association between Self-Reported Childhood Sexual Abuse and Adverse Psychosocial Outcomes: Results from a Twin Study. *Arch. Gen. Psychiatry* **59**:139. [4]

Network Pathway Analysis Subgroup of Psychiatric Genomics Consortium. 2015. Psychiatric Genome-Wide Association Study Analyses Implicate Neuronal, Immune and Histone Pathways. *Nat. Neurosci.* **18**:199–209. [1, 11]

Ni, G., J. Zeng, J. A. Revez, et al. 2021. A Comparison of Ten Polygenic Score Methods for Psychiatric Disorders Applied across Multiple Cohorts. *Biol. Psychiatry* **90**:611–620. [13]

Nicholas, C. R., J. Chen, Y. Tang, et al. 2013. Functional Maturation of Hpsc-Derived Forebrain Interneurons Requires an Extended Timeline and Mimics Human Neural Development. *Cell Stem Cell* **12**:573–586. [7]

Niemi, M. E. K., H. C. Martin, D. L. Rice, et al. 2018. Common Genetic Variants Contribute to Risk of Rare Severe Neurodevelopmental Disorders. *Nature* **562**:268–271. [3, 9, 13]

Nonnenmacher, M., W. Wang, M. A. Child, et al. 2021. Rapid Evolution of Blood-Brain-Barrier-Penetrating AAV Capsids by RNA-Driven Biopanning. *Mol. Ther. Methods Clin. Dev.* **20**:366–378. [6]

Noor, A., L. Dupuis, K. Mittal, et al. 2015. 15q11.2 Duplication Encompassing Only the *UBE3A* Gene Is Associated with Developmental Delay and Neuropsychiatric Phenotypes. *Hum. Mutat.* **36**:689–693. [5]

Nott, A., I. R. Holtman, N. G. Coufal, et al. 2019. Brain Cell Type-Specific Enhancer-Promoter Interactome Maps and Disease-Risk Association. *Science* **366**:1134–1139. [10]

Nowakowski, T. J., A. Bhaduri, A. A. Pollen, et al. 2017. Spatiotemporal Gene Expression Trajectories Reveal Developmental Hierarchies of the Human Cortex. *Science* **358**:1318–1323. [11]

O'Brien, H. E., E. Hannon, M. J. Hill, et al. 2018. Expression Quantitative Trait Loci in the Developing Human Brain and Their Enrichment in Neuropsychiatric Disorders. *Genome Biol.* **19**:194. [11]

Ochoa, D., M. Karim, M. Ghoussaini, et al. 2022. Human Genetics Evidence Supports Two-Thirds of the 2021 FDA-Approved Drugs. *Nat. Rev. Drug Discov.* **21**:551. [8]

O'Connor, L. J., A. P. Schoech, F. Hormozdiari, et al. 2019. Extreme Polygenicity of Complex Traits Is Explained by Negative Selection. *Am. J. Hum. Genet.* **105**:456–476. [3]

Oetjens, M. T., M. A. Kelly, A. C. Sturm, C. L. Martin, and D. H. Ledbetter. 2019. Quantifying the Polygenic Contribution to Variable Expressivity in Eleven Rare Genetic Disorders. *Nat. Commun.* **10**:4897. [13]

Okano, H., K. Hikishima, A. Iriki, and E. Sasaki. 2012. The Common Marmoset as a Novel Animal Model System for Biomedical and Neuroscience Research Applications. *Semin. Fetal Neonatal Med.* **17**:336–340. [5]

Oldham, M. C., G. Konopka, K. Iwamoto, et al. 2008. Functional Organization of the Transcriptome in Human Brain. *Nat. Neurosci.* **11**:1271–1282. [11]

Olney, J. W., J. W. Newcomer, and N. B. Farber. 1999. NMDA Receptor Hypofunction Model of Schizophrenia. *J. Psychiatr. Res.* **33**:523–533. [11]

Onishi, K., S. S. Kikuchi, T. Abe, T. Tokuhara, and T. Shimogori. 2022. Molecular Cell Identities in the Mediodorsal Thalamus of Infant Mice and Marmoset. *J. Comp. Neurol.* **530**:963–977. [5]

Orlando, L. A., C. Voils, C. R. Horowitz, et al. 2019. Ignite Network: Response of Patients to Genomic Medicine Interventions. *Mol. Genet. Genomic Med.* **7**:e636. [13]

Ormond, K. E., M. Y. Laurino, K. Barlow-Stewart, et al. 2018. Genetic Counseling Globally: Where Are We Now? *Am. J. Med. Genet. B Neuropsychiatr. Genet.* **178**:98–107. [15]

O'Roak, B. J., H. A. Stessman, E. A. Boyle, et al. 2014. Recurrent *de Novo* Mutations Implicate Novel Genes Underlying Simplex Autism Risk. *Nat. Commun.* **5**:5595. [7]

O'Roak, B. J., L. Vives, W. Fu, et al. 2012a. Multiplex Targeted Sequencing Identifies Recurrently Mutated Genes in Autism Spectrum Disorders. *Science* **338**:1619–1622. [7]

O'Roak, B. J., L. Vives, S. Girirajan, et al. 2012b. Sporadic Autism Exomes Reveal a Highly Interconnected Protein Network of *de Novo* Mutations. *Nature* **485**:246–250. [11]

O'Sullivan, J. W., S. Raghavan, C. Marquez-Luna, et al. 2022. Polygenic Risk Scores for Cardiovascular Disease: A Scientific Statement from the American Heart Association. *Circulation* **146**:e93–e118. [13]

Overwater, I. E., A. B. Rietman, S. E. Mous, et al. 2019. A Randomized Controlled Trial with Everolimus for IQ and Autism in Tuberous Sclerosis Complex. *Neurology* **93**:e200–e209. [6]

Owen, M. J., H. J. Williams, and M. C. O'Donovan. 2009. Schizophrenia Genetics: Advancing on Two Fronts. *Curr. Opin. Genet. Dev.* **19**:266–270. [5]

Page, S. C., S. R. Sripathy, F. Farinelli, et al. 2022. Electrophysiological Measures from Human iPSC-Derived Neurons Are Associated with Schizophrenia Clinical Status and Predict Individual Cognitive Performance. *PNAS* **119**:e2109395119. [8]

Pain, O., F. Dudbridge, A. G. Cardno, et al. 2018. Genome-Wide Analysis of Adolescent Psychotic-Like Experiences Shows Genetic Overlap with Psychiatric Disorders. *Am. J. Med. Genet. B Neuropsychiatr. Genet.* **177**:416–425. [2]

Pain, O., A. C. Gillett, J. C. Austin, L. Folkersen, and C. M. Lewis. 2022a. A Tool for Translating Polygenic Scores onto the Absolute Scale Using Summary Statistics. *Eur. J. Hum. Genet.* **30**:339–348. [13]

Pain, O., K. Hodgson, V. Trubetskoy, et al. 2022b. Identifying the Common Genetic Basis of Antidepressant Response. *Biol. Psychiatry Glob. Open Sci.* **2**:115–126. [12, 14]

Pak, C., T. Danko, V. R. Mirabella, et al. 2021. Cross-Platform Validation of Neurotransmitter Release Impairments in Schizophrenia Patient-Derived NRXN1-Mutant Neurons. *PNAS* **118**:e2025598118. [1]

Pak, C., T. Danko, Y. Zhang, et al. 2015. Human Neuropsychiatric Disease Modeling Using Conditional Deletion Reveals Synaptic Transmission Defects Caused by Heterozygous Mutations in NRXN1. *Cell Stem Cell* **17**:316–328. [5, 7]

Palmer, D. S., D. P. Howrigan, S. B. Chapman, et al. 2022. Exome Sequencing in Bipolar Disorder Identifies AKAP11 as a Risk Gene Shared with Schizophrenia. *Nat. Genet.* **54**:541–547. [3, 7]

Palmer, M. J., A. J. Irving, G. R. Seabrook, D. E. Jane, and G. L. Collingridge. 1997. The Group I mGlu Receptor Agonist Dhpg Induces a Novel Form of LTD in the CA1 Region of the Hippocampus. *Neuropharmacol.* **36**:1517–1532. [5]

Pankevich, D. E., B. M. Altevogt, J. Dunlop, F. H. Gage, and S. E. Hyman. 2014. Improving and Accelerating Drug Development for Nervous System Disorders. *Neuron* **84**:546–553. [6]

Pardiñas, A. F., P. Holmans, A. J. Pocklington, et al. 2018. Common Schizophrenia Alleles Are Enriched in Mutation-Intolerant Genes and in Regions under Strong Background Selection. *Nat. Genet.* **50**:381–389. [7, 10]

Pardiñas, A. F., M. Nalmpanti, A. J. Pocklington, et al. 2019. Pharmacogenomic Variants and Drug Interactions Identified through the Genetic Analysis of Clozapine Metabolism. *Am. J. Psychiatry* **176**:477–486. [4]

Pardiñas, A. F., M. J. Owen, and J. T. R. Walters. 2021. Pharmacogenomics: A Road Ahead for Precision Medicine in Psychiatry. *Neuron* **109**:3914–3929. [13]

Parellada, M., Á. Andreu-Bernabeu, M. Burdeus, et al. 2023. In Search of Biomarkers to Guide Interventions in Autism Spectrum Disorder: A Systematic Review. *Am. J. Psychiatry* **180**:23–40. [5]

Parikshak, N. N., M. J. Gandal, and D. H. Geschwind. 2015. Systems Biology and Gene Networks in Neurodevelopmental and Neurodegenerative Disorders. *Nat. Rev. Genet.* **16**:441–458. [11]

Parikshak, N. N., R. Luo, A. Zhang, et al. 2013. Integrative Functional Genomic Analyses Implicate Specific Molecular Pathways and Circuits in Autism. *Cell* **155**:1008–1021. [3, 5, 11]

Parikshak, N. N., V. Swarup, T. G. Belgard, et al. 2016. Genome-Wide Changes in Incrna, Splicing, and Regional Gene Expression Patterns in Autism. *Nature* **540**:423–427. [11]

Park, C. Y., J. Zhou, A. K. Wong, et al. 2021. Genome-Wide Landscape of RNA-Binding Protein Target Site Dysregulation Reveals a Major Impact on Psychiatric Disorder Risk. *Nat. Genet.* **53**:166–173. [11]

Pasaniuc, B., and A. L. Price. 2017. Dissecting the Genetics of Complex Traits Using Summary Association Statistics. *Nat. Rev. Genet.* **18**:117–127. [9]

Paşca, A. M., S. A. Sloan, L. E. Clarke, et al. 2015. Functional Cortical Neurons and Astrocytes from Human Pluripotent Stem Cells in 3D Culture. *Nat. Methods* **12**:671–678. [7]

Paşca, S. P. 2019. Assembling Human Brain Organoids. *Science* **363**:126. [7]

Paşca, S. P., P. Arlotta, H. S. Bateup, et al. 2022. A Nomenclature Consensus for Nervous System Organoids and Assembloids. *Nature* **609**:907–910. [5]

Paşca, S. P., T. Portmann, I. Voineagu, et al. 2011. Using iPSC-Derived Neurons to Uncover Cellular Phenotypes Associated with Timothy Syndrome. *Nat. Med.* **17**:1657–1662. [7]

Patch, C., and A. Middleton. 2018. Genetic Counselling in the Era of Genomic Medicine. *Br. Med. Bull.* **126**:27–36. [12]

Paulsen, B., S. Velasco, A. J. Kedaigle, et al. 2022. Autism Genes Converge on Asynchronous Development of Shared Neuron Classes. *Nature* **602**:268–273. [7]

Pearce, M., L. Garcia, A. Abbas, et al. 2022. Association between Physical Activity and Risk of Depression: A Systematic Review and Meta-Analysis. *JAMA Psychiatry* **79**:550–559. [13]

Pearl, R. L., and M. S. Lebowitz. 2014. Beyond Personal Responsibility: Effects of Causal Attributions for Overweight and Obesity on Weight-Related Beliefs, Stigma, and Policy Support. *Psychol. Health* **29**:1176–1191. [14]

Peay, H. L., and J. C. Austin. 2011. How to Talk with Families About Genetics and Psychiatric Illness. New York: W. W. Norton. [15]

Peca, J., C. Feliciano, J. T. Ting, et al. 2011. Shank3 Mutant Mice Display Autistic-Like Behaviours and Striatal Dysfunction. *Nature* **472**:437–442. [7]

Peck, L., K. Borle, L. Folkersen, and J. Austin. 2022. Why Do People Seek out Polygenic Risk Scores for Complex Disorders, and How Do They Understand and React to Results? *Eur. J. Hum. Genet.* **30**:81–87. [12, 13, 15]

Penagarikano, O., B. S. Abrahams, E. I. Herman, et al. 2011. Absence of CNTNAP2 Leads to Epilepsy, Neuronal Migration Abnormalities, and Core Autism-Related Deficits. *Cell* **147**:235–246. [7]

Penner-Goeke, S., M. Bothe, N. Kappelmann, et al. 2022. *Preprint*: Assessment of Glucocorticoid-Induced Enhancer Activity of Esnp Regions Using Starr-Seq Reveals Novel Molecular Mechanisms in Psychiatric Disorders. *MedRxiv* 22275090. [8]

Pereira, S., K. A. Muñoz, B. J. Small, et al. 2022. Psychiatric Polygenic Risk Scores: Child and Adolescent Psychiatrists' Knowledge, Attitudes, and Experiences. *Am. J. Med. Genet. B Neuropsychiatr. Genet.* **189**:293–302. [12]

Perkins, D. O., L. Olde Loohuis, J. Barbee, et al. 2020. Polygenic Risk Score Contribution to Psychosis Prediction in a Target Population of Persons at Clinical High Risk. *Am. J. Psychiatry* **177**:155–163. [13]

Pers, T. H., J. M. Karjalainen, Y. Chan, et al. 2015. Biological Interpretation of Genome-Wide Association Studies Using Predicted Gene Functions. *Nat. Commun.* **6**:5890. [11]

Persons, J. B. 1986. The Advantages of Studying Psychological Phenomena Rather Than Psychiatric Diagnoses. *Am. Psychol.* **41**:1252–1260. [2]

Petersen, A. H., and T. Lange. 2020. What Is the Causal Interpretation of Sibling Comparison Designs? *Epidemiology* **31**:75–81. [4]

Peterson, R. E., N. Cai, A. W. Dahl, et al. 2018. Molecular Genetic Analysis Subdivided by Adversity Exposure Suggests Etiologic Heterogeneity in Major Depression. *Am. J. Psychiatry* **175**:545–554. [2]

Petrazzini, B. O., K. Chaudhary, C. Marquez-Luna, et al. 2022. Coronary Risk Estimation Based on Clinical Data in Electronic Health Records. *J. Am. Coll. Cardiol.* **79**:1155–1166. [13]

Peyrot, W. J., D. I. Boomsma, B. W. Penninx, and N. R. Wray. 2016. Disease and Polygenic Architecture: Avoid Trio Design and Appropriately Account for Unscreened Control Subjects for Common Disease. *Am. J. Hum. Genet.* **98**:382–391. [2]

Peyrot, W. J., and A. L. Price. 2021. Identifying Loci with Different Allele Frequencies among Cases of Eight Psychiatric Disorders Using CC-GWAS. *Nat. Genet.* **53**:445–454. [2]

Pino, M. G., K. A. Rich, and S. J. Kolb. 2021. Update on Biomarkers in Spinal Muscular Atrophy. *Biomark. Insights* **16**:11772719211035643. [5]

Pintacuda, G., Y.-H. H. Hsu, K. Tsafou, et al. 2021. *Preprint*: Interaction Studies of Risk Proteins in Human Induced Neurons Reveal Convergent Biology and Novel Mechanisms Underlying Autism Spectrum Disorders. *medRxiv* 21264575. [11]

Pinto, D., A. T. Pagnamenta, L. Klei, et al. 2010. Functional Impact of Global Rare Copy Number Variation in Autism Spectrum Disorders. *Nature* **466**:368–372. [11]

Plomin, R. 2014. Genotype-Environment Correlation in the Era of DNA. *Behav. Genet.* **44**:629–638. [2]

Polderman, T. J., B. Benyamin, C. A. de Leeuw, et al. 2015. Meta-Analysis of the Heritability of Human Traits Based on Fifty Years of Twin Studies. *Nat. Genet.* **47**:702–709. [7]

Polioudakis, D., L. de la Torre-Ubieta, J. Langerman, et al. 2019. A Single-Cell Transcriptomic Atlas of Human Neocortical Development during Mid-Gestation. *Neuron* **103**:785–801. [11]

Polygenic Risk Score Task Force of the Intl. Common Disease Alliance. 2021. Responsible Use of Polygenic Risk Scores in the Clinic: Potential Benefits, Risks and Gaps. *Nat. Med.* **27**:1876–1884. [13]

Popejoy, A. B., D. I. Ritter, K. Crooks, et al. 2018. The Clinical Imperative for Inclusivity: Race, Ethnicity, and Ancestry (REA) in Genomics. *Hum. Mutat.* **39**:1713–1720. [3]

Power, R. A., S. Kyaga, R. Uher, et al. 2013. Fecundity of Patients with Schizophrenia, Autism, Bipolar Disorder, Depression, Anorexia Nervosa, or Substance Abuse vs Their Unaffected Siblings. *JAMA Psychiatry* **70**:22–30. [3]

Pratt, B. M., and H. Won. 2022. Advances in Profiling Chromatin Architecture Shed Light on the Regulatory Dynamics Underlying Brain Disorders. *Semin. Cell Dev. Biol.* **121**:153–160. [10]

Privé, F., B. J. Vilhjálmsson, H. Aschard, and M. G. B. Blum. 2019. Making the Most of Clumping and Thresholding for Polygenic Scores. *Am. J. Hum. Genet.* **105**:1213–1221. [13]

Prohl, A. K., B. Scherrer, X. Tomas-Fernandez, et al. 2019. Reproducibility of Structural and Diffusion Tensor Imaging in the Tacern Multi-Center Study. *Front. Integr. Neurosci.* **13**:24. [5]

Psaty, B. M., C. J. O'Donnell, V. Gudnason, et al. 2009. Cohorts for Heart and Aging Research in Genomic Epidemiology (Charge) Consortium: Design of Prospective Meta-Analyses of Genome-Wide Association Studies from 5 Cohorts. *Circ. Cardiovasc. Genet.* **2**:73–80. [8]

PsychENCODE Consortium, S. Akbarian, C. Liu, et al. 2015. The Psychencode Project. *Nat. Neurosci.* **18**:1707–1712. [5, 8, 11]

Purcell, S. M., J. L. Moran, M. Fromer, et al. 2014. A Polygenic Burden of Rare Disruptive Mutations in Schizophrenia. *Nature* **506**:185–190. [7, 11]

Purves, K. L., J. R. I. Coleman, S. M. Meier, et al. 2020. A Major Role for Common Genetic Variation in Anxiety Disorders. *Mol. Psychiatry* **25**:3292–3303. [3]

Qi, L. S., M. H. Larson, L. A. Gilbert, et al. 2013. Repurposing CRISPR as an RNA-Guided Platform for Sequence-Specific Control of Gene Expression. *Cell* **152**:1173–1183. [5]

Qian, X., H. N. Nguyen, M. M. Song, et al. 2016. Brain-Region-Specific Organoids Using Mini-Bioreactors for Modeling Zikv Exposure. *Cell* **165**:1238–1254. [7]

Qiu, Y., T. Arbogast, S. M. Lorenzo, et al. 2019. Oligogenic Effects of 16p11.2 Copy-Number Variation on Craniofacial Development. *Cell Rep.* **28**:3320–3328. [5]

Quaid, K. A., S. R. Aschen, C. L. Smiley, and J. I. Nurnberger. 2001. Perceived Genetic Risks for Bipolar Disorder in a Patient Population: An Exploratory Study. *J. Genet. Counsel.* **10**:41–51. [15]

Quinn, V., B. Meiser, A. Wilde, et al. 2014. Preferences Regarding Targeted Education and Risk Assessment in People with a Family History of Major Depressive Disorder. *J. Genet. Counsel.* **23**:785–795. [15]

Rabani, M., L. Pieper, G. L. Chew, and A. F. Schier. 2017. A Massively Parallel Reporter Assay of 3'UTR Sequences Identifies *in Vivo* Rules for mRNA Degradation. *Mol. Cell* **68**:1083–1094. [8]

Rajarajan, P., T. Borrman, W. Liao, et al. 2018. Neuron-Specific Signatures in the Chromosomal Connectome Associated with Schizophrenia Risk. *Science* **362**:eaat4311. [7]

Rajkumar, A. P., B. Poonkuzhali, A. Kuruvilla, M. Jacob, and K. S. Jacob. 2013. Clinical Predictors of Serum Clozapine Levels in Patients with Treatment-Resistant Schizophrenia. *Int. Clin. Psychopharmacol.* **28**:50–56. [4]

Ramaswami, G., H. Won, M. J. Gandal, et al. 2020. Integrative Genomics Identifies a Convergent Molecular Subtype That Links Epigenomic with Transcriptomic Differences in Autism. *Nat. Commun.* **11**:4873. [11]

Raznahan, A., H. Won, D. C. Glahn, and S. Jacquemont. 2022. Convergence and Divergence of Rare Genetic Disorders on Brain Phenotypes: A Review. *JAMA Psychiatry* **79**:818–828. [1]

Readhead, B., B. J. Hartley, B. J. Eastwood, et al. 2018. Expression-Based Drug Screening of Neural Progenitor Cells from Individuals with Schizophrenia. *Nat. Commun.* **9**:4412. [7]

Rees, E., H. D. J. Creeth, H. G. Hwu, et al. 2021. Schizophrenia, Autism Spectrum Disorders and Developmental Disorders Share Specific Disruptive Coding Mutations. *Nat. Commun.* **12**:5353. [7]

Reid, N. J., D. G. Brockman, C. Elisabeth Leonard, R. Pelletier, and A. V. Khera. 2021. Concordance of a High Polygenic Score Among Relatives: Implications for Genetic Counseling and Cascade Screening. *Circ. Genom. Precis. Med.* **14**:e003262. [13]

Resta, R. G. 1997. The Historical Perspective: Sheldon Reed and 50 Years of Genetic Counseling. *J. Genet. Counsel.* **6**:375–377. [15]

———. 2006. Defining and Redefining the Scope and Goals of Genetic Counseling. *Am. J. Med. Genet. C Semin. Med. Genet.* **142**:269–275. [15]

Resta, R. G., B. B. Biesecker, R. L. Bennett, et al. 2006. A New Definition of Genetic Counseling: National Society of Genetic Counselors' Task Force Report. *J. Genet. Counsel.* **15**:77–83. [12, 15]

Reveley, A. 1985. Genetic Counselling for Schizophrenia. *Br. J. Psychiatry* **147**:107–112. [15]

Rimfeld, K., M. Malanchini, T. Spargo, et al. 2019. Twins Early Development Study: A Genetically Sensitive Investigation into Behavioral and Cognitive Development from Infancy to Emerging Adulthood. *Twin Res. Hum. Genet.* **22**:508–513. [2]

Rinaldi, C., and M. J. A. Wood. 2018. Antisense Oligonucleotides: The Next Frontier for Treatment of Neurological Disorders. *Nat. Rev. Neurol.* **14**:9–21. [5]

Ripke, S., C. O'Dushlaine, K. Chambert, et al. 2013. Genome-Wide Association Analysis Identifies 13 New Risk Loci for Schizophrenia. *Nat. Genet.* **45**:1150–1159. [9]

Ritchie, M. D., E. R. Holzinger, R. Li, S. A. Pendergrass, and D. Kim. 2015. Methods of Integrating Data to Uncover Genotype-Phenotype Interactions. *Nat. Rev. Genet.* **16**:85–97. [11]

Rizzardi, L. F., P. F. Hickey, V. Rodriguez DiBlasi, et al. 2019. Neuronal Brain-Region-Specific DNA Methylation and Chromatin Accessibility Are Associated with Neuropsychiatric Trait Heritability. *Nat. Neurosci.* **22**:307–316. [11]

Robins, C., Y. Liu, W. Fan, et al. 2021. Genetic Control of the Human Brain Proteome. *Am. J. Hum. Genet.* **108**:400–410. [11]

Robinson, E. B., K. E. Samocha, J. A. Kosmicki, et al. 2014. Autism Spectrum Disorder Severity Reflects the Average Contribution of *de Novo* and Familial Influences. *PNAS* **111**:15161–15165. [9]

Rodrigues, S. M., E. P. Bauer, C. R. Farb, G. E. Schafe, and J. E. LeDoux. 2002. The Group I Metabotropic Glutamate Receptor mGluR5 Is Required for Fear Memory Formation and Long-Term Potentiation in the Lateral Amygdala. *J. Neurosci.* **22**:5219–5229. [5]

Ronald, A., N. de Bode, and T. J. Polderman. 2021. Systematic Review: How the Attention-Deficit/Hyperactivity Disorder Polygenic Risk Score Adds to Our Understanding of ADHD and Associated Traits. *J. Am. Acad. Child Adolesc. Psychiatry* **60**:1234–1277. [2]

Ronald, A., H. Larsson, H. Anckarsater, and P. Lichtenstein. 2011. A Twin Study of Autism Symptoms in Sweden. *Mol. Psychiatry* **16**:1039–1047. [2]

Rosenberg, A. B., R. P. Patwardhan, J. Shendure, and G. Seelig. 2015. Learning the Sequence Determinants of Alternative Splicing from Millions of Random Sequences. *Cell* **163**:698–711. [8]

Rosenthal, D., I. Goldberg, B. Jacobsen, et al. 1974. Migration, Heredity, and Schizophrenia. *Psychiatry* **37**:321–339. [4]

Rotaru, D. C., G. M. van Woerden, I. Wallaard, and Y. Elgersma. 2018. Adult *Ube3a* Gene Reinstatement Restores the Electrophysiological Deficits of Prefrontal Cortex Layer 5 Neurons in a Mouse Model of Angelman Syndrome. *J. Neurosci.* **38**:8011–8030. [5]

Roussos, P., P. Katsel, K. L. Davis, L. J. Siever, and V. Haroutunian. 2012. A System-Level Transcriptomic Analysis of Schizophrenia Using Postmortem Brain Tissue Samples. *Arch. Gen. Psychiatry* **69**:1205–1213. [11]

Roussos, P., A. C. Mitchell, G. Voloudakis, et al. 2014. A Role for Noncoding Variation in Schizophrenia. *Cell Rep.* **9**:1417–1429. [7]

Ruan, Y., Y. F. Lin, Y. A. Feng, et al. 2022. Improving Polygenic Prediction in Ancestrally Diverse Populations. *Nat. Genet.* **54**:573–580. [13]

Ruderfer, D. M., A. W. Charney, B. Readhead, et al. 2016. Polygenic Overlap between Schizophrenia Risk and Antipsychotic Response: A Genomic Medicine Approach. *Lancet Psychiatry* **3**:350–357. [7]

Ruth, K. S., F. R. Day, J. Tyrrell, et al. 2020. Using Human Genetics to Understand the Disease Impacts of Testosterone in Men and Women. *Nat. Med.* **26**:252–258. [9]

Ruzzo, E. K., L. Perez-Cano, J. Y. Jung, et al. 2019. Inherited and *de Novo* Genetic Risk for Autism Impacts Shared Networks. *Cell* **178**:850–866. [7]

Ryan, J., A. Virani, and J. C. Austin. 2015. Ethical Issues Associated with Genetic Counseling in the Context of Adolescent Psychiatry. *Appl. Transl. Genom.* **5**:23–29. [12]

Sabo, A., D. Murdock, S. Dugan, et al. 2020. Community-Based Recruitment and Exome Sequencing Indicates High Diagnostic Yield in Adults with Intellectual Disability. *Mol. Genet. Genomic Med.* **8**:e1439. [12]

Saby, J. N., T. A. Benke, S. U. Peters, et al. 2021. Multisite Study of Evoked Potentials in Rett Syndrome. *Ann. Neurol.* **89**:790–802. [5]

Sahin, M., S. R. Jones, J. A. Sweeney, et al. 2018. Discovering Translational Biomarkers in Neurodevelopmental Disorders. *Nat. Rev. Drug Discov.* **18**:235–236. [5, 6]

Sahin, M., and M. Sur. 2015. Genes, Circuits, and Precision Therapies for Autism and Related Neurodevelopmental Disorders. *Science* **350**:aab3897. [6]

Sakai, Y., C. A. Shaw, B. C. Dawson, et al. 2011. Protein Interactome Reveals Converging Molecular Pathways among Autism Disorders. *Sci. Transl. Med.* **3**:86ra49. [11]

Sánchez Fernández, I., T. Loddenkemper, M. Gaínza-Lein, B. R. Sheidley, and A. Poduri. 2019. Diagnostic Yield of Genetic Tests in Epilepsy: A Meta-Analysis and Cost-Effectiveness Study. *Neurology* **92**:e418–428. [12]

Sanders, S. J., A. J. Campbell, J. R. Cottrell, et al. 2018. Progress in Understanding and Treating SCN2A-Mediated Disorders. *Trends Neurosci.* **41**:442–456. [3, 5]

Sanders, S. J., X. He, A. J. Willsey, et al. 2015. Insights into Autism Spectrum Disorder Genomic Architecture and Biology from 71 Risk Loci. *Neuron* **87**:1215–1233. [5–7, 11]

Sanders, S. J., M. T. Murtha, A. R. Gupta, et al. 2012. *De Novo* Mutations Revealed by Whole-Exome Sequencing Are Strongly Associated with Autism. *Nature* **485**:237–241. [7]

Sanders, S. J., B. M. Neale, H. Huang, et al. 2017. Whole Genome Sequencing in Psychiatric Disorders: The WGSPD Consortium. *Nat. Neurosci.* **20**:1661–1668. [3, 5]

Sanders, S. J., M. Sahin, J. Hostyk, et al. 2019. A Framework for the Investigation of Rare Genetic Disorders in Neuropsychiatry. *Nat. Med.* **25**:1477–1487. [6]

Sanderson, E., M. M. Glymour, M. V. Holmes, et al. 2022. Mendelian Randomization. *Nat. Rev. Meth. Primers* **2**:6. [4]

Sandweiss, A. J., V. L. Brandt, and H. Y. Zoghbi. 2020. Advances in Understanding of Rett Syndrome and MECP2 Duplication Syndrome: Prospects for Future Therapies. *Lancet Neurol.* **19**:689–698. [1]

Sanghani, H. R., A. Jagannath, T. Humberstone, et al. 2021. Patient Fibroblast Circadian Rhythms Predict Lithium Sensitivity in Bipolar Disorder. *Mol. Psychiatry* **26**:5252–5265. [8, 9]

Sanson, K. R., R. E. Hanna, M. Hegde, et al. 2018. Optimized Libraries for CRISPR-Cas9 Genetic Screens with Multiple Modalities. *Nat. Commun.* **9**:5416. [7]

Saragosa-Harris, N. M., N. Chaku, N. MacSweeney, et al. 2022. A Practical Guide for Researchers and Reviewers Using the ABCD Study and Other Large Longitudinal Datasets. *Dev. Cogn. Neurosci.* **55**:101115. [2]

Sariaslan, A., L. Arseneault, H. Larsson, P. Lichtenstein, and S. Fazel. 2020. Risk of Subjection to Violence and Perpetration of Violence in Persons with Psychiatric Disorders in Sweden. *JAMA Psychiatry* **77**:359–367. [4]

Sariaslan, A., A. Kääriälä, J. Pitkänen, et al. 2021a. Long-Term Health and Social Outcomes in Children and Adolescents Placed in out-of-Home Care. *JAMA Pediatr.* **176**:e214324. [4]

Sariaslan, A., J. Mikkonen, M. Aaltonen, et al. 2021b. No Causal Associations between Childhood Family Income and Subsequent Psychiatric Disorders, Substance Misuse and Violent Crime Arrests: A Nationwide Finnish Study of >650 000 Individuals and Their Siblings. *Int. J. Epidemiol.* **50**:1628–1638. [4]

Sasaki, E., H. Suemizu, A. Shimada, et al. 2009. Generation of Transgenic Non-Human Primates with Germline Transmission. *Nature* **459**:523–527. [5]

Satterstrom, F. K., J. A. Kosmicki, J. Wang, et al. 2020. Large-Scale Exome Sequencing Study Implicates Both Developmental and Functional Changes in the Neurobiology of Autism. *Cell* **180**:568–584.e523. [3, 5–7, 11]

Satterstrom, F. K., R. K. Walters, T. Singh, et al. 2019. Autism Spectrum Disorder and Attention Deficit Hyperactivity Disorder Have a Similar Burden of Rare Protein-Truncating Variants. *Nat. Neurosci.* **22**:1961–1965. [3]

Savatt, J. M., and S. M. Myers. 2021. Genetic Testing in Neurodevelopmental Disorders. *Front. Pediatr.* **9**:526779. [12]

Sawiak, S. J., Y. Shiba, L. Oikonomidis, et al. 2018. Trajectories and Milestones of Cortical and Subcortical Development of the Marmoset Brain from Infancy to Adulthood. *Cerebral Cortex* **28**:4440–4453. [8]

Schaefer, G. B., N. J. Mendelsohn, and Professional Practice and Guidelines Committee. 2013. Clinical Genetics Evaluation in Identifying the Etiology of Autism Spectrum Disorders: 2013 Guideline Revisions. *Genet. Med.* **15**:399–407. [13]

Schaid, D. J., W. Chen, and N. B. Larson. 2018. From Genome-Wide Associations to Candidate Causal Variants by Statistical Fine-Mapping. *Nat. Rev. Genet.* **19**:491–504. [8]

Schizophrenia Working Group of the Psychiatric Genomics Consortium. 2014. Biological Insights from 108 Schizophrenia-Associated Genetic Loci. *Nature* **511**:421–427. [8]

Schmid, R. S., X. Deng, P. Panikker, et al. 2021. CRISPR/Cas9 Directed to the *Ube3a* Antisense Transcript Improves Angelman Syndrome Phenotype in Mice. *J. Clin. Invest.* **131**:e142574. [5]

Schork, A. J., H. Won, V. Appadurai, et al. 2019. A Genome-Wide Association Study of Shared Risk across Psychiatric Disorders Implicates Gene Regulation during Fetal Neurodevelopment. *Nat. Neurosci.* **22**:353–361. [2, 7, 11]

Schrode, N., S. M. Ho, K. Yamamuro, et al. 2019. Synergistic Effects of Common Schizophrenia Risk Variants. *Nat. Genet.* **51**:1475–1485. [7, 8]

Schulte, S., M. Gries, A. Christmann, and K.-H. Schäfer. 2021. Using Multielectrode Arrays to Investigate Neurodegenerative Effects of the Amyloid-Beta Peptide. *Bioelectron. Med.* **7**:15. [8]

Sebat, J., B. Lakshmi, D. Malhotra, et al. 2007. Strong Association of *de Novo* Copy Number Mutations with Autism. *Science* **316**:445–449. [3, 7]

Segura, À. G., A. Martinez-Pinteño, P. Gassó, et al. 2022. Metabolic Polygenic Risk Scores Effect on Antipsychotic-Induced Metabolic Dysregulation: A Longitudinal Study in a First Episode Psychosis Cohort. *Schizophr. Res.* **244**:101–110. [13]

Seibert, T. M., C. C. Fan, Y. Wang, et al. 2018. Polygenic Hazard Score to Guide Screening for Aggressive Prostate Cancer: Development and Validation in Large Scale Cohorts. *BMJ* **360**:j5757. [13]

Sekar, A., A. R. Bialas, H. de Rivera, et al. 2016. Schizophrenia Risk from Complex Variation of Complement Component 4. *Nature* **530**:177–183. [3, 5, 11]

Sellgren, C. M., J. Gracias, B. Watmuff, et al. 2019. Increased Synapse Elimination by Microglia in Schizophrenia Patient-Derived Models of Synaptic Pruning. *Nat. Neurosci.* **22**:374–385. [7]

Selten, J.-P., E. Cantor-Graae, J. Slaets, and R. S. Kahn. 2002. Ødegaard's Selection Hypothesis Revisited: Schizophrenia in Surinamese Immigrants to the Netherlands. *Am. J. Psychiatry* **159**:669–671. [4]

Selten, J.-P., J. P. J. Slaets, and R. S. Kahn. 1997. Schizophrenia in Surinamese and Dutch Antillean Immigrants to the Netherlands: Evidence of an Increased Incidence. *Psychol. Med.* **27**:807–811. [4]

Selzam, S., J. R. I. Coleman, A. Caspi, T. E. Moffitt, and R. Plomin. 2018. A Polygenic P Factor for Major Psychiatric Disorders. *Transl. Psychiatry* **8**:205. [2]

Selzam, S., S. J. Ritchie, J. B. Pingault, et al. 2019. Comparing Within- and between-Family Polygenic Score Prediction. *Am. J. Hum. Genet.* **105**:351–363. [2]

Semaka, A., and J. Austin. 2019. Patient Perspectives on the Process and Outcomes of Psychiatric Genetic Counseling: An Empowering Encounter. *J. Genet. Couns.* **28**:856–868. [12, 15]

Sey, N. Y. A., B. Hu, M. Iskhakova, et al. 2022. Chromatin Architecture in Addiction Circuitry Identifies Risk Genes and Potential Biological Mechanisms Underlying Cigarette Smoking and Alcohol Use Traits. *Mol. Psychiatry* **27**:3085–3094. [10]

Sey, N. Y. A., B. Hu, W. Mah, et al. 2020. A Computational Tool (H-MAGMA) for Improved Prediction of Brain-Disorder Risk Genes by Incorporating Brain Chromatin Interaction Profiles. *Nat. Neurosci.* **23**:583–593. [7, 8, 10]

Shah, J. L., J. Scott, P. D. McGorry, et al. 2020. Transdiagnostic Clinical Staging in Youth Mental Health: A First International Consensus Statement. *World Psychiatry* **19**:233–242. [8]

Shakoor, S., H. M. Zavos, C. M. Haworth, et al. 2016. Association between Stressful Life Events and Psychotic Experiences in Adolescence: Evidence for Gene–Environment Correlations. *Br. J. Psychiatry* **208**:532–538. [2]

Shao, Z., H. Noh, W. Bin Kim, et al. 2019. Dysregulated Protocadherin-Pathway Activity as an Intrinsic Defect in Induced Pluripotent Stem Cell-Derived Cortical Interneurons from Subjects with Schizophrenia. *Nat. Neurosci.* **22**:229–242. [7]

Shcheglovitov, A., O. Shcheglovitova, M. Yazawa, et al. 2013. SHANK3 and IGF1 Restore Synaptic Deficits in Neurons from 22q13 Deletion Syndrome Patients. *Nature* **503**:267–271. [7]

Shima, Y., K. Sugino, C. M. Hempel, et al. 2016. A Mammalian Enhancer Trap Resource for Discovering and Manipulating Neuronal Cell Types. *eLife* **5**:e13503. [7]

Shitamukai, A., D. Konno, and F. Matsuzaki. 2011. Oblique Radial Glial Divisions in the Developing Mouse Neocortex Induce Self-Renewing Progenitors Outside the Germinal Zone That Resemble Primate Outer Subventricular Zone Progenitors. *J. Neurosci.* **31**:3683–3695. [7]

Sieberts, S. K., T. M. Perumal, M. M. Carrasquillo, et al. 2020. Large eQTL Meta-Analysis Reveals Differing Patterns between Cerebral Cortical and Cerebellar Brain Regions. *Sci. Data* **7**:1–11. [3]

Sigström, R., K. Kowalec, L. Jonsson, et al. 2022. Association between Polygenic Risk Scores and Outcome of ECT. *Am. J. Psychiatry* **179**:844–852. [13]

Sigurdsson, T., K. L. Stark, M. Karayiorgou, J. A. Gogos, and J. A. Gordon. 2010. Impaired Hippocampal-Prefrontal Synchrony in a Genetic Mouse Model of Schizophrenia. *Nature* **464**:763–767. [7]

Silbereis, J. C., S. Pochareddy, Y. Zhu, M. Li, and N. Sestan. 2016. The Cellular and Molecular Landscapes of the Developing Human Central Nervous System. *Neuron* **89**:248–268. [11]

Silva-Santos, S., G. M. van Woerden, C. F. Bruinsma, et al. 2015. *Ube3a* Reinstatement Identifies Distinct Developmental Windows in a Murine Angelman Syndrome Model. *J. Clin. Invest.* **125**:2069–2076. [5]

Singh, T., M. I. Kurki, D. Curtis, et al. 2016. Rare Loss-of-Function Variants in Setd1a Are Associated with Schizophrenia and Developmental Disorders. *Nat. Neurosci.* **19**:571–577. [7]

Singh, T., T. Poterba, D. Curtis, et al. 2022. Rare Coding Variants in Ten Genes Confer Substantial Risk for Schizophrenia. *Nature* **604**:509–516. [1–3, 5, 7, 11]

Singh, T., and M. Rajput. 2006. Misdiagnosis of Bipolar Disorder. *Psychiatry* **3**:57–63. [13]

Sinnett, S. E., E. Boyle, C. Lyons, and S. J. Gray. 2021. Engineered microRNA-Based Regulatory Element Permits Safe High-Dose Minimecp2 Gene Therapy in Rett Mice. *Brain* **144**:3005–3019. [6]

Sinnett, S. E., and S. J. Gray. 2017. Recent Endeavors in MECP2 Gene Transfer for Gene Therapy of Rett Syndrome. *Discov. Med.* **24**:153–159. [6]

Sinnott-Armstrong, N., S. Naqvi, M. Rivas, and J. K. Pritchard. 2021. GWAS of Three Molecular Traits Highlights Core Genes and Pathways Alongside a Highly Polygenic Background. *eLife* **10**:e58615. [9]

Skene, N. G., J. Bryois, T. E. Bakken, et al. 2018. Genetic Identification of Brain Cell Types Underlying Schizophrenia. *Nat. Genet.* **50**:825–833. [7, 8, 11]

Slatkin, M. 2008. Exchangeable Models of Complex Inherited Diseases. *Genetics* **179**:2253–2261. [9]

Smoller, J. W., N. Craddock, K. Kendler, et al. 2013. Erratum: Identification of Risk Loci with Shared Effects on Five Major Psychiatric Disorders: A Genome-Wide Analysis. *Lancet* **381**:1371–1379. [2]

So, H. C., and P. C. Sham. 2017. Exploring the Predictive Power of Polygenic Scores Derived from Genome-Wide Association Studies: A Study of 10 Complex Traits. *Bioinformatics* **33**:886–892. [13]

Song, M., M. P. Pebworth, X. Yang, et al. 2020. Cell-Type-Specific 3D Epigenomes in the Developing Human Cortex. *Nature* **587**:644–649. [10]

Sperber, N. R., O. M. Dong, M. C. Roberts, et al. 2021. Strategies to Integrate Genomic Medicine into Clinical Care: Evidence from the Ignite Network. *J. Pers. Med.* **11**:647. [13]

Spiess, K., and H. Won. 2020. Regulatory Landscape in Brain Development and Disease. *Curr. Opin. Genet. Dev.* **65**:53–60. [10]

Spratt, P. W. E., R. Ben-Shalom, C. M. Keeshen, et al. 2019. The Autism-Associated Gene Scn2a Contributes to Dendritic Excitability and Synaptic Function in the Prefrontal Cortex. *Neuron* **103**:673–685. [5, 7]

Srivastava, S., J. A. Love-Nichols, K. A. Dies, et al. 2019. Meta-Analysis and Multidisciplinary Consensus Statement: Exome Sequencing Is a First-Tier Clinical Diagnostic Test for Individuals with Neurodevelopmental Disorders. *Genet. Med.* **21**:2413–2421. [6, 13]

Stahl, E. A., G. Breen, A. J. Forstner, et al. 2019. Genome-Wide Association Study Identifies 30 Loci Associated with Bipolar Disorder. *Nat. Genet.* **51**:793–803. [2]

Stancer, H. C., and D. K. Wagener. 1984. Genetic Counselling: Its Need in Psychiatry and the Directions It Gives for Future Research. *Can. J. Psychiatry* **29**:289–294. [15]

Stein, M. B., D. F. Levey, Z. Cheng, et al. 2021. Genome-Wide Association Analyses of Post-Traumatic Stress Disorder and Its Symptom Subdomains in the Million Veteran Program. *Nat. Genet.* **53**:174–184. [2]

Steinberg, S., S. Gudmundsdottir, G. Sveinbjornsson, et al. 2017. Truncating Mutations in Rbm12 Are Associated with Psychosis. *Nat. Genet.* **49**:1251–1254. [7]

Stern, S., S. Linker, K. C. Vadodaria, M. C. Marchetto, and F. H. Gage. 2018. Prediction of Response to Drug Therapy in Psychiatric Disorders. *Open Biol.* **8**:180031. [7]

Stevenson, A., D. Akena, R. E. Stroud, et al. 2019. Neuropsychiatric Genetics of African Populations-Psychosis (NeuroGAP-Psychosis): A Case-Control Study Protocol and GWAS in Ethiopia, Kenya, South Africa and Uganda. *BMJ Open* **9**:e025469. [2]

Steyerberg, E. W., A. J. Vickers, N. R. Cook, et al. 2010. Assessing the Performance of Prediction Models: A Framework for Traditional and Novel Measures. *Epidemiology* **21**:128–138. [13]

Stoker, T. B., K. E. R. Andresen, and R. A. Barker. 2021. Hydrocephalus Complicating Intrathecal Antisense Oligonucleotide Therapy for Huntington's Disease. *Mov. Disord.* **36**:263–264. [6]

Stoll, G., O. P. H. Pietilainen, B. Linder, et al. 2013. Deletion of TOP3beta, a Component of FMRP-Containing Mrnps, Contributes to Neurodevelopmental Disorders. *Nat. Neurosci.* **16**:1228–1237. [2]

Südhof, T. C. 2008. Neuroligins and Neurexins Link Synaptic Function to Cognitive Disease. *Nature* **455**:903–911. [5]

———. 2017a. Molecular Neuroscience in the 21st Century: A Personal Perspective. *Neuron* **96**:536–541. [7]

———. 2017b. Synaptic Neurexin Complexes: A Molecular Code for the Logic of Neural Circuits. *Cell* **171**:745–769. [5]

———. 2018. Towards an Understanding of Synapse Formation. *Neuron* **100**:276–293. [11]

Sugathan, A., M. Biagioli, C. Golzio, et al. 2014. CHD8 Regulates Neurodevelopmental Pathways Associated with Autism Spectrum Disorder in Neural Progenitors. *PNAS* **111**:E4468–E4477. [11]

Sullivan, P. F. 2005. The Genetics of Schizophrenia. *PLOS Med.* **2**:e212. [5]

———. 2013. Questions About DISC1 as a Genetic Risk Factor for Schizophrenia. *Mol. Psychiatry* **18**:1050–1052. [7]

Sullivan, P. F., A. Agrawal, C. M. Bulik, et al. 2018. Psychiatric Genomics: An Update and an Agenda. *Am. J. Psychiatry* **175**:15–27. [1]

Sullivan, P. F., and D. H. Geschwind. 2019. Defining the Genetic, Genomic, Cellular, and Diagnostic Architectures of Psychiatric Disorders. *Cell* **177**:162–183. [7, 11]

Sun, L., L. Pennells, S. Kaptoge, et al. 2021. Polygenic Risk Scores in Cardiovascular Risk Prediction: A Cohort Study and Modelling Analyses. *PLOS Med.* **18**:e1003498. [13]

Suvrathan, A., C. A. Hoeffer, H. Wong, E. Klann, and S. Chattarji. 2010. Characterization and Reversal of Synaptic Defects in the Amygdala in a Mouse Model of Fragile X Syndrome. *PNAS* **107**:11591–11596. [5]

Szklarczyk, D., A. L. Gable, K. C. Nastou, et al. 2021. The String Database in 2021: Customizable Protein-Protein Networks, and Functional Characterization of User-Uploaded Gene/Measurement Sets. *Nucleic Acids Res.* **49**:D605–D612. [11]

Takahashi, K., K. Tanabe, M. Ohnuki, et al. 2007. Induction of Pluripotent Stem Cells from Adult Human Fibroblasts by Defined Factors. *Cell* **131**:861–872. [7]

Takata, A., N. Matsumoto, and T. Kato. 2017. Genome-Wide Identification of Splicing QTLs in the Human Brain and Their Enrichment among Schizophrenia-Associated Loci. *Nat. Commun.* **8**:14519. [11]

Takata, A., B. Xu, I. Ionita-Laza, et al. 2014. Loss-of-Function Variants in Schizophrenia Risk and Setd1a as a Candidate Susceptibility Gene. *Neuron* **82**:773–780. [7]

Talkowski, M. E., J. A. Rosenfeld, I. Blumenthal, et al. 2012. Sequencing Chromosomal Abnormalities Reveals Neurodevelopmental Loci That Confer Risk across Diagnostic Boundaries. *Cell* **149**:525–537. [7]

Tamura, S., A. D. Nelson, P. W. E. Spratt, et al. 2022. *Preprint*: CRISPR Activation Rescues Abnormalities in *SCN2A* Haploinsufficiency-Associated Autism Spectrum Disorder. *bioRxiv* 486483. [5]

Taniguchi, H., M. He, P. Wu, et al. 2011. A Resource of Cre Driver Lines for Genetic Targeting of GABAergic Neurons in Cerebral Cortex. *Neuron* **71**:995–1013. [7]

Tansey, K. E., M. Guipponi, X. Hu, et al. 2013. Contribution of Common Genetic Variants to Antidepressant Response. *Biol. Psychiatry* **73**:679–682. [13]

Tansey, K. E., E. Rees, D. E. Linden, et al. 2016. Common Alleles Contribute to Schizophrenia in CNV Carriers. *Mol. Psychiatry* **21**:1153. [7]

Taylor, M. J., D. Freeman, S. Lundstrom, H. Larsson, and A. Ronald. 2022. Heritability of Psychotic Experiences in Adolescents and Interaction with Environmental Risk. *JAMA Psychiatry* **79**:889–897. [2]

Tewhey, R., D. Kotliar, D. S. Park, et al. 2016. Direct Identification of Hundreds of Expression-Modulating Variants Using a Multiplexed Reporter Assay. *Cell* **165**:1519–1529. [8]

Thakore, P. I., A. M. D'Ippolito, L. Song, et al. 2015. Highly Specific Epigenome Editing by CRISPR-Cas9 Repressors for Silencing of Distal Regulatory Elements. *Nat. Methods* **12**:1143–1149. [7]

Thomas, K. R., and M. R. Capecchi. 1987. Site-Directed Mutagenesis by Gene Targeting in Mouse Embryo-Derived Stem Cells. *Cell* **51**:503–512. [5]

Thompson, P. M., N. Jahanshad, L. Schmaal, et al. 2022. The Enhancing Neuroimaging Genetics through Meta-Analysis Consortium: 10 Years of Global Collaborations in Human Brain Mapping. *Hum. Brain Mapp.* **43**:15–22. [8]

Thomson, J. A., J. Itskovitz-Eldor, S. S. Shapiro, et al. 1998. Embryonic Stem Cell Lines Derived from Human Blastocysts. *Science* **282**:1145–1147. [7]

Thygesen, J. H., K. Wolfe, A. McQuillin, et al. 2018 Neurodevelopmental Risk Copy Number Variants in Adults with Intellectual Disabilities and Comorbid Psychiatric Disorders. *Br. J. Psychiatry* **212**:287–294. [12]

Tian, R., M. A. Gachechiladze, C. H. Ludwig, et al. 2019. CRISPR Interference-Based Platform for Multimodal Genetic Screens in Human iPSC-Derived Neurons. *Neuron* **104**:239–255. [7]

Till, S. M., A. Asiminas, A. D. Jackson, et al. 2015. Conserved Hippocampal Cellular Pathophysiology but Distinct Behavioural Deficits in a New Rat Model of FXS. *Hum. Mol. Genet.* **24**:5977–5984. [5]

Tillotson, R., J. Selfridge, M. V. Koerner, et al. 2017. Radically Truncated MeCP2 Rescues Rett Syndrome-Like Neurological Defects. *Nature* **550**:398–401. [6]

Timshel, P. N., J. J. Thompson, and T. H. Pers. 2020. Genetic Mapping of Etiologic Brain Cell Types for Obesity. *eLife* **9**:e55851. [9]

Tomioka, I., T. Maeda, H. Shimada, et al. 2010. Generating Induced Pluripotent Stem Cells from Common Marmoset (*Callithrix jacchus*) Fetal Liver Cells Using Defined Factors, Including Lin28. *Genes Cells* **15**:959–969. [5]

Townsley, K. G., K. J. Brennand, and L. M. Huckins. 2020. Massively Parallel Techniques for Cataloguing the Regulome of the Human Brain. *Nat. Neurosci.* **23**:1509–1521. [7]

Townsley, K. G., A. Li, P. J. M. Deans, et al. 2022. *Preprint*: Convergent Impact of Schizophrenia Risk Genes. *bioRxiv* 486286. [7]

Toyonaga, T., A. Fesharaki-Zadeh, S. M. Strittmatter, R. E. Carson, and Z. Cai. 2022. PET Imaging of Synaptic Density: Challenges and Opportunities of Synaptic Vesicle Glycoprotein 2a PET in Small Animal Imaging. *Front. Neurosci.* **16**:787404. [8]

Tremblay, I., A. Janvier, and A. M. Laberge. 2018. Paediatricians Underuse Recommended Genetic Tests in Children with Global Developmental Delay. *Paediatr. Child Health* **23**:e156–e162. [12]

Tremblay, J., M. Haloui, R. Attaoua, et al. 2021. Polygenic Risk Scores Predict Diabetes Complications and Their Response to Intensive Blood Pressure and Glucose Control. *Diabetologia* **64**:2012–2025. [13]

Treutlein, B., O. Gokce, S. R. Quake, and T. C. Südhof. 2014. Cartography of Neurexin Alternative Splicing Mapped by Single-Molecule Long-Read mRNA Sequencing. *PNAS* **111**:E1291–E1299. [11]

Tromp, A., B. Mowry, and J. Giacomotto. 2021. Neurexins in Autism and Schizophrenia-a Review of Patient Mutations, Mouse Models and Potential Future Directions. *Mol. Psychiatry* **26**:747–760. [5]

Trubetskoy, V., A. F. Pardinas, T. Qi, et al. 2022. Mapping Genomic Loci Implicates Genes and Synaptic Biology in Schizophrenia. *Nature* **604**:502–508. [3, 7–9, 11–13]

Trujillo, C. A., R. Gao, P. D. Negraes, et al. 2019. Complex Oscillatory Waves Emerging from Cortical Organoids Model Early Human Brain Network Development. *Cell Stem Cell* **25**:558–569. [5]

Truong, T. K., A. Kenneson, A. R. Rosen, and R. H. Singh. 2021. Genetic Referral Patterns and Responses to Clinical Scenarios: A Survey of Primary Care Providers and Clinical Geneticists. *J. Prim. Care Comm. Health* **12**:21501327211046734. [12]

Tsai, P. T., C. Hull, Y. Chu, et al. 2012. Autistic-Like Behaviour and Cerebellar Dysfunction in Purkinje Cell Tsc1 Mutant Mice. *Nature* **488**:647–651. [6]

Tsai, P. T., S. Rudolph, C. Guo, et al. 2018. Sensitive Periods for Cerebellar-Mediated Autistic-Like Behaviors. *Cell Rep.* **25**:357–367. [5, 6]

Tsuda, Y., J. Saruwatari, and N. Yasui-Furukori. 2014. Meta-Analysis: The Effects of Smoking on the Disposition of Two Commonly Used Antipsychotic Agents, Olanzapine and Clozapine. *BMJ Open* **4**:e004216. [4]

Turissini, M., T. Mercer, J. Baenziger, et al. 2020. Developing Ethical and Sustainable Global Health Educational Exchanges for Clinical Trainees: Implementation and Lessons Learned from the 30-Year Academic Model Providing Access to Healthcare (AMPATH) Partnership. *Ann. Glob. Health* **86**:137. [2]

Turley, P., M. N. Meyer, N. Wang, et al. 2021. Problems with Using Polygenic Scores to Select Embryos. *N. Engl. J. Med.* **385**:78–86. [13, 14]

Turnwald, B. P., J. P. Goyer, D. Z. Boles, et al. 2019. Learning One's Genetic Risk Changes Physiology Independent of Actual Genetic Risk. *Nat. Hum. Behav.* **3**:48–56. [15]

Tyler, J., S. W. Choi, and M. Tewari. 2020. Real-Time, Personalized Medicine through Wearable Sensors and Dynamic Predictive Modeling: A New Paradigm for Clinical Medicine. *Curr. Opin. Syst. Biol.* **20**:17–25. [5]

Udler, M. S., M. I. McCarthy, J. C. Florez, and A. Mahajan. 2019. Genetic Risk Scores for Diabetes Diagnosis and Precision Medicine. *Endocr. Rev.* **40**:1500–1520. [9]

Uebbing, S., J. Gockley, S. K. Reilly, et al. 2021. Massively Parallel Discovery of Human-Specific Substitutions That Alter Enhancer Activity. *PNAS* **118**:e2007049118. [7, 8]

Uezu, A., D. J. Kanak, T. W. A. Bradshaw, et al. 2016. Identification of an Elaborate Complex Mediating Postsynaptic Inhibition. *Science* **353**:1123–1129. [11]

Uhlmann, W. R., J. L. Schuette, and B. Yashar, eds. 2010. A Guide to Genetic Counseling. Hoboken: John Wiley and Sons. [15]

Ure, K., H. Lu, W. Wang, et al. 2016. Restoration of Mecp2 Expression in GABAergic Neurons Is Sufficient to Rescue Multiple Disease Features in a Mouse Model of Rett Syndrome. *eLife* **5**:e14198. [5]

Urresti, J., P. Zhang, P. Moran-Losada, et al. 2021. Cortical Organoids Model Early Brain Development Disrupted by 16p11.2 Copy Number Variants in Autism. *Mol. Psychiatry* **26**:7560–7580. [5]

Valassina, N., S. Brusco, A. Salamone, et al. 2022. *Scn1a* Gene Reactivation after Symptom Onset Rescues Pathological Phenotypes in a Mouse Model of Dravet Syndrome. *Nat. Commun.* **13**:161. [5]

van Alten, S., B. W. Domingue, T. Galama, and A. T. Marees. 2022. *Preprint*: Reweighting the UK Biobank to Reflect Its Underlying Sampling Population Substantially Reduces Pervasive Selection Bias Due to Volunteering. *medRxiv* 22275048. [2]

Van den Adel, B., A. Inglis, and J. Austin. 2022. An Internship in Psychiatric Genetic Counseling: Impact on Genetic Counseling Graduates' Practice and Career Choices. *J. Genet. Counsel.* **31**:1071–1079. [15]

van der Wijst, M. G. P., D. H. de Vries, H. Brugge, H.-J. Westra, and L. Franke. 2018. An Integrative Approach for Building Personalized Gene Regulatory Networks for Precision Medicine. *Genome Med.* **10**:96. [11]

van Loo, H. M., P. de Jonge, J. W. Romeijn, R. C. Kessler, and R. A. Schoevers. 2012. Data-Driven Subtypes of Major Depressive Disorder: A Systematic Review. *BMC Med.* **10**:156. [2]

Van Nostrand, E. L., P. Freese, G. A. Pratt, et al. 2020. A Large-Scale Binding and Functional Map of Human RNA-Binding Proteins. *Nature* **583**:711–719. [11]

Van Os, J., D. J. Castle, N. Takei, G. Der, and R. M. Murray. 1996. Psychotic Illness in Ethnic Minorities: Clarification from the 1991 Census. *Psychol. Med.* **26**:203–208. [4]

Vassena, E., J. Deraeve, and W. H. Alexander. 2017. Predicting Motivation: Computational Models of Pfc Can Explain Neural Coding of Motivation and Effort-Based Decision-Making in Health and Disease. *J. Cogn. Neurosci.* **29**:1633–1645. [2]

Vatine, G. D., R. Barrile, M. J. Workman, et al. 2019. Human iPSC-Derived Blood-Brain Barrier Chips Enable Disease Modeling and Personalized Medicine Applications. *Cell Stem Cell* **24**:995–1005. [7]

Veach, P. M. C., D. M. Bartels, and B. S. LeRoy. 2007. Coming Full Circle: A Reciprocal-Engagement Model of Genetic Counseling Practice. *J. Genet. Counsel.* **16**:713–728. [15]

Velasco, S., A. J. Kedaigle, S. K. Simmons, et al. 2019. Individual Brain Organoids Reproducibly Form Cell Diversity of the Human Cerebral Cortex. *Nature* **570**:523–527. [5, 7]

Velmeshev, D., L. Schirmer, D. Jung, et al. 2019. Single-Cell Genomics Identifies Cell Type-Specific Molecular Changes in Autism. *Science* **364**:685–689. [5, 11]

Vickers, A. J., B. Van Calster, and E. W. Steyerberg. 2016. Net Benefit Approaches to the Evaluation of Prediction Models, Molecular Markers, and Diagnostic Tests. *BMJ* **352**:i6. [13]

Visscher, P. M., W. G. Hill, and N. R. Wray. 2008. Heritability in the Genomics Era: Concepts and Misconceptions. *Nat. Rev. Genet.* **9**:255–266. [7]

Vodopivec, M., S. Laporsek, J. Stare, and M. Vodopivec. 2021. The Effects of Unemployment on Health, Hospitalizations, and Mortality: Evidence from Administrative Data. *SSRN IZA Disc. Paper* **14318**:1–53. [4]

Voineagu, I., X. Wang, P. Johnston, et al. 2011. Transcriptomic Analysis of Autistic Brain Reveals Convergent Molecular Pathology. *Nature* **474**:380–384. [11]

Volpato, V., J. Smith, C. Sandor, et al. 2018. Reproducibility of Molecular Phenotypes after Long-Term Differentiation to Human iPSC-Derived Neurons: A Multi-Site Omics Study. *Stem Cell Rep.* **11**:897–911. [6]

Wainberg, M., G. R. Jacobs, M. di Forti, and S. J. Tripathy. 2021. Cannabis, Schizophrenia Genetic Risk, and Psychotic Experiences: A Cross-Sectional Study of 109,308 Participants from the UK Biobank. *Transl. Psychiatry* **11**:211. [13]

Wainger, B. J., E. Kiskinis, C. Mellin, et al. 2014. Intrinsic Membrane Hyperexcitability of Amyotrophic Lateral Sclerosis Patient-Derived Motor Neurons. *Cell Rep.* **7**:1–11. [5, 6]

Walker, R. L., G. Ramaswami, C. Hartl, et al. 2019. Genetic Control of Expression and Splicing in Developing Human Brain Informs Disease Mechanisms. *Cell* **179**:750–771.e722. [3, 10, 11]

Wang, B., A. M. Mezlini, F. Demir, et al. 2014. Similarity Network Fusion for Aggregating Data Types on a Genomic Scale. *Nat. Methods* **11**:333–337. [11]

Wang, B. S., R. Sarnaik, and J. Cang. 2010. Critical Period Plasticity Matches Binocular Orientation Preference in the Visual Cortex. *Neuron* **65**:246–256. [5]

Wang, D., S. Liu, J. Warrell, et al. 2018. Comprehensive Functional Genomic Resource and Integrative Model for the Human Brain. *Science* **362**:eaat8464. [3, 8, 10, 11]

Wang, D., P. W. L. Tai, and G. Gao. 2019. Adeno-Associated Virus Vector as a Platform for Gene Therapy Delivery. *Nat. Rev. Drug Discov.* **18**:358–378. [6]

Wang, X., and D. B. Goldstein. 2020. Enhancer Domains Predict Gene Pathogenicity and Inform Gene Discovery in Complex Disease. *Am. J. Hum. Genet.* **106**:215–233. [10]

Wang, X., J. W. Tsai, B. LaMonica, and A. R. Kriegstein. 2011. A New Subtype of Progenitor Cell in the Mouse Embryonic Neocortex. *Nat. Neurosci.* **14**:555–561. [7]

Wang, Y., K. Tsuo, M. Kanai, B. M. Neale, and A. R. Martin. 2022. Challenges and Opportunities for Developing More Generalizable Polygenic Risk Scores. *Annu. Rev. Biomed. Data Sci.* **5**:293–320. [13]

Ward, J., N. Graham, R. J. Strawbridge, et al. 2018. Polygenic Risk Scores for Major Depressive Disorder and Neuroticism as Predictors of Antidepressant Response: Meta-Analysis of Three Treatment Cohorts. *PLOS ONE* **13**:e0203896. [13, 14]

Warren, C. R., C. E. Jaquish, and C. A. Cowan. 2017. The Nextgen Genetic Association Studies Consortium: A Foray into *in Vitro* Population Genetics. *Cell Stem Cell* **20**:431–433. [8]

Watanabe, K., S. Stringer, O. Frei, et al. 2019a. A Global Overview of Pleiotropy and Genetic Architecture in Complex Traits. *Nat. Genet.* **51**:1339–1348. [7, 8]

Watanabe, K., E. Taskesen, A. van Bochoven, and D. Posthuma. 2017. Functional Mapping and Annotation of Genetic Associations with Fuma. *Nat. Commun.* **8**:1826. [11]

Watanabe, K., M. Umićević Mirkov, C. A. de Leeuw, M. P. van den Heuvel, and D. Posthuma. 2019b. Genetic Mapping of Cell Type Specificity for Complex Traits. *Nat. Commun.* **10**:3222. [10, 11]

Weiner, D. J., S. Gazal, E. B. Robinson, and L. J. O'Connor. 2022a. Partitioning Gene-Mediated Disease Heritability without eQTLs. *Am. J. Hum. Genet.* **109**:405–416. [3]

Weiner, D. J., E. Ling, S. Erdin, et al. 2022b. Statistical and Functional Convergence of Common and Rare Genetic Influences on Autism at Chromosome 16p. *Nat. Genet.* **54**:1630–1639. [3]

Weiner, D. J., E. M. Wigdor, S. Ripke, et al. 2017. Polygenic Transmission Disequilibrium Confirms That Common and Rare Variation Act Additively to Create Risk for Autism Spectrum Disorders. *Nat. Genet.* **49**:978–985. [7]

Weiss, L. A., Y. Shen, J. M. Korn, et al. 2008. Association between Microdeletion and Microduplication at 16p11.2 and Autism. *N. Engl. J. Med.* **358**:667–675. [5]

Weissbrod, O., M. Kanai, H. Shi, et al. 2022. Leveraging Fine-Mapping and Multipopulation Training Data to Improve Cross-Population Polygenic Risk Scores. *Nat. Genet.* **54**:450–458. [13]

Werling, D. M., H. Brand, J.-Y. An, et al. 2018. An Analytical Framework for Whole-Genome Sequence Association Studies and Its Implications for Autism Spectrum Disorder. *Nat. Genet.* **50**:727–736. [3]

Werling, D. M., S. Pochareddy, J. Choi, et al. 2020. Whole-Genome and RNA Sequencing Reveal Variation and Transcriptomic Coordination in the Developing Human Prefrontal Cortex. *Cell Rep.* **31**:107489. [3, 10, 11]

Werner-Lin, A., J. L. M. McCoyd, and B. A. Bernhardt. 2019. Actions and Uncertainty: How Prenatally Diagnosed Variants of Uncertain Significance Become Actionable. Looking for the Psychosocial Impacts of Genomic Information, Special Report. *Hastings Cent. Rep.* **49**:S61–S71. [14]

Whalen, S., and K. S. Pollard. 2019. Most Chromatin Interactions Are Not in Linkage Disequilibrium. *Genome Res.* **29**:334–343. [8]

Wheat, R., M. Vess, and P. Holte. 2022. Genetic Risk Information Influences Risk-Taking Behavior. *Soc. Cogn.* **40**:387–395. [14]

Wickstrom, J., C. Farmer, L. Green Snyder, et al. 2021. Patterns of Delay in Early Gross Motor and Expressive Language Milestone Attainment in Probands with Genetic Conditions versus Idiopathic ASD from Sfari Registries. *J. Child Psychol. Psychiatry* **62**:1297–1307. [3]

Wilhelm, K., B. Meiser, P. B. Mitchell, et al. 2009. Issues Concerning Feedback About Genetic Testing and Risk of Depression. *Br. J. Psychiatry* **194**:404–410. [14, 15]

Williams, M. S. 2019. Early Lessons from the Implementation of Genomic Medicine Programs. *Annu. Rev. Genomics Hum. Genet.* **20**:389–411. [13]

Williams, M. S., C. O. Taylor, N. A. Walton, et al. 2019. Genomic Information for Clinicians in the Electronic Health Record: Lessons Learned from the Clinical Genome Resource Project and the Electronic Medical Records and Genomics Network. *Front. Genet.* **10**:1059. [13]

Willsey, A. J., M. T. Morris, S. Wang, et al. 2018. The Psychiatric Cell Map Initiative: A Convergent Systems Biological Approach to Illuminating Key Molecular Pathways in Neuropsychiatric Disorders. *Cell* **174**:505–520. [11]

Willsey, A. J., S. J. Sanders, M. Li, et al. 2013. Coexpression Networks Implicate Human Midfetal Deep Cortical Projection Neurons in the Pathogenesis of Autism. *Cell* **155**:997–1007. [3, 5]

Willsey, H. R., C. R. T. Exner, Y. Xu, et al. 2021. Parallel *in Vivo* Analysis of Large-Effect Autism Genes Implicates Cortical Neurogenesis and Estrogen in Risk and Resilence. *Neuron* **109**:788–804. [7]

Windrem, M. S., M. Osipovitch, Z. Liu, et al. 2017. Human iPSC Glial Mouse Chimeras Reveal Glial Contributions to Schizophrenia. *Cell Stem Cell* **21**:195–208. [7]

Wingo, T. S., Y. Liu, E. S. Gerasimov, et al. 2021. Brain Proteome-Wide Association Study Implicates Novel Proteins in Depression Pathogenesis. *Nat. Neurosci.* **24**:810–817. [11]

Wolter, J. M., H. Mao, G. Fragola, et al. 2020. Cas9 Gene Therapy for Angelman Syndrome Traps *Ube3a-Ats* Long Non-Coding RNA. *Nature* **587**:281–284. [5, 6]

Won, H., L. de la Torre-Ubieta, J. L. Stein, et al. 2016. Chromosome Conformation Elucidates Regulatory Relationships in Developing Human Brain. *Nature* **538**:523–527. [10]

Wortmann, S. B., M. M. Oud, M. Alders, et al. 2022. How to Proceed after "Negative" Exome: A Review on Genetic Diagnostics, Limitations, Challenges, and Emerging New Multiomics Techniques. *J. Inherit. Metab. Dis.* **45**:663–681. [12]

Wray, N. R., T. Lin, J. Austin, et al. 2021. From Basic Science to Clinical Application of Polygenic Risk Scores: A Primer. *JAMA Psychiatry* **78**:101–109. [12, 13, 15]

Wray, N. R., and R. Maier. 2014. Genetic Basis of Complex Genetic Disease: The Contribution of Disease Heterogeneity to Missing Heritability. *Curr. Epidemiol. Rep.* **1**:220–227. [2, 9]

Wray, N. R., S. Ripke, M. Mattheisen, et al. 2018a. Genome-Wide Association Analyses Identify 44 Risk Variants and Refine the Genetic Architecture of Major Depression. *Nat. Genet.* **50**:668–681. [7, 15]

Wray, N. R., C. Wijmenga, P. F. Sullivan, J. Yang, and P. M. Visscher. 2018b. Common Disease Is More Complex Than Implied by the Core Gene Omnigenic Model. *Cell* **173**:1573–1580. [7, 9]

Wu, Y., Z. Zheng, P. M. Visscher, and J. Yang. 2017. Quantifying the Mapping Precision of Genome-Wide Association Studies Using Whole-Genome Sequencing Data. *Genome Biol.* **18**:86. [8]

Xiang, Y., Y. Tanaka, B. Cakir, et al. 2019. Hesc-Derived Thalamic Organoids Form Reciprocal Projections When Fused with Cortical Organoids. *Cell Stem Cell* **24**:487–497. [7]

Xu, M.-Q., W.-S. Sun, B.-X. Liu, et al. 2009. Prenatal Malnutrition and Adult Schizophrenia: Further Evidence from the 1959-1961 Chinese Famine. *Schizophr. Bull.* **35**:568–576. [4]

Xu, X., A. B. Wells, D. R. O'Brien, A. Nehorai, and J. D. Dougherty. 2014. Cell Type-Specific Expression Analysis to Identify Putative Cellular Mechanisms for Neurogenetic Disorders. *J. Neurosci.* **34**:1420–1431. [11]

Yamazaki, Y., C. Echigo, M. Saiki, et al. 2011. Tool-Use Learning by Common Marmosets (*Callithrix jacchus*). *Exp. Brain Res.* **213**:63–71. [5]

Yang, C., F. H. G. Farias, L. Ibanez, et al. 2021. Genomic Atlas of the Proteome from Brain, Csf and Plasma Prioritizes Proteins Implicated in Neurological Disorders. *Nat. Neurosci.* **24**:1302–1312. [3]

Yang, J., S. H. Lee, M. E. Goddard, and P. M. Visscher. 2011. Gcta: A Tool for Genome-Wide Complex Trait Analysis. *Am. J. Hum. Genet.* **88**:76–82. [2]

Yang, S., and X. Zhou. 2022. Pgs-Server: Accuracy, Robustness and Transferability of Polygenic Score Methods for Biobank Scale Studies. *Brief. Bioinform.* **23**:bbac039. [2]

Yengo, L., S. Vedantam, E. Marouli, et al. 2022. *Preprint*: A Saturated Map of Common Genetic Variants Associated with Human Height from 5.4 Million Individuals of Diverse Ancestries. *bioRxiv* 475305. [2]

Yeo, N. C., A. Chavez, A. Lance-Byrne, et al. 2018. An Enhanced CRISPR Repressor for Targeted Mammalian Gene Regulation. *Nat. Methods* **15**:611–616. [10]

Yi, F., T. Danko, S. C. Botelho, et al. 2016. Autism-Associated SHANK3 Haploinsufficiency Causes Ih Channelopathy in Human Neurons. *Science* **352**:aaf2669. [7]

Yilmaz, M., E. Yalcin, J. Presumey, et al. 2021. Overexpression of Schizophrenia Susceptibility Factor Human Complement C4A Promotes Excessive Synaptic Loss and Behavioral Changes in Mice. *Nat. Neurosci.* **24**:214–224. [1]

Yoshimizu, T., J. Q. Pan, A. E. Mungenast, et al. 2015. Functional Implications of a Psychiatric Risk Variant within CACNA1C in Induced Human Neurons. *Mol. Psychiatry* **20**:162–169. [7]

Yu, A. W., J. D. Peery, and H. Won. 2021. Limited Association between Schizophrenia Genetic Risk Factors and Transcriptomic Features. *Genes* **12**:1062. [10]

Yu, D. X., F. P. Di Giorgio, J. Yao, et al. 2014. Modeling Hippocampal Neurogenesis Using Human Pluripotent Stem Cells. *Stem Cell Rep.* **2**:295–310. [7]

Zaneva, M., C. Guzman-Holst, A. Reeves, and L. Bowes. 2022. The Impact of Monetary Poverty Alleviation Programs on Children's and Adolescents' Mental Health: A Systematic Review and Meta-Analysis across Low-, Middle-, and High-Income Countries. *J. Adolesc. Health* **71**:147–156. [4]

Zebrowski, A. M., D. E. Ellis, F. K. Barg, et al. 2019. Qualitative Study of System-Level Factors Related to Genomic Implementation. *Genet. Med.* **21**:1534–1540. [13]

Zeier, Z., L. L. Carpenter, N. H. Kalin, et al. 2018. Clinical Implementation of Pharmacogenetic Decision Support Tools for Antidepressant Drug Prescribing. *Am. J. Psychiatry* **175**:873–886. [13]

Zeng, B., J. Bendl, R. Kosoy, et al. 2022. Multi-Ancestry eQTL Meta-Analysis of Human Brain Identifies Candidate Causal Variants for Brain-Related Traits. *Nat. Genet.* **54**:161–169. [8, 10]

Zeng, J., A. Xue, L. Jiang, et al. 2021. Widespread Signatures of Natural Selection across Human Complex Traits and Functional Genomic Categories. *Nat. Commun.* **12**:1164. [1, 9]

Zeng, L. H., L. Xu, D. H. Gutmann, and M. Wong. 2008. Rapamycin Prevents Epilepsy in a Mouse Model of Tuberous Sclerosis Complex. *Ann. Neurol.* **63**:444–453. [6]

Zerres, K., and S. Rudnik-Schöneborn. 1995. Natural History in Proximal Spinal Muscular Atrophy. Clinical Analysis of 445 Patients and Suggestions for a Modification of Existing Classifications. *Arch. Neurol.* **52**:518–523. [5]

Zhang, J. P., D. Robinson, J. Yu, et al. 2019. Schizophrenia Polygenic Risk Score as a Predictor of Antipsychotic Efficacy in First-Episode Psychosis. *Am. J. Psychiatry* **176**:21–28. [7, 13, 14]

Zhang, S., H. Zhang, M. P. Forrest, et al. 2021. *Preprint*: Multiple Genes in cis Mediate the Effects of a Single Chromatin Accessibility Variant on Aberrant Synaptic Development and Function in Human Neurons. *bioRxiv* 472229. [7]

Zhang, T., L. Xu, X. Tang, et al. 2020a. Real-World Effectiveness of Antipsychotic Treatment in Psychosis Prevention in a 3-Year Cohort of 517 Individuals at Clinical High Risk from the Sharp (Shanghai at Risk for Psychosis). *Aust. N. Z. J. Psychiatry* **54**:696–706. [13]

Zhang, Y., H. T. Yang, K. Kadash-Edmondson, et al. 2020b. Regional Variation of Splicing QTLs in Human Brain. *Am. J. Hum. Genet.* **107**:196. [3]

Zhang, Z., S. G. Marro, Y. Zhang, et al. 2018. The Fragile X Mutation Impairs Homeostatic Plasticity in Human Neurons by Blocking Synaptic Retinoic Acid Signaling. *Sci. Transl. Med.* **10**:eaar4338. [7]

Zheutlin, A. B., J. Dennis, R. Karlsson Linner, et al. 2019. Penetrance and Pleiotropy of Polygenic Risk Scores for Schizophrenia in 106,160 Patients across Four Health Care Systems. *Am. J. Psychiatry* **176**:846–855. [1, 7, 13]

Zhu, H., L. Shang, and X. Zhou. 2020. A Review of Statistical Methods for Identifying Trait-Relevant Tissues and Cell Types. *Front. Genet.* **11**:587887. [9]

Zhu, Y., A. M. M. Sousa, T. Gao, et al. 2018. Spatiotemporal Transcriptomic Divergence across Human and Macaque Brain Development. *Science* **362**:eaat8077. [8]

Zierhut, H. A., K. M. Shannon, D. L. Cragun, and S. A. Cohen. 2016. Elucidating Genetic Counseling Outcomes from the Perspective of Genetic Counselors. *J. Genet. Counsel.* **25**:993–1001. [15]

Zoghbi, H. Y. 2003. Postnatal Neurodevelopmental Disorders: Meeting at the Synapse? *Science* **302**:826–830. [11]

Zolkowska, K., E. Cantor-Graae, and T. F. McNeil. 2001. Increased Rates of Psychosis among Immigrants to Sweden: Is Migration a Risk Factor for Psychosis? *Psychol. Med.* **31**:669–678. [4]

Zylka, M. J. 2020. Prenatal Treatment Path for Angelman Syndrome and Other Neurodevelopmental Disorders. *Autism Res.* **13**:11–17. [5]

Subject Index

Strüngmann Forum Report Series*

Intrusive Thinking: From Molecules to Free Will
Edited by Peter W. Kalivas and Martin P. Paulus
ISBN: 9780262542371

Deliberate Ignorance: Choosing Not to Know
edited by Ralph Hertwig and Christoph Engel
ISBN 9780262045599

Youth Mental Health: A Paradigm for Prevention and Early Intervention
Edited by Peter J. Uhlhaas and Stephen J. Wood
ISBN: 9780262043977

The Neocortex
Edited by Wolf Singer, Terrence J. Sejnowski and Pasko Rakic
ISBN: 9780262043243

Interactive Task Learning: Humans, Robots, and Agents Acquiring New Tasks through Natural Interactions
Edited by Kevin A. Gluck and John E. Laird
ISBN: 9780262038829

Agrobiodiversity: Integrating Knowledge for a Sustainable Future
Edited by Karl S. Zimmerer and Stef de Haan
ISBN: 9780262038683

Rethinking Environmentalism: Linking Justice, Sustainability, and Diversity
Edited by Sharachchandra Lele, Eduardo S. Brondizio, John Byrne, Georgina M. Mace and Joan Martinez-Alier
ISBN: 9780262038966

Emergent Brain Dynamics: Prebirth to Adolescence
Edited by April A. Benasich and Urs Ribary
ISBN: 9780262038638

The Cultural Nature of Attachment: Contextualizing Relationships and Development
Edited by Heidi Keller and Kim A. Bard
ISBN (Hardcover): 9780262036900 ISBN (ebook): 9780262342865
Winner of the Ursula Gielen Global Psychology Book Award

Investors and Exploiters in Ecology and Economics: Principles and Applications
edited by Luc-Alain Giraldeau, Philipp Heeb and Michael Kosfeld
ISBN (Hardcover): 9780262036122 ISBN (eBook): 9780262339797

Computational Psychiatry: New Perspectives on Mental Illness
edited by A. David Redish and Joshua A. Gordon
ISBN: 9780262035422

---

* Available at https://mitpress.mit.edu/books/series/strungmann-forum-reports

Complexity and Evolution: Toward a New Synthesis for Economics
edited by David S. Wilson and Alan Kirman
ISBN: 9780262035385

The Pragmatic Turn: Toward Action-Oriented Views in Cognitive Science
edited by Andreas K. Engel, Karl J. Friston and Danica Kragic
ISBN: 9780262034326

Translational Neuroscience: Toward New Therapies
edited by Karoly Nikolich and Steven E. Hyman
ISBN: 9780262029865

Trace Metals and Infectious Diseases
edited by Jerome O. Nriagu and Eric P. Skaar
ISBN 9780262029193

Pathways to Peace: The Transformative Power of Children and Families
edited by James F. Leckman, Catherine Panter-Brick and Rima Salah,
ISBN 9780262027984

Rethinking Global Land Use in an Urban Era
edited by Karen C. Seto and Anette Reenberg
ISBN 9780262026901

Schizophrenia: Evolution and Synthesis
edited by Steven M. Silverstein, Bita Moghaddam and Til Wykes,
ISBN 9780262019620

Cultural Evolution: Society, Technology, Language, and Religion
edited by Peter J. Richerson and Morten H. Christiansen,
ISBN 9780262019750

Language, Music, and the Brain: A Mysterious Relationship
edited by Michael A. Arbib
ISBN 9780262019620

Evolution and the Mechanisms of Decision Making
edited by Peter Hammerstein and Jeffrey R. Stevens
ISBN 9780262018081

Cognitive Search: Evolution, Algorithms, and the Brain
edited by Peter M. Todd, Thomas T. Hills and Trevor W. Robbins,
ISBN 9780262018098

Animal Thinking: Contemporary Issues in Comparative Cognition
edited by Randolf Menzel and Julia Fischer
ISBN 9780262016636

Disease Eradication in the 21st Century: Implications for Global Health
edited by Stephen L. Cochi and Walter R. Dowdle
ISBN 9780262016735

Better Doctors, Better Patients, Better Decisions: Envisioning Health Care 2020
edited by Gerd Gigerenzer and J. A. Muir Gray
ISBN 9780262016032

Dynamic Coordination in the Brain: From Neurons to Mind
edited by Christoph von der Malsburg, William A. Phillips and Wolf Singer,
ISBN 9780262014717

Linkages of Sustainability
edited by Thomas E. Graedel and Ester van der Voet
ISBN 9780262013581

Biological Foundations and Origin of Syntax
edited by Derek Bickerton and Eörs Szathmáry
ISBN 9780262013567

Clouds in the Perturbed Climate System: Their Relationship to Energy Balance, Atmospheric Dynamics, and Precipitation
edited by Jost Heintzenberg and Robert J. Charlson
ISBN 9780262012874
Winner of the Atmospheric Science Librarians International Choice Award

Better Than Conscious? Decision Making, the Human Mind, and Implications For Institutions
edited by Christoph Engel and Wolf Singer
ISBN 978-0-262-19580-5